Operative Techniques in Vascular Surgery

Operative Techniques in Vascular Surgery

edited by

JOHN J. BERGAN, M.D.

Magerstadt Professor of Surgery
and Chief, Division of Vascular Surgery
Northwestern University Medical School
Chicago, Illinois

and

JAMES S. T. YAO, M.D., Ph.D.

Professor of Surgery
and Director, Blood Flow Laboratory
Northwestern University Medical School
Chicago, Illinois

Grune & Stratton
A Subsidiary of Harcourt Brace Jovanovich, Publishers
New York London Toronto Sydney San Francisco

Grune & Stratton, Inc.
111 Fifth Avenue
New York, New York 10003

Distributed in the United Kingdom by
Academic Press, Inc. (London) Ltd.
24/28 Oval Road, London NW 1

Library of Congress Catalog Number 80-24811
International Standard Book Number 0-8089-1334-4
Printed in the United States of America

Contents

Foreword

This book is relatively unique, both in concept and in execution. This volume is based on a symposium in vascular surgery that has been carefully developed by Dr. John J. Bergan and Dr. James S. T. Yao. The symposium has served as a model for others by virtue of its precise planning and the excellence of its faculty.

This year, the symposium is devoted to the technical aspects of vascular surgery, and includes both aortic and venous surgery, as well as the operative approach to portal hypertension. The book has been divided into appropriate sections, such as surgery of the aorta, cerebral revascularization, surgery of the aortic branches, and other well chosen areas of surgical treatment of vascular disease. The authors of each chapter have contributed significantly to the advancement of vascular surgery in the particular areas to which they have been assigned. The participation by H. H. G. Eastcott, Roger Greenhalgh, and Henner Muller-Wiefel has added an international scope to the symposium. It is a tribute to the authors, as well as to Dr. Bergan and Dr. Yao that the volume is available at the time of the symposium. In addition, this book should be of great interest to vascular surgeons throughout the country.

John M. Beal, M.D.
Elcock Professor of Surgery
Chairman, Department of Surgery
Northwestern University Medical School

Preface

This book in intended to be practical. It is recognized that treatment, which is that part of surgery that changes as time passes, is evanescent. Nevertheless, success of operative procedures is dependent upon technical perfection, whatever the operation may be. Such technical perfection is literally in the hands of the surgeon. He brings with him to the operating room skill, knowledge, and a personality that allows him to control the operation in hours of calm and in moments of chaos.

A volume cannot contribute to a surgeon's skill, nor can it modify his personality. It cannot make him a more capable leader of his operating team. On the other hand, a volume can bring to him the best thoughts from the most reliable authorities relative to technical performance of the operation itself. This is done in the pages that follow.

In the modern era, surgery of aortic aneurysms was a most significant technical advance. Surgery of the aorta remains the keystone of vascular surgery as practiced in the 1980s. Therefore, it is appropriate to bring together the thoughts on treatment of aortic aneurysms as stated so clearly by Jesse Thompson of Dallas, Stanley Crawford of Houston, Richard Kempczinski of Cincinnati, and H. H. G. Eastcott of London. While the latter contributors speak of aortic occlusion, rather than aneurysm surgery, the problems in management of aortic disease are similar in both instances. Some thoughts on elective and urgent aneurysm resection are contributed by Bergan, speaking for the Northwestern University vascular group.

Surgery of the intra-abdominal aortic branches demands technical perfection. It is appropriate, therefore, to include the thoughts of Richard Dean of Nashville and James Stanley of Ann Arbor, who stand preeminent in the field of renal revascularization. William Ehrenfeld of San Francisco describes the techniques worked out in his very large experience with *ex-vivo* repair of the renal artery. Similarly, operations for acute and chronic mesenteric ischemia have been a long time interest of the Northwestern group, and their approaches to these problems are illustrated and described.

Revascularization of the lower extremity has been characterized in modern times by exploration of more and more distal anastomoses. The entire field is exceedingly well discussed by Muller-Wiefel of Dusseldorf, Frank Veith of New York, and Roger Greenhalgh of London. The techniques described by them are nicely complemented by descriptions of sequential bypass grafting, as enumerated by William Flinn of the Northwestern group; composite arterial grafting, as described by Jonathan Towne of Milwaukee; and a well-crafted description of care of peripheral aneurysms by Robert Hobson of Newark.

Extra-anatomic reconstructions are useful in a variety of situations, none of which are simple and some of which are extremely complex. Therefore, the clear description of the axillofemoral bypass by Robert Rutherford of Denver and the knowledgeable exposition by Preston Flanigan of the University of Illinois on femorofemoral grafting are most helpful.

Jesse Thompson of Dallas stands preeminent in the field of cerebral revascularization. Therefore, it is appropriate to include his description of his method of carotid endarterectomy. Alternative methods of cerebral revascularization and technical advances in carotid surgery are the focus of William Baker's discussion. Preston Flanigan has very clearly described his methods of subclavian-carotid anastomosis for cerebral ischemia, and W. H. Edwards of Nashville has succinctly described his methods of vertebral artery reconstructive surgery. Indications have appeared for external carotid endarterectomy. The special technical problems associated with this procedure are described and their management detailed by Charles O'Mara of Johns Hopkins University.

Upper extremity arterial reconstruction has become a particular interest of a small group of surgeons. Among these are William Flinn of the Northwestern group and David Roos of Denver. Their descriptions of upper extremity bypass procedures, transaxillary sympathectomy, the first rib resection comprise a concise segment on surgery of the vasculature of the upper extremity.

Complications of arterial surgery are with us always. Therefore, it is appropriate to include within this volume thoughts about technique in management of graft complications. Among these is a description of the methods of management of aortoenteric fistula by Victor Bernhard of Milwaukee; of the infected aortic graft by Roger Smith of the Henry Ford Hospital, Detroit; of the technique of obturator bypass by Ralph DePalma, now of Reno; and an interesting, innovative technique of distal profunda femoris bypass, also by Dr. DePalma. One problem of distal reconstructive surgery is that redo operations are frequently necessary. These can be approached in a simplified fashion, as described by James Yao, writing from the Northwestern vascular group.

Reconstructive surgery of the venous system is now possible. In this regard, Andrew Dale's technique of crossover grafting is included in this book, as are Robert Kistner's description of venous valve repair and Luis Queral's contribution on venous valve transposition. The Iowa City group's innovative approach to creation of spiral grafts is described by Creighton Wright and, in a section on surgery of portal hypertension, the mesocaval shunt is described by John Cameron of the Johns Hopkins Hospital, the LeVeen shunt by its inventor, now in Charleston, South Carolina, the Sugiura procedure of gastroesophageal devascularization by George Johnson of Chapel Hill, and the interesting mesoatrial shunt for Budd-Chiari syndrome by Cameron of Baltimore.

The strength of these presentations is the authority that each surgeon brings to his description of his technical modifications of standard procedures. Although no book can include all of the operations now being done, a book on vascular surgery in 1980 can include a description of a large proportion of them. This book does this, and it is hoped that it will go far toward supplying the needs of surgeons in training, and even contribute thoughts to experienced surgeons who always look for a new way to speed and simplify operative approaches to solution of vascular problems.

John J. Bergan
James S. T. Yao

Contributors

William H. Baker, M.D.

Professor and Chief, Section of Peripheral Vascular Surgery
Stritch School of Medicine, Loyola University Medical Center, Maywood, Illinois

John J. Bergan, M.D.

Magerstadt Professor of Surgery and Chief, Division of Vascular Surgery
Northwestern University Medical School, Chicago, Illinois

Victor M. Bernhard, M.D.

Professor of Surgery
The Medical College of Wisconsin, Milwaukee, Wisconsin

John L. Cameron, M.D.

Professor of General and Thoracic Surgery
The Johns Hopkins University School of Medicine, Baltimore, Maryland

E. Stanley Crawford, M.D.

Professor of Surgery
Baylor College of Medicine, The Methodist Hospital, Houston, Texas

W. Andrew Dale, M.D.

Professor of Clinical Surgery
Vanderbilt University School of Medicine, Nashville, Tennessee

Richard H. Dean, M.D.

Associate Professor of Surgery and Head, Division of Vascular Surgery
Vanderbilt University School of Medicine, Nashville, Tennessee

Richard G. DePalma, M.D.

Professor and Chairman, Department of Surgery
University of Nevada School of Medical Sciences, Reno, Nevada

Donald B. Doty, M.D.

Professor of Surgery, Division of Thoracic and Cardiovascular Surgery
The University of Iowa Hospitals and Clinics, Iowa City, Iowa

H. H. G. Eastcott, M.S., F.R.C.S., F.A.C.S. (Hon.), F.R.A.C.S. (Hon.)

Consultant Surgeon
St. Mary's Hospital, London, England

William H. Edwards, M.D.

Associate Professor of Surgery
Vanderbilt University Medical Center and St. Thomas Hospital, Nashville, Tennessee

William K. Ehrenfeld, M.D.

Professor of Surgery
University of California School of Medicine, San Francisco, California

Eugene B. Ferris, M.D.

Department of Vascular Surgery, Straub Clinic and
Department of Surgery, John A. Burns School of Medicine, University of Hawaii, Honolulu, Hawaii

D. Preston Flanigan, M.D.

Assistant Professor of Surgery and Director, Vascular Surgical Services and Blood Flow Laboratories
Abraham Lincoln School of Medicine, University of Illinois Medical Center, Chicago, Illinois

William R. Flinn, M.D.

Assistant Professor of Surgery
Northwestern University Medical School, Chicago, Illinois

R.M. Greenhalgh, M.A., M. Chir., F.R.C.S.

Senior Lecturer in Surgery and Honorary Consultant Surgeon
Charing Cross Hospital Medical School, London, England

Sushil K. Gupta, M.D.

Assistant Professor of Surgery
Montefiore Hospital-Albert Einstein College of Medicine, New York, New York

John P. Harris, M.D.

Jobst Fellow in Peripheral Vascular Surgery
Northwestern University Medical School, Chicago, Illinois

Robert W. Hobson, II, M.D.

Professor of Surgery and Director, Division of Vascular Surgery
New Jersey Medical School, College of Medicine and Dentistry of New Jersey, Newark, New Jersey

Zafar Jamil, M.D.

Assistant Professor of Surgery, Division of Vascular Surgery
New Jersey Medical School, College of Medicine and Dentistry of New Jersey, Newark, New Jersey

George Johnson, Jr., M.D.

Roscoe B. G. Cowper Professor of Surgery and Chief, Division of General Surgery
University of North Carolina School of Medicine, Chapel Hill, North Carolina

Blair A. Keagy, M.D.

Department of Cardiovascular and Thoracic Surgery
Geisinger Medical Center, Danville, Pennsylvania

Richard F. Kempczinski, M.D.

Associate Professor of Surgery and Chief, Vascular Service
University of Cincinnati College of Medicine, Cincinnati, Ohio

Terry A. King, M.D.

Department of Surgery
Case Western Reserve University, Cleveland, Ohio

Robert L. Kistner, M.D.

Associate Professor of Surgery,
John A. Burns School of Medicine, University of Hawaii
and Department of Vascular Surgery,
Straub Clinic, Honolulu, Hawaii

Harry H. LeVeen, M.D.

Professor of Surgery
Medical University of South Carolina, Charleston, South Carolina

Thomas G. Lynch, M.D.

Assistant Professor of Surgery
New Jersey Medical School, Newark, New Jersey

Joseph L. Mulherin, Jr., M.D.

Assistant Clinical Professor of Surgery
Vanderbilt University Medical Center and St. Thomas Hospital, Nashville, Tennessee

Prof. Dr. med. Henner Muller-Wiefel

Chief, Vascular Surgical Clinic
St. Johannes-Hospital, Dusseldorf, West Germany

Charles S. O'Mara, M.D.

Assistant Professor of Surgery
The Johns Hopkins University School of Medicine, Baltimore, Maryland

Luis A. Queral, M.D.

Assistant Professor of Surgery
University of Maryland School of Medicine, Baltimore, Maryland

Robert S. Rhodes, M.D.

Department of Surgery
Case Western Reserve University School of Medicine, Cleveland, Ohio

David B. Roos, M.D.

Associate Clinical Professor of Surgery
University of Colorado School of Medicine, Denver, Colorado

Neil D. Rudo, M.D.

Fellow in Peripheral Vascular Surgery
Northwestern University Medical School, Chicago, Illinois

Robert B. Rutherford, M.D.

Professor of Surgery
University of Colorado School of Medicine, Denver, Colorado

Salwa A. Saleh, M.D.

Assistant Professor of Anesthesiology
Baylor College of Medicine and The Methodist Hospital, Houston, Texas

Oscar Salvatierra, Jr., M.D.

Associate Professor of Surgery and Urology and Chief, Transplant Service
University of California School of Medicine, San Francisco, California

Roger F. Smith, M.D.

Clinical Professor of Surgery, University of Michigan
Head, Division of Vascular Surgery, Henry Ford Hospital, Detroit, Michigan

James C. Stanley, M.D.

Professor of Surgery and Head, Division of Peripheral Vascular Surgery
University of Michigan Medical School, Ann Arbor, Michigan

Ronald J. Stoney, M.D.

Associate Professor of Surgery
University of California School of Medicine, San Francisco, California

Jesse E. Thompson, M.D.

Attending Surgeon and Director of Graduate Education in Vascular Surgery
Baylor University Medical Center, Dallas, Texas

Jonathan B. Towne, M.D.

Associate Professor of Surgery
The Medical College of Wisconsin, Milwaukee, Wisconsin

Frank J. Veith, M.D.

Professor of Surgery and Chief of Vascular Surgery
Montefiore Hospital-Albert Einstein College of Medicine, New York, New York

Walter M. Whitehouse, Jr., M.D.

Assistant Professor of Surgery, Division of Peripheral Vascular Surgery
University of Michigan Medical School, Ann Arbor, Michigan

Creighton B. Wright, M.D.

Professor of Surgery, Division of Thoracic and Cardiovascular Surgery
University of Iowa Hospitals and Clinics, Iowa City, Iowa

James S. T. Yao, M.D., Ph.D.

Professor of Surgery and Director, Blood Flow Laboratory
Northwestern University Medical School, Chicago, Illinois

Operative Techniques in Vascular Surgery

SURGERY OF THE AORTA

Technique of Aortic Aneurysm Resection

John J. Bergan, William R. Flinn, Neil D. Rudo, John P. Harris, James S. T. Yao

Ultimately, three factors influence a decision about surgery in patients with an abdominal aortic aneurysm. These are the patient's age, the size of the aneurysm, and the associated medical conditions. It is acknowledged that aortic aneurysms are potentially lethal and that their behavior is unpredictable.[1] Age is not normally a contraindication to abdominal aortic aneurysm surgery, but it becomes a relative consideration at the extremes encountered in persons with dilation of the aorta. Over age 70, associated medical conditions become increasingly important. Among these, pulmonary insufficiency is the most troublesome, renal insufficiency the most overemphasized, and senility the most philosophically important. When myocardial ischemia is present, judgment must be exercised to choose between operative risk and risk of death from rupture of the aneurysm.[2] It is thought that a 5- to 6-cm transverse diameter of an aneurysm divides those lesions that can be watched expectantly from those that must be operated upon.[3] However, most vascular surgeons feel that the presence of an abdominal aortic aneurysm is reason enough for its resection.[4] (It must be recognized that ultrasound evaluation of aneurysms underestimates their actual size.)

A patient with an aneurysm 6 cm or less in diameter has a 75 percent chance of surviving 1 year and a 50 percent chance of surviving 5 years without surgery. These figures are reversed in patients with aneurysms greater than 6 cm in diameter. Such patients have a 50 percent chance of surviving 1 year and a 6 percent chance of surviving 5 years. Death from aneurysm rupture will occur in 43 percent of all the patients.

Supported in part by the Conrad Jobst Foundation and the Northwestern University Vascular Research Fund.

ELECTIVE ANEURYSM RESECTION

Surgical preparation begins when the patient with an abdominal aortic aneurysm enters the hospital several days in advance of operation. Pulmonary ventilatory function is assessed and therapy given as needed. Smoking is prohibited and carboxyhemoglobin determination is added to the routine list of laboratory examinations. Aortography is performed if the institution has a capable angiographer. Nothing is to be gained from preoperative digitalization or bowel preparation. Mannitol is not used in preoperative preparation of the patient, but an overnight infusion of 1000 ml of noncolloidal fluid is given. An antibiotic effective against staphylococcus and Escherichia coli is started 24 hours prior to surgery and continued through 3 days postoperatively. An arterial line, a central venous catheter and a catheter in the urinary bladder are placed after induction of general anesthesia. The Swann-Ganz catheter monitor is necessary only in patients with proven ventricular dysfunction.

Transverse abdominal incisions render this operation needlessly complex. A vertical midline incision to be closed in a single layer is made from xiphoid to pubis. A total abdominal exploration is done, with careful attention being turned to each organ system before examination of the retroperitoneum. Unanticipated lesions should be found prior to resection of the aneurysm and appropriate surgical judgment exercised.[7]

The transverse colon and mesocolon are reflected upward. The small bowel is reflected to the right and upward. The ligament of Treitz and the superior duodenal attachments are incised, and the inferior mesenteric vein is divided. The retroperitoneum is opened distally to expose the bifurcation of the iliac arteries. Systemic heparin is given in a dose of 0.6 to 1.0 mg/kg of body weight.

After a decision is made as to whether or not a bifurcation graft will be utilized, the iliac arteries are clamped to prevent distal embolization. It is felt to be important to occlude the distal circulation prior to manipulation of the aneurysm or the aorta superior to it.

Following distal clamping, attention is turned to the superior portion of the aneurysm. Retroperitoneal fibroareolar and lymphatic tissues are incised to expose the aortic wall, which then is encircled with an index finger and clamped with any of the many aortic clamps. Several options are now available to the operating surgeon. If the aneurysm is large and associated large iliac aneurysms are also present, the surgeon may elect to do an aortobifemoral graft. If this technique is chosen, it is only necessary to oversew the neck of the aneurysm after transecting the aorta. There is no need to open the sac, evacuate the clot, or otherwise extend the operation further. The aortobifemoral graft is led parallel and usually medial to the aneurysm. The femoral graft limbs are led through the retroperitoneum in a conventional fashion, much as in reconstructions for occlusive disease. The only difference is that the femoral arteries are transected prior to anastomosis.

If the aneurysm is of moderate size and affects one or both common iliac arteries, it may be elected to extend the bifurcation graft to the external iliac arteries. These can be dissected free and skeletonized at any time prior to opening the aortic aneurysm itself. If, on the other hand, a tube graft is to be done, then simple crossclamping of the common iliac arteries without further dissection may be the technique of choice. Figures 1 through 6 show the simplest form of the aneurysm replacement.

Fig. 1. In emergency situations, proximal aortic control can be obtained with the aortic compressor. Otherwise, the upper aorta is exposed by incising the ligament of Treitz, mobilizing the duodenum to the patient's right, and incising the fibroareolar tissue to the aorta and encircling the aorta with a finger. The compressor can be applied in the region of the renal arteries, as shown, or in the lesser omental sac. (Reprinted with persmission.[8])

Fig. 2. Distal iliac artery clamping is performed without mobilization of the iliac arteries if the patient's aneurysm is confined to the aorta itself. Following this, the aneurysm is incised and laminated clot evacuated. (Reprinted with permission.[8])

Fig. 3. After opening the aortic sac widely, inferior mesenteric artery back-bleeding is noted. This and lumbar arterial orifices are suture closed. (Reprinted with permission.[8])

Fig. 4. After completion of the proximal suture line and near total completion of the distal suture line, the aorta and graft are flushed from above and below. (Reprinted with permission.[8])

Fig. 5. Following completion of the anastomoses, the aortic wall is imbricated over the graft to obliterate all dead space and assure hemostasis in the retroperitoneum. (Reprinted with permission.[8])

Fig. 6. A two-layer aortic wall imbrication is useful when the aneurysmal sac is large and redundant. (Reprinted with permission.[8])

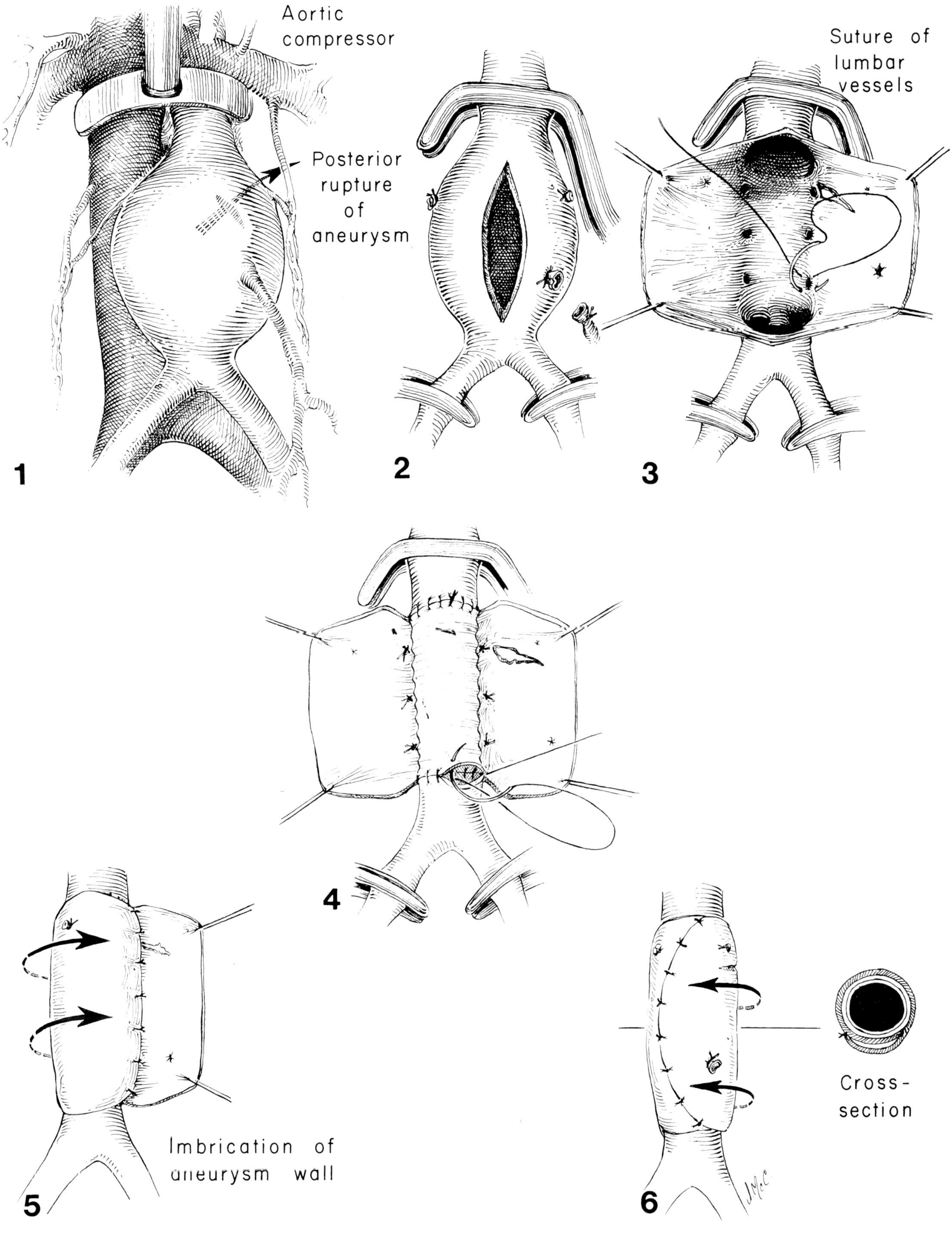
Aortic
compressor
Posterior
rupture
of
aneurysm
Suture of
lumbar
vessels
1
2
3
4
Imbrication of
aneurysm wall
5
Cross-
section
6

Elective surgery for aortic aneurysm is only slightly different.[6] If the aneurysm is small and modest in size, the aortic wall is incised vertically after aortic crossclamping, and the inferior mesenteric artery back-bleeding is noted and crossclamped. A suture ligature can be applied for hemostasis. Individual lumbar arteries back-bleeding into the aortic aneurysm sac can be transfixed with interrupted figure-eight sutures. Loose laminated thrombus is removed, but there is no need to do an endarterectomy of the aortic wall. While the thrombus within aortic aneurysms has been found in many instances to contain bacteria, this is of no clinical importance. Graft infection following elective aortic aneurysm surgery is an extremely rare occurrence.

A graft ranging in size from 19 to 22 mm is sewn end-to-end to the proximal aortic stump with a running continuous 3–0 prolene suture. This is started on the back wall and carried to the anterior aspect of the aorta, where one end is tied to the other. Distally, the graft is sewn in place without transecting the aorta. Special care is taken to include full-thickness aortic wall in the posterior suture line. The aorta and the graft are flushed prior to closing of the distal anastomosis. Once hemostasis is attained following completion of the suture line, distal blood flow is restored in four steps: (1) to one internal iliac artery, (2) to the ipsilateral external iliac artery, (3) to the contralateral internal iliac artery, and (4) to the ipsilateral external iliac artery. During all of these maneuvers, blood pressure is carefully monitored.

ANEURYSM RESECTION IN EMERGENCY CIRCUMSTANCES

A patient with a suspected rupturing abdominal aortic aneurysm should be moved to the operating room. Large-bore intravenous cannulas are placed in the upper extremities, and the bladder is catheterized. Blood is drawn for typing, crossmatching, and preliminary laboratory testing. The patient's abdomen is prepped and draped, and surgical instruments are assembled. After this is done, the anesthetist may induce anesthesia.

The operation may need to be started immediately upon induction of anesthesia, since at this time the patient may lapse into deep shock. As indicated in Figure 1, following opening of the abdomen an aortic compressor can be placed against the aorta and that vessel closed by pressure against the vertebral bodies.[5] Such aortic pressure can be applied in the lesser omental sac between the liver and the stomach or directly upon the aorta above the renal arteries after superior retraction of the omentum and mesocolon. Once the aortic compressor is in place, attention can be turned to incising the fibroareolar tissue around the aorta inferior to the renal arteries, and an aortic clamp is placed. The patient should be heparinized shortly after induction of anesthesia so that arrest of blood flow will not cause thrombosis in the stagnant lower circulation.

Following aortic crossclamping, the procedure proceeds much as in elective aortic surgery. Distal control is obtained by clamping the iliac arteries without skeletonizing them. If the aneurysm involves only the aorta, a tube graft is placed. If small- to moderate-sized iliac aneurysms are present, a bifurcation graft is utilized with connection to the iliac artery bifurcations. If, on the other hand, the aortic aneurysm is large and large common iliac and hypogastric aneurysms are present, the reconstruction is to the common femoral arteries, with trapping of all of the aneurysms by excluding them from the circulation.

Following elective or emergency aortic aneurysm resection, it is wise to leave the endotracheal tube in place until the patient is responsive and postoperative blood gas values are obtained and evaluated. It is important to control the patient's blood pressure within the normal range, not allowing hypotension or hypertension to occur. Similarly, urine output must be maintained with adequate intravenous fluid therapy and diuretics as indicated.

REFERENCES

1. Estes JE Jr: Abdominal aortic aneurysm: A study of 102 cases. Circulation 2:258, 1950
2. Baker AG Jr, Roberts B: Long-term survival following abdominal aortic aneurysmectomy. JAMA 212:445, 1970
3. Szilagyi DE, Elliott JP, Smith RF: Clinical fate of the patient with asymptomatic abdominal aortic aneurysm and unfit for surgical treatment. Arch Surg 104:600, 1972
4. Bernstein EF, Fisher JC, Varco RL: Is excision the optimum treatment for all abdominal aortic aneurysms? Surgery 61:83, 1967
5. Conn J Jr, Trippel OH, Bergan JJ: A new atraumatic aortic occluder. Surgery 64:1158, 1968
6. Johnson G Jr, McDevitt NB, Proctor HJ, Mandel SR, Peacock JB: Emergent or elective operation for symptomatic abdominal aortic aneurysm. Arch Surg 115:51, 1980
7. Swanson RJ, Littooy FN, Hunt TK, Stoney RJ: Laparotomy as a precipitating factor in the rupture of intra-abdominal aneurysms. Arch Surg 115:299, 1980
8. Bergan JS, Yao JST: Modern management of abdominal aortic aneurysms. Surg Clin North Am 54:175–193, 1974

Aortic Occlusion: Treatment by Grafting

H. H. G. Eastcott

Without doubt, the reconstruction of the occluded abdominal aorta and the iliac arteries is the most generally successful of the major vascular surgical procedures, and probably the safest, if the operator has had sufficient experience in general abdominal surgery and a minimum of one year's vascular training in a busy unit. He or she must be prepared to undertake either aortofemoral bypass grafting or the technically more demanding aortoiliac endarterectomy with patch grafting. The decision as to which of these will be chosen will often not be made until the surgical exposure has been completed.

EXPOSURE (FIG. 1A–D)

In the writer's opinion, the advantages of the long median left paraumbilical incision far outweigh its drawbacks. Generous exposure of the whole abdomen, best access to the difficult upper and lower ends of the vascular procedure, and freedom from restriction in the choice of reconstructive method more than balance the greater patient comfort, somewhat reduced incidence of chest complications, and shorter period of ileus that the transverse transperitoneal and the oblique extraperitoneal incisions both offer. The former is unsuitable for self-retaining retraction, and the latter entails serious limitation in the exposure of the right iliac artery as well as of the abdominal aorta itself above the inferior mesenteric, which is necessarily on stretch. Helsby and Moosa[1], however, have reported favorably on the left lateral extraperitoneal approach, which, in their experience, was followed by fewer postoperative complications (just under 17 percent, compared with 29 percent when the peritoneum was opened).

Similar considerations apply for whether to pack the intestines over to the right beneath the deep blade of the self-retaining retractor (Goligher's pattern is ideal for abdominal vascular surgery), or alternatively to lift the mid-gut loop out of the abdomen, placing it in a plastic bag that rests on the right costal margin without tension on the mesentery. Mobilization of the caecum and ascending colon is usually necessary except in obese patients or where the proximal aortic surgical procedure is likely to be difficult. Again, in the writer's experience, this maneuver has not apparently led to any increase in postoperative ileus.

Locating and mobilizing the occluded aorta may be difficult, particularly in obese patients and in non-Caucasian subjects, in whom dense and rather vascular periaortic adhesions are often found. Without the pulsations to guide the surgeon to the line of the aorta, the aorta can readily be found by incising the posterior peritoneum along a line that runs vertically between the left margin of the duodenum and the inferior mesenteric vein (Fig. 1C). The duodenum is then mobilized to the right, a much simpler process than in some cases of abdominal aortic aneurysm; the left renal vein and the vena cava are identified (Fig. 1D).

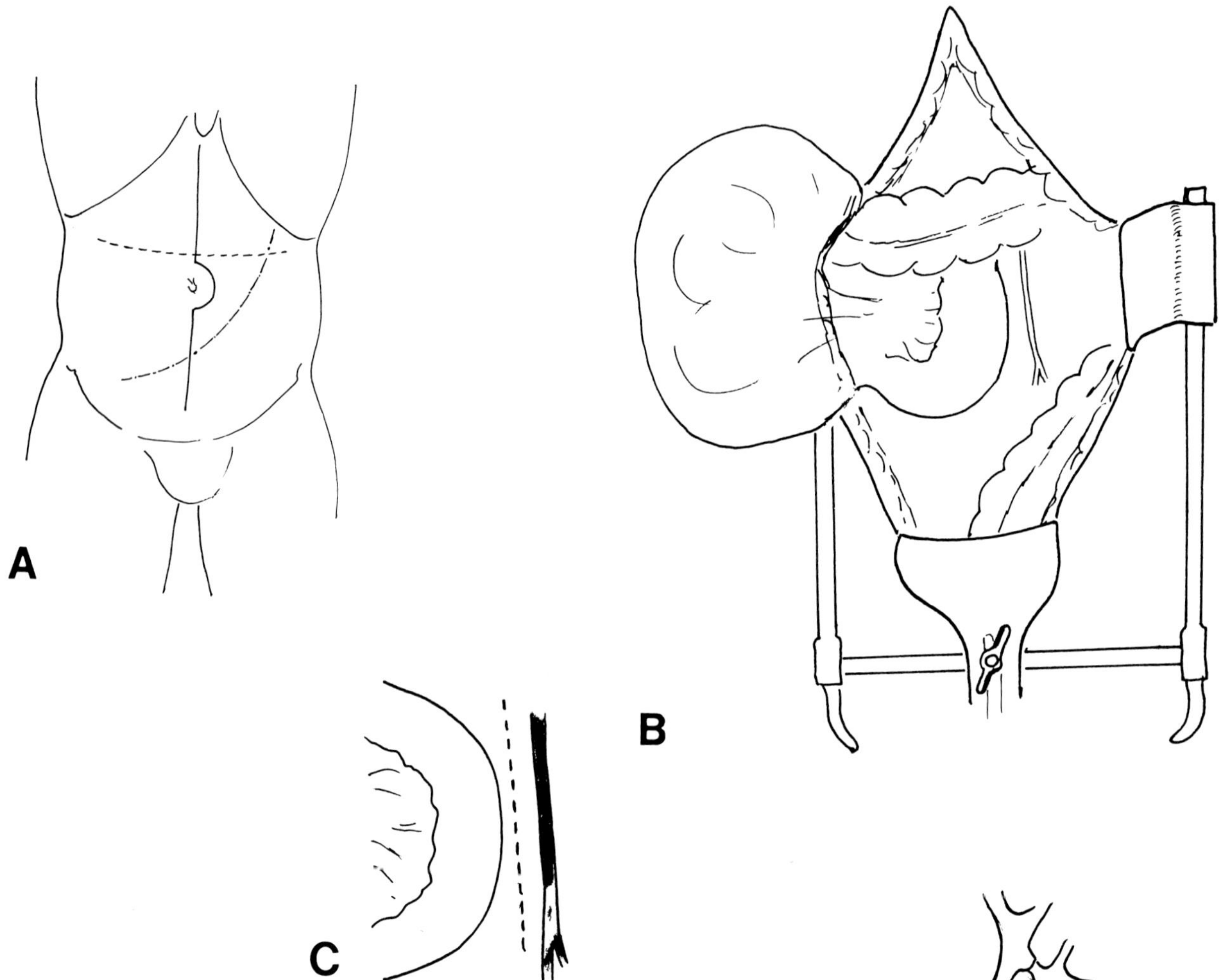

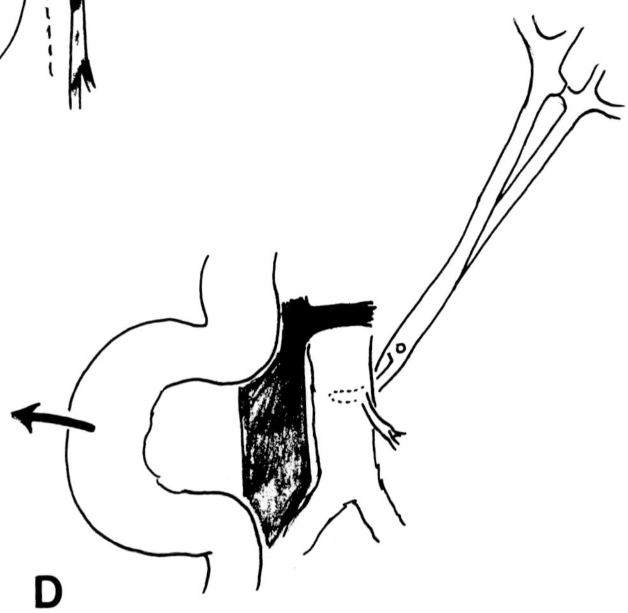

Fig. 1. Exposure of the aortoiliac region.
(A) Three possible incisions. The median paraumbilical is most generally useful and heals well.
(B) Exposure of the posterior abdominal wall, often requiring exenteration of the mid-gut loop.
(C) Line of posterior peritoneal incision over aorta.
(D) Reflection of duodenum and first stage in aortic mobilization.

Deciding the type of reconstruction is now necessary. Much will depend upon the extent and severity of the occluding lesion.

Complete aortic occlusion with extensive iliac disease	Aorto-femoral bypass with proximal transection.
Diffuse, incomplete aortic occlusion, external iliacs affected	Aorto-femoral bypass without transection.
Localised aorto-iliac lesion	Endarterectomy.

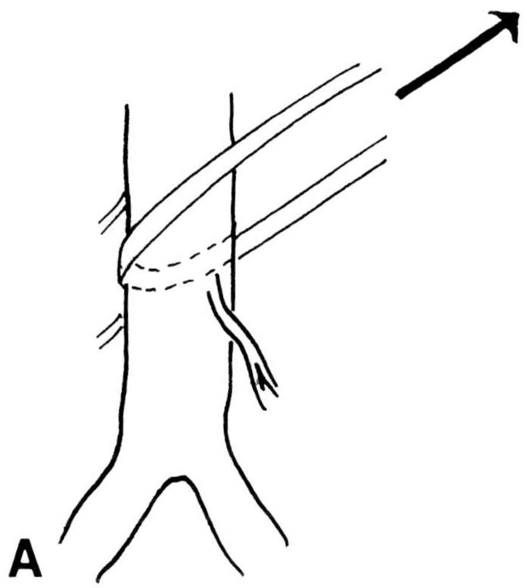

Where endarterectomy has been chosen, the aortoiliac mobilization is continued (Fig. 2A–D). After passing cholecystectomy forceps gently beneath the aorta, avoiding any nearby lumbar arteries, a nylon tape is placed (Fig. 2A and B), and traction upon it exposes the lumbar arteries, aided by gentle Lahey swab dissection. This process is completed on both the right and the left sides until the lumbars are ready for clipping. A careful watch should be kept for transversely running veins, although these are smaller and less adherent than with aneurysms in this area. An alternative method of posterior control is shown in Figure 2D.

If, at this stage in the operation, it is decided that the case is more suitable for aortofemoral bypass, the abdominal stage should be taken no further until exposure of the common femorals has been made. In many instances, this will have been the plan at the outset so that the groin dissection can be made first, with the advantage that the abdominal exposure need not be lost when the surgeon must turn to the lower dissection.

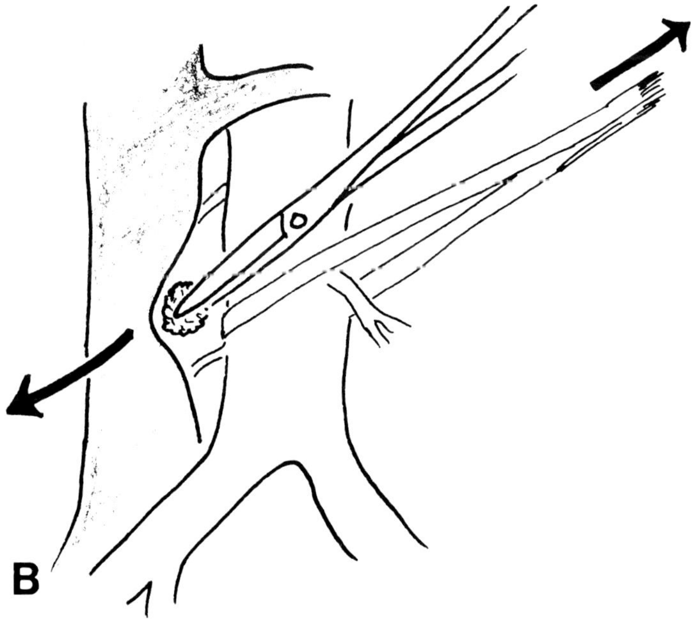

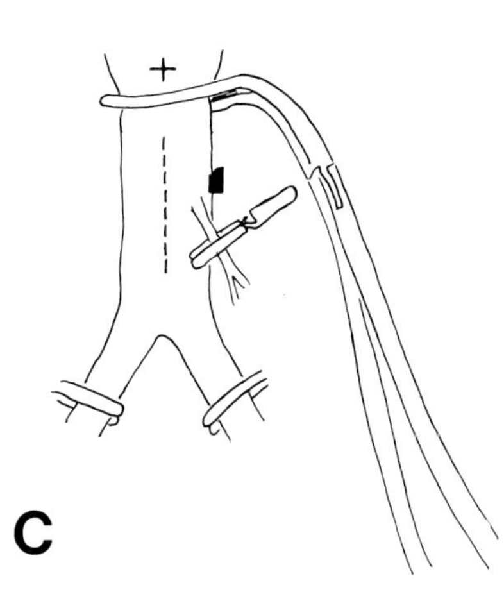

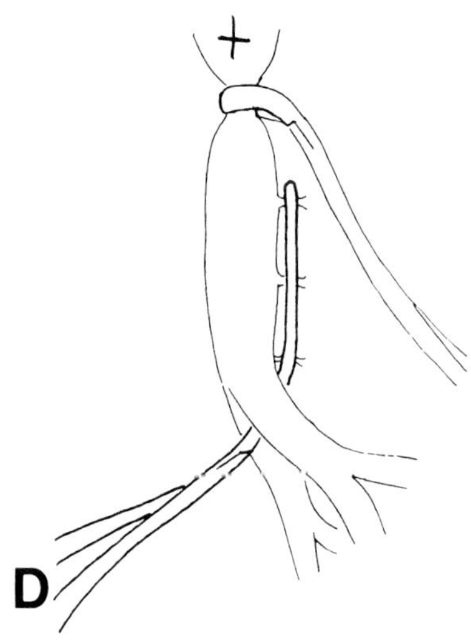

Fig. 2. Control of aorta.
(A) Tape sling beneath mid-aorta.
(B) Exposure of lumbar branches.
(C) Clamping the aorta and its branches.
(D) Posterior clamping of partly mobilized aorta.

Clamping the aorta and its branches. There are many different ways of doing this. It is the writer's general preference to mobilize the whole of the segment to be clamped and isolated. In this way complete hemostasis can be ensured, without which the preparation and reconstruction cannot be as perfect as it should be.

Clamping in situ is quicker and simpler but may leave atheromas beyond the clamps, some of which may be loose and can give rise to an atheroembolism, which passes down the less-affected iliac and lower limb arteries into the pedal arches, where it is totally inaccessible and may result in the condition known as "trash foot."

One method of avoiding this serious complication in partly occluded, loosely atheromatous cases (in which it is most likely to occur) is to place the distal clamps first, perhaps before the aortic dissection, or at least before the grosser movements and adjustments of the main proximal aortic clamp, which could so easily displace material in this highly turbulent segment.[2]

ENDARTERECTOMY VS BYPASS

A final decision must now be made, and while indications are not within the scope of this article, nevertheless the choice must sometimes await inspection of the fully exposed lesion. While safety must always be the first consideration, effectiveness of operation is axiomatic.

Some of the factors that should be taken into account are shown in Table 1. Brewster and Darling[3] have written well on this topic.

Table 1.

Endarterectomy	Bypass
Technically more difficult	Easier operation
Primary failure common	Seldom needs early revision
Late results good	Branch occlusion common under five years
Revision easier	Revision more difficult

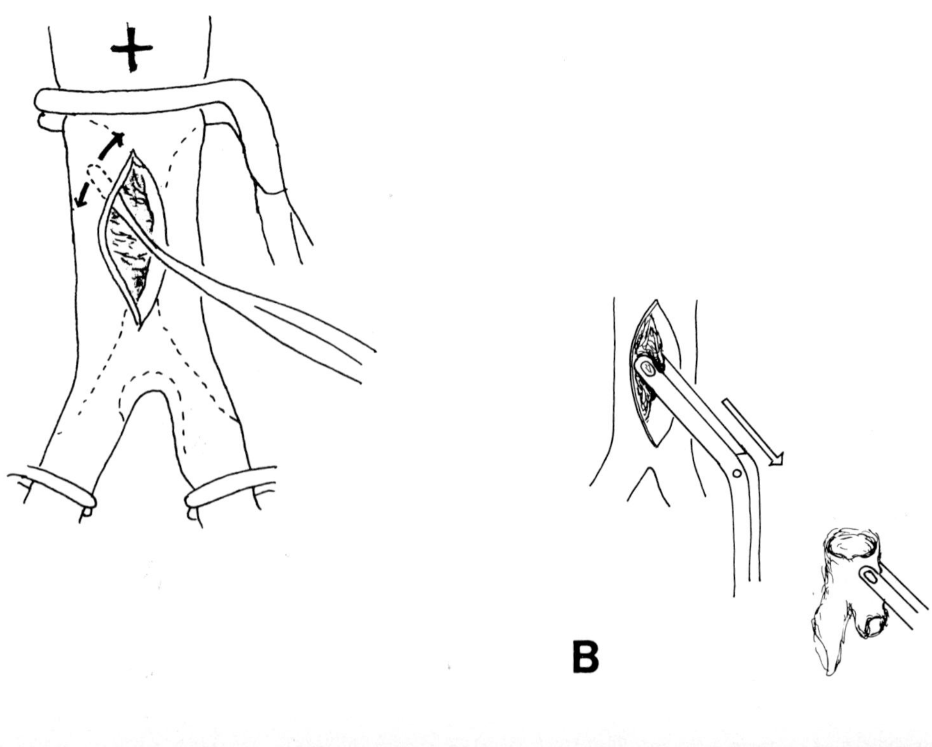

A B

ENDARTERECTOMY TECHNIQUE (FIG. 3A–D)

Localized aortic occlusion may require only one aortotomy. Whereas aortoiliac endarterectomy will require at least two openings (Fig. 3D). It is absolutely essential that the distal end of the lesion be fully seen and, if necessary, sutured into place.

A firmly made longitudinal incision into the arterial wall divides the adventitia and the medial remnant, within which lies the atheromatous, endarterectomy plug, sometimes with calcification, which, however, with care can usually be cleanly extracted. The true plane of the endarterectomy is usually clear and well defined, and can be easily developed and followed using a Watson Cheyne probe-pointed dissector (Fig. 3A). The aortic plug can be grasped with Luc's forceps and removed (Fig. 3B). Any remaining loose shreds or flaps should be gently peeled free with fine nontoothed dissecting forceps (Fig. 3C). This may open up the occluded orifice of an unclipped lumbar artery, which will then require separate control behind the aorta.

Patch grafting is usually essential for the iliac opening or across the bifurcation, although not always for a simple aortic repair. Choice of material will depend upon whether or not heparin has been used and, if so, the dosage chosen. Most vascular surgeons appreciate the latitude that systemic heparinization provides, particularly in complicated cases with multiple lesions, which will require a fairly prolonged clamping time. For simpler, well-localized cases, a small dose (eg 25 mg) or none are satisfactory. Even with such a dose and correct reversal using protamine sulphate in twice the dosage of heparin, there is often free bleeding through the mesh of a plain knitted patch, although less with velour material. Woven patches allow little bleeding but are harder to insert.

The insertion technique is simple, made so by use of lateral traction sutures at the midpoint of the two sides of the arteriotomy. The patch is cut to size and sutured in place using multifilament polyester material where the arterial remnant is strong; polypropylene is more suitable when the wall is thinner.

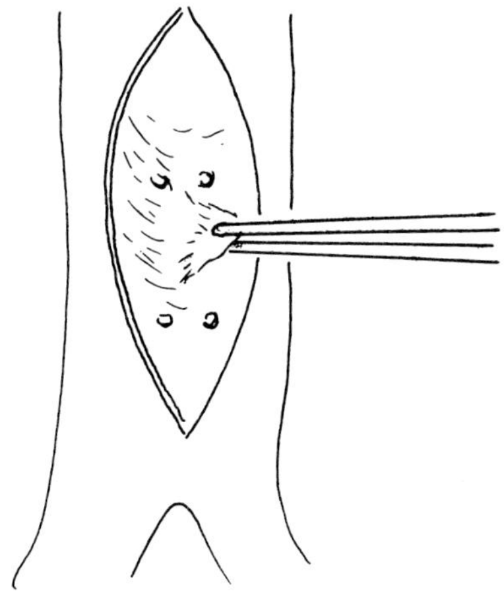

C

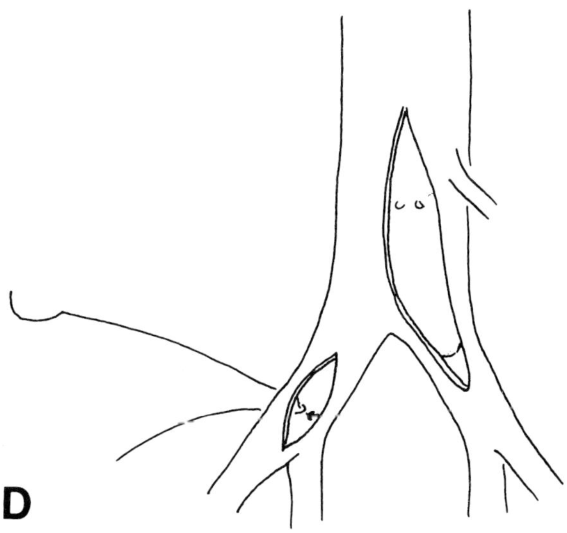

D

Fig. 3. Aortoiliac endarterectomy.
(A) Defining the plane of endarterectomy.
(B) Extraction of aortic plug.
(C) Removal of remnants of atheroma.
(D) A full view must be obtained of the distal-cut intimal edge.

Aortofemoral bypass grafting (Fig. 4A–E)

For the end-to-side method in most general use, the aorta is prepared and endarterectomized as described above. This method has the merits of preserving potentially important branches, including the inferior mesenteric and the lumbars, and is technically easier than transection and end-to-end anastomosis. One absolute indication for transection is the development of uncontrolled bleeding behind the aorta.

The technique advised is to divide the aorta at least 3 or 4 cm below the left renal vein (Fig 4A). This will be possible without clamping in the juxtarenal occlusion case to which this method is ideally suited. Any remaining lumbar branches on the upper stump can be ligated and divided now, and the stump itself can, if wished, be transposed forwards in front of the left renal vein, giving an ideal view for the endarterectomy and anastomoty stages.

With careful probe dissection, preserving a good thickness of aortic wall for subsequent suturing, the risk of renal embolism is small, for the thrombus is usually firm and cupped at its upper face and will be ejected free and intact. Nevertheless the writer prefers to control the renals either by direct finger pressure or by applying soft bulldog clips. Sometimes intra-aortic instrumentation is necessary if the force of the aortic outflow is small. Remaining material should be gently grasped with curved forceps while maintaining aortic compression at the renal level with the left hand.

The femoral exposure is by the standard longitudinal technique as in femoropopliteal bypass grafting. Care is taken to avoid unnecessary damage to lymphatic structures, which can sometimes result in lymph fistula during early recovery from the operation. Likewise, the internal saphenous vein should be preserved, since it may well be required later for coronary or femoropopliteal bypass.

Construction of the tunnel is best performed as soon as the aortic exposure is complete and before the heparin has been given. Care should be taken not to damage the small tributaries to the iliac vein, which if torn at their confluence with the main vein, can cause increasing venous bleeding from the tunnel, which may require division of the abdominal wall between the groin and laparotomy incisions before control can be obtained, and which may lead to a major venous insufficiency problem that will mar the recovery and spoil the end result. Provided the tunneling is gentle, using the two index fingers and directing them well lateral to the line of the vein (Fig. 4B), this serious accident should be easily avoided.

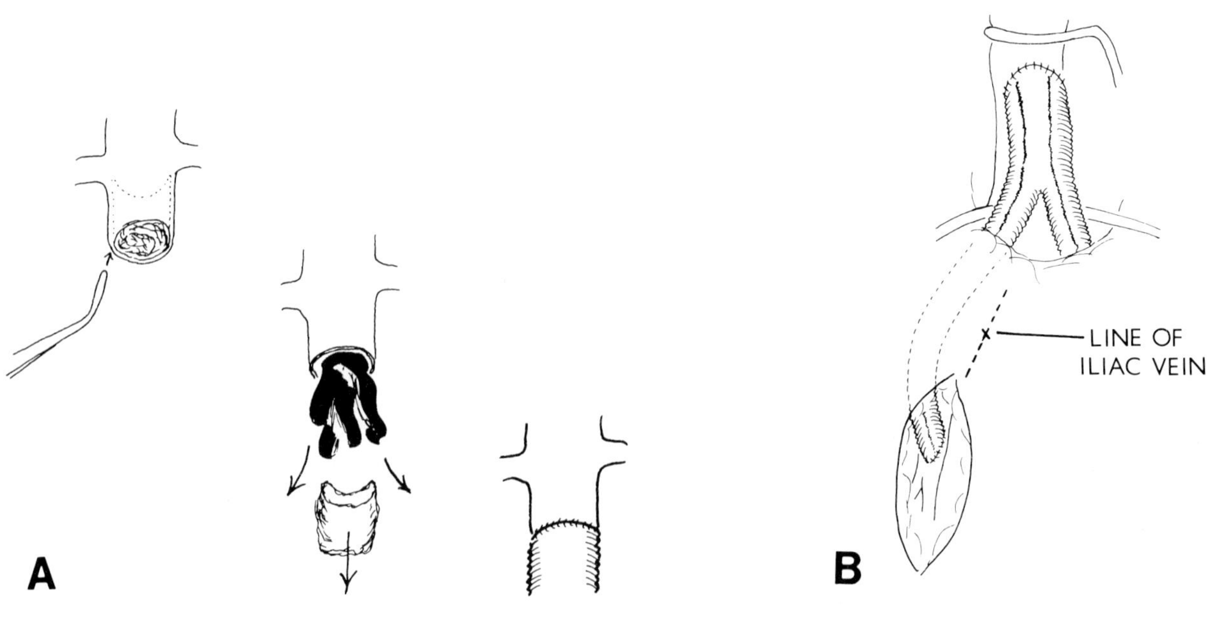

THE FEMORAL ANASTOMOSIS

Many surgeons now favor a routine femoral endarterectomy and profundoplasty before making the lower anastomosis. The writer would restrict this, however, to cases of severe atheromatous irregularity or instability with superficial femoral occlusion and a demonstrably narrowed profunda orifice with poor back flow. The reason for this conservatism is the generally increased prevalence of false aneurysm late after the operation, almost always in the groin and most probably due to a compliance mismatch between the stiff and thrusting dacron graft and the already diseased and now further weakened common femoral artery.[4] The graft should be under sufficient but not excessive tension (too much tension may itself be an accessory to the development of false aneurysm[5]).

The actual anastomosis has no special features, except for the risk in some cases of displacement of a lateral atheromatous plaque into the lumen by injudicious suturing methods. Larger bites, placed from within the lumen, should avoid this major mishap.

The aortic clamp is momentarily released to check the inflow. Both lower anastomoses should spurt strongly through the short remaining open segment in the upper lateral quarter of the suture line left for this purpose. The graft is then flushed through one of these openings with dilute heparin-saline solution, and the two anastomoses are completed, while the anaesthetist gives protamine, as already described.

With a standard woven Dacron graft, which is the writer's preference (except when profundaplasty has been required), there should be little bleeding. There will be more if one of the knitted grafts has been used, though less with velour material. If much blood appears to be coming down from the previously dry tunnel, it is most likely to be coming from the interstices of the fabric, and the aortic clamp should be replaced for diminishing intervals until the oozing is checked.

Vacuum drainage of the groins should be avoided unless a minor slow ooze persists, which may happen in some patients after heparin reversal, from all the tissues of the operative field. The writer does not hesitate to give an antifibrinolytic agent such as epsilon aminocaproic acid in such circumstances.

C

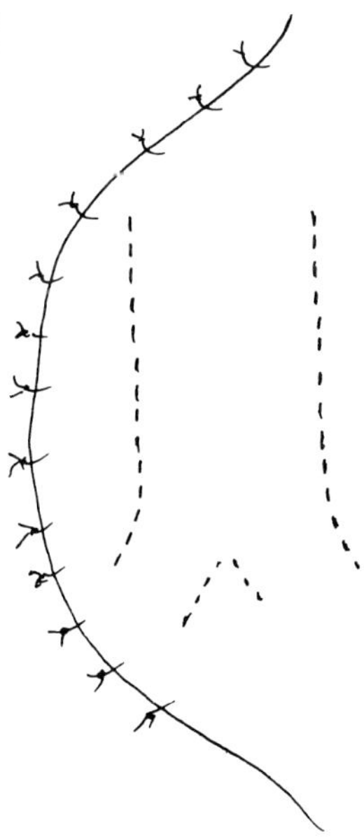

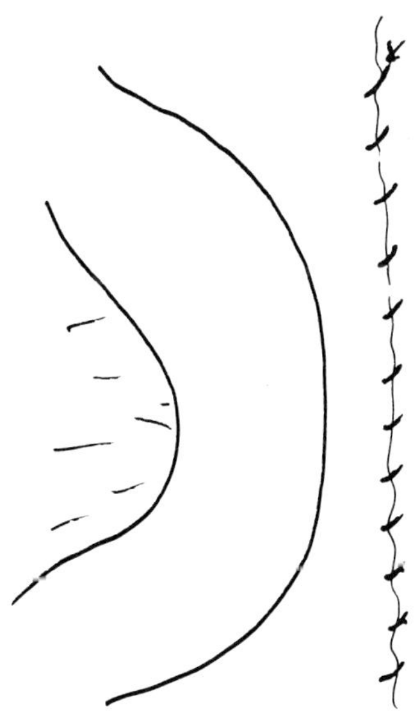

Fig. 4. Aortofemoral bypass and closure.
(A) Extracting juxtarenal aortic plug.
(B) Correct placement of bifurcation graft.
(C) Posterior peritoneal repair.
(D) Wound closure. P = parietal peritoneum, P.R.S. = posterior rectus sheath. A.R.S. = anterior rectus sheath.
(E) Tying of tension sutures over gauze roll

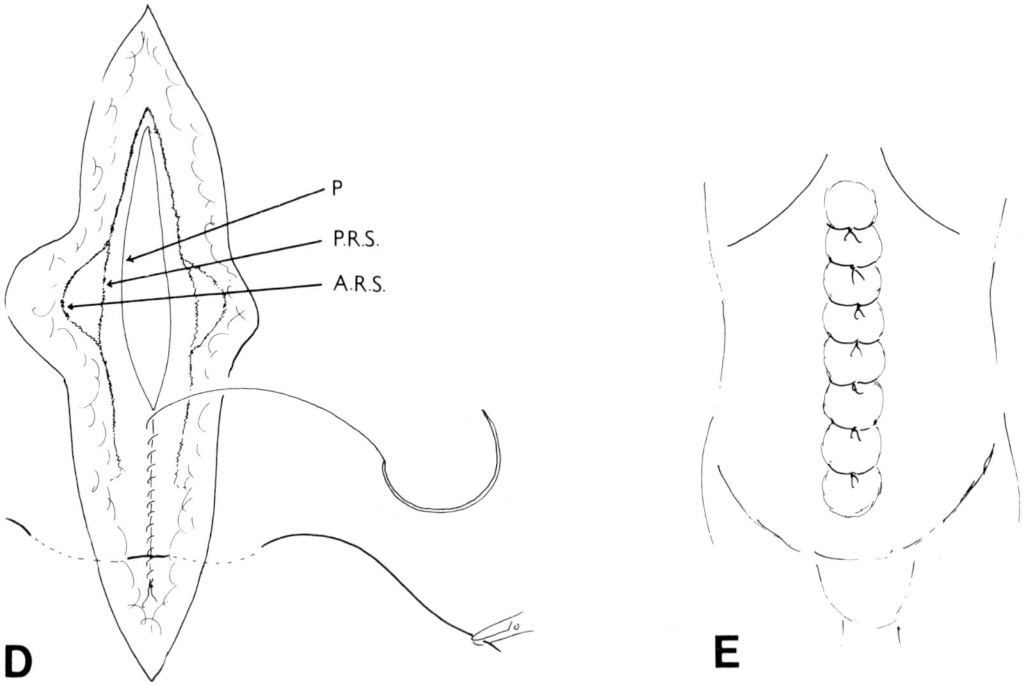

Wound Closure (Fig. 4)

The graft must be covered, if possible with the left leaf of posterior peritoneum (Fig. 4C) and the duodenum is replaced. The parietal peritoneum is repaired with 2-0 polypropylene on a large 5/8 or Moynihan type of hand needle. The same suture is used as a continuous stitch also for the aponeurotic repair, after placing six to eight deep subaponeurotic tension stitches, left long for subsequent tying over a long gauze roll or pad.

Since adopting this closure seven years ago, the writer has not had any cases of burst abdomen after abdominal aortic operation.

Final Procedures in Operating Room

A nasogastric tube and urinary catheter are inserted. Elderly subjects and those with cardiorespiratory problems should also have a central venous pressure line.

REFERENCES

1. Helsby R, Moossa AR: Aorto-iliac reconstruction with a special reference to the extraperitoneal approach. Br J Surg 62; 596, 1975
2. Starr DS, Lawrie GM, Weatherford SC, Morris GC: Prevention of distal embolism during arterial reconstruction. Am J Surg 138: 764, 1979
3. Brewster DC, Darling RC: Optimal methods of aortoiliac reconstruction. Surgery 84: 739, 1978
4. Baird RN, Kidson IG, L'Itaien GJ, Abbott WM: Dynamic compliance of arterial grafts. Am J Physiol 233: H568, 1977
5. Christensen RD, Bernatz PE: Anastomotic aneurysms involving the femoral artery. Proc Mayo Clin 47: 313, 1972

An End-to-end, Interrupted Technique for Aortic Anastomosis: An Alternate Approach

Richard F. Kempczinski

The long-term durability and functional improvement following bypass surgery from the aorta to the iliac or femoral arteries have made it one of the most popular and important procedures in the vascular surgeon's armamentarium.[1] The end-to-side technique for aortic anastomosis, as described in the chapter by Eastcott remains the most popular approach for this part of the operation because of the ease and rapidity with which it can be performed and because it leaves the host aorta undisturbed as an alternate source of distal blood flow should the graft subsequently thrombose or become infected and have to be removed. However, when the abdominal aorta is aneurysmal or totally occluded to the level of the renal arteries, an end-to-end anastomosis to the infrarenal aorta is necessary. Over the past six years, we have performed aortic anastomosis using an interrupted, end-to-end technique in more than 150 cases, reserving the end-to-side approach for situations in which the aorta is unusually small or there are anomalous visceral vessels that would have to be reimplanted. We feel the advantages of this technique can be summarized as follows:

1. It results in hemodynamically superior inflow into the graft.
2. It avoids competitive flow through the distal aorta, thus maximizing graft flow.
3. It prevents dissemination of atheromatous emboli from the diseased aorta to the lower extremities.[2]
4. It facilitates closure of the retroperitoneum over the aortic anastomosis, thus preventing duodenal erosion and fistula formation.
5. It permits a meticulous thromboendarterectomy of the proximal aorta when necessary, and a secure anastomosis despite the apparent fragility of the remaining aortic wall.
6. It results in a threefold reduction in late graft limb failure.[3]

We employ this technique routinely in elective aortic bypass surgery. However, to those surgeons who still prefer the end-to-side technique, we can recommend it as an alternate approach, especially in those circumstances where endarterectomy of the infrarenal aorta must be performed.

TECHNIQUE

The aorta is approached through a standard midline incision. The intestines are reflected to the patient's right and the retroperitoneum over the aorta is incised in the usual fashion. The infrarenal aorta is completely mobilized from the level of the left renal vein to the origin of the inferior mesenteric artery and carefully encircled with a renal pedicle clamp. A sterile shoestring is passed around the aorta. Traction on the shoestring and blunt dissection along the lateral, aortic wall will usually reveal a single pair of lumbar arteries originating at this level. These are divided between ligatures, and a segment of infrarenal aorta, 3 to 4 cm in length, is thus effectively mobilized (Fig. 1).

In most patients, the juxtarenal aorta will be patent and relatively soft. We routinely prefer anastomosis at this level even if the more distal aorta is patent, since this segment is likely to be relatively disease-free and to remain so, thus, insuring good long-term inflow for the graft. Prior to dividing the aorta, a knitted, Dacron, double-velour graft of appropriate size is selected. The patient is systemically heparinized with 1 mg/kg of beef-lung heparin administered through the central venous line. After allowing 1 to 2 minutes to elapse for adequate circulation of the heparin, 150 cc of blood are withdrawn from the infrarenal aorta, using a 50-cc syringe with an 18-gauge needle. The blood is placed in a sterile kidney basin on the operative field and used to preclot the Dacron graft. Gentle pressure over the needle-puncture site on the aorta will usually satisfactorily control any bleeding. This maneuver is performed prior to aortic clamping to minimize the duration of aortic occlusion.

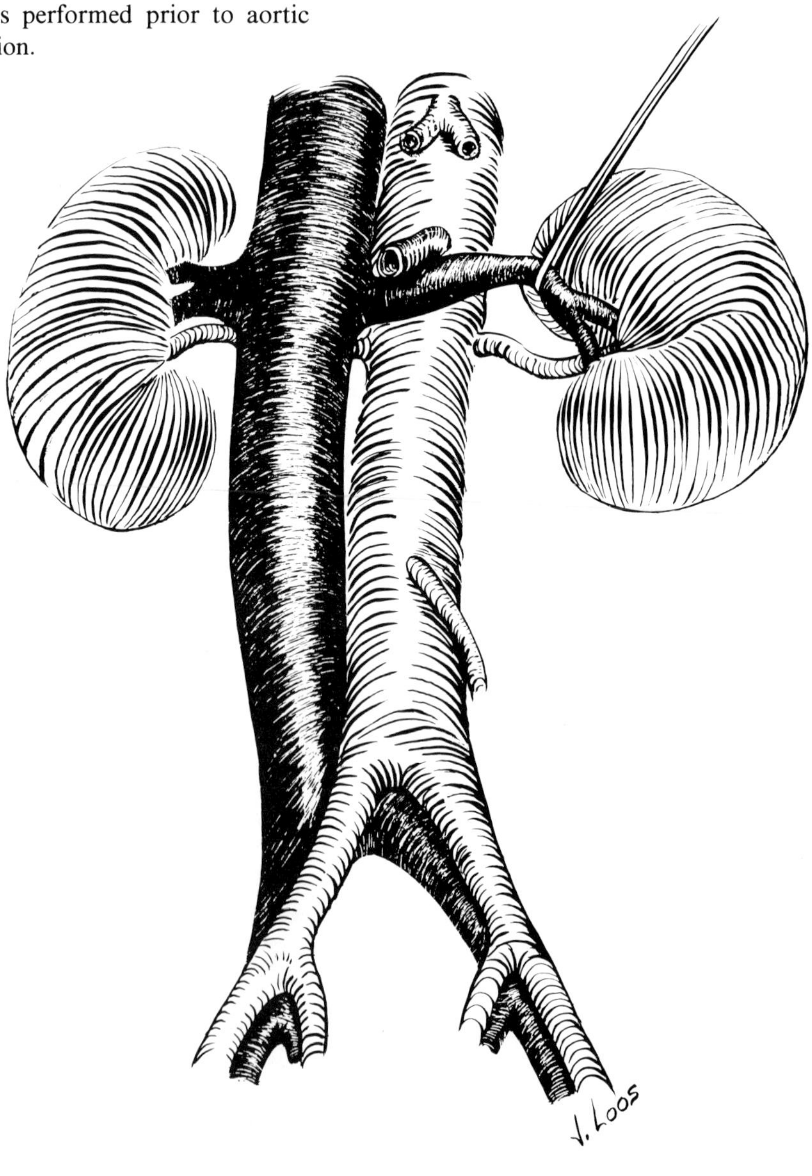

Fig. 1 Skeletonization of the aorta gives adequate exposure for ultimate grafting.

The aortic portion of the Dacron graft is trimmed to a length of 5 to 7 cm. A straight clamp is applied to it, and it is immersed in the basin of blood. Using two 50-cc Toomey syringes, the surgeon and the assistant draw blood from the basin and force it repeatedly through the iliac limbs of the bifurcation graft (Fig. 2). After repeating this maneuver for 15 to 20 minutes depending on the porosity of the Dacron graft selected, it will begin to distend and show resistance to the efflux of blood, indicating that the preclotting process has been completed. The use of heparinized blood to preclot Dacron grafts results in a thin, more durable, less thrombogenic flow surface and has been used successfully by several other surgeons with equally good results.[4,5]

Following completion of the preclotting process, the graft is carefully evacuated of any luminal blood and inspected to ensure that there are no fibrin strands or thrombi retained within the lumen. Clamps are applied to the distal iliac limbs, and the graft is replaced in the preclotting basin.

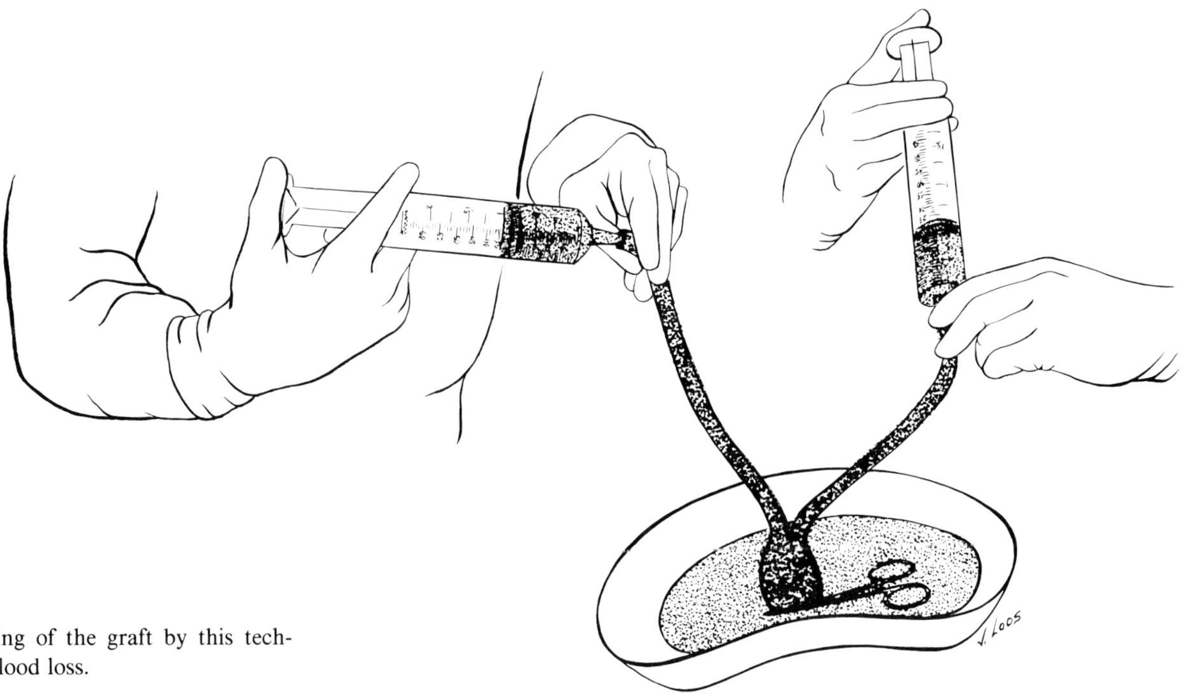

Fig. 2. Preclotting of the graft by this technique decreases blood loss.

If the infrarenal aorta is completely thrombosed or extensively calcified, thus precluding the application of standard vascular clamps, intraluminal balloon occlusion of the aorta is used to gain proximal control. This can be accomplished by threading a small Foley catheter with a 30-cc balloon through the proposed aortic graft. If the infrarenal aorta is still patent but calcified, it is temporarily controlled by manually compressing the aorta against the lumbar spine above the renal arteries. A transverse aortotomy is then made through the anterior half of the aorta 2 to 3 cm below the renal artery, and the Foley catheter is passed into a suprarenal position. If, on the other hand, the juxtarenal aorta is totally thrombosed, the aortotomy can be made without proximal compression, and the Foley catheter can usually be threaded directly through the luminal thrombus into the proximal patent portion of the aorta. The balloon is inflated with saline and pulled down so that both the aorta and the renal arteries are satisfactorily occluded (Fig. 3). A thromboendarterectomy of the infrarenal aorta is then readily performed. Following this maneuver, graft anastomosis can be completed using the Foley catheter to maintain aortic control. However, since this increases the period of renal ischemia, it should be replaced, when feasible, by an infrarenal aortic clamp.

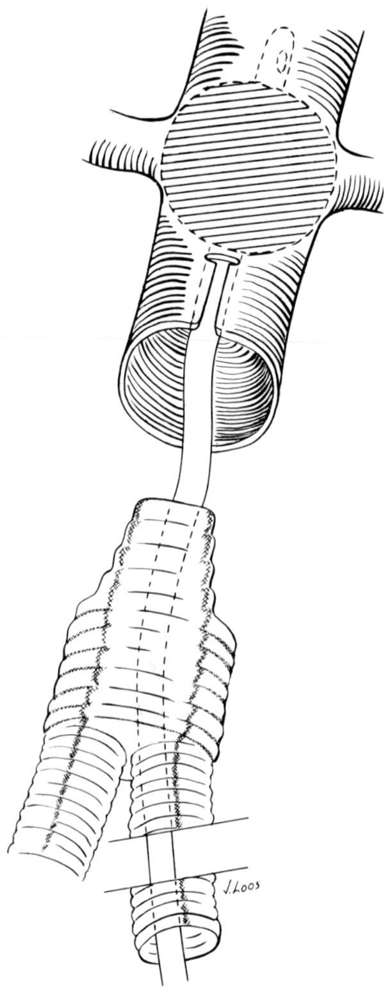

Fig. 3. Balloon occlusion of the suprarenal aorta allows juxtarenal endarterectomy to be performed.

When the juxtarenal aorta is soft and patent, it is elevated, and aortic clamps are applied immediately below the renal artery and above the inferior mesenteric artery. The aorta is transected approximately 1 cm above the distal clamp and is oversewn with a running 3–0 braided suture. A segment of aorta need not be excised. If the juxtarenal aorta is small in caliber, as is frequently the case in patients with occlusive disease, the length of the anastomosis is increased by making an anterior aortotomy of 1 to $1\frac{1}{2}$ cm. The most proximal portion of this aortotomy is widened with a T extension, 3 to 4 mm in length (Fig. 4). Following oversewing of the distal aortic segment, that clamp can be removed, thus improving exposure for the proximal anastomosis.

If the juxtarenal aorta is severely diseased or calcified, thromboendarterectomy is performed at this level without fear of compromising the subsequent aortic anastomosis. We feel this maneuver is important not only to facilitate anastomosis but also to maintain long-term patency of the aortic inflow (Fig. 5). The proximal clamp should not be released to flush the aorta until the posterior row of the anastomosis has been placed, lest the aorta retract, resulting in loss of proximal control.

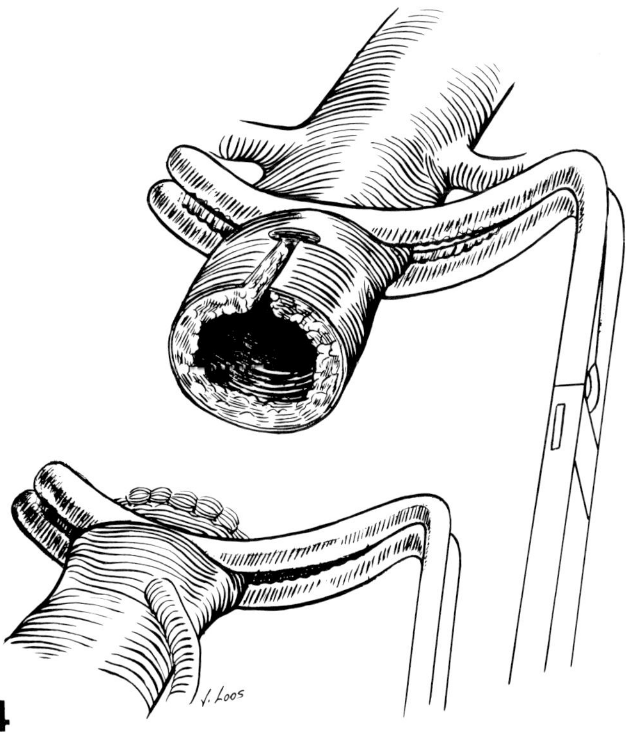

4

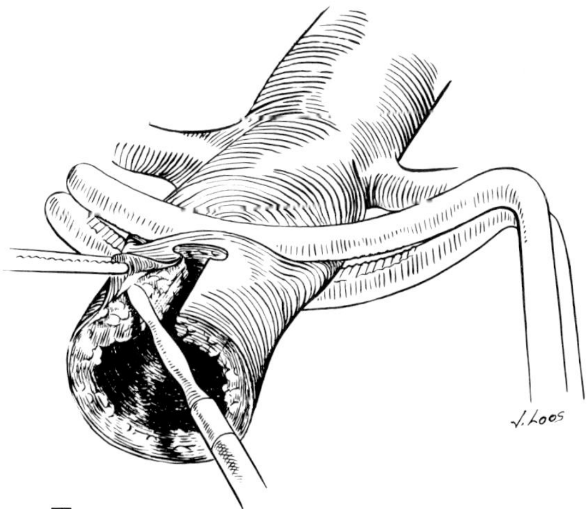

5

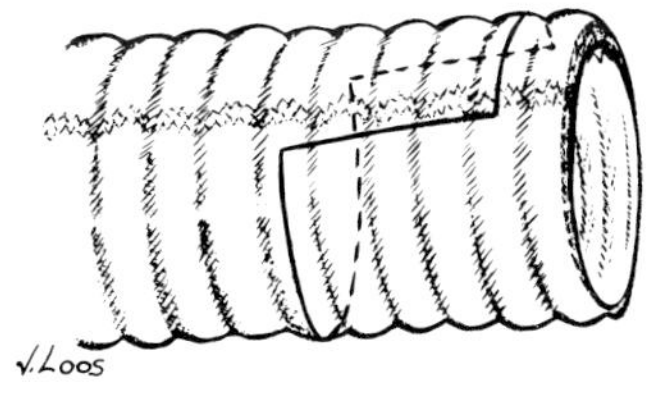

6

Figs. 4, 5, 6. Aortoplasty according to the technique shown allows widening of the proximal anastomosis.

The graft is then trimmed to match the aortotomy (Fig. 6). We employ 3-0 braided Dacron sutures for all anastomoses between prosthesis and aorta. The suture line is begun in the center of the posterior aortic wall. A horizontal mattress technique is employed. Both needles are passed through the Dacron graft from outside to inside with a space of 5 to 6 mm between them, then through corresponding points on the aortic wall, posteriorly, and finally through an individual 7-mm square pledget of Teflon felt (Fig. 7). The two ends of the suture are grasped with a hemostat and the needles cut off. The second suture is placed, in identical fashion, immediately adjacent to the first. By leaving little or no space between sutures and doing all traveling within each suture, a secure blood-tight anastomosis will result. Suturing of the posterior row is facilitated by placing the aortic graft on the patient's chest wall with the distal limbs pointing towards the head (Fig. 8). Once the 180 degrees of the posterior row are complete, the graft is guided into place and the sutures are each individually tied against the Teflon pledget, which prevents them from pulling through the aortic wall, and the excess suture is cut. Seven to nine stitches are generally required for this half of the anastomosis.

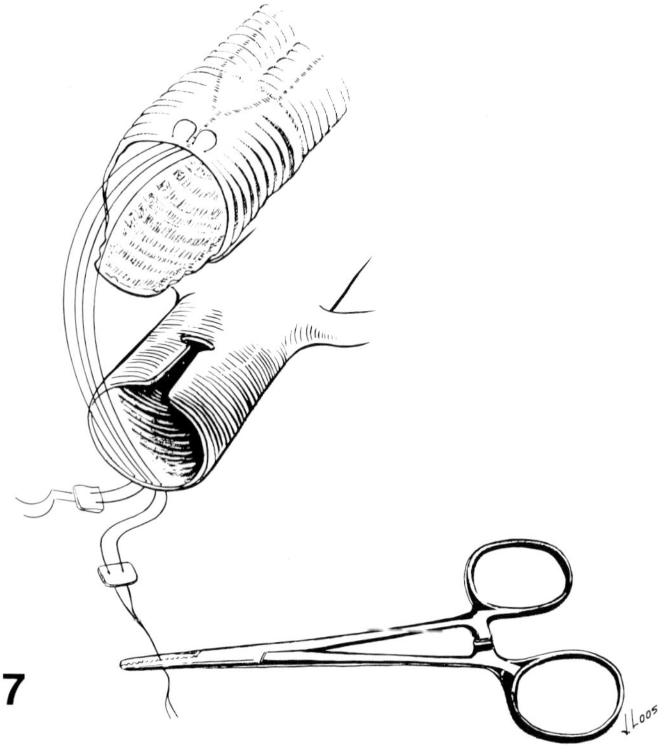

7

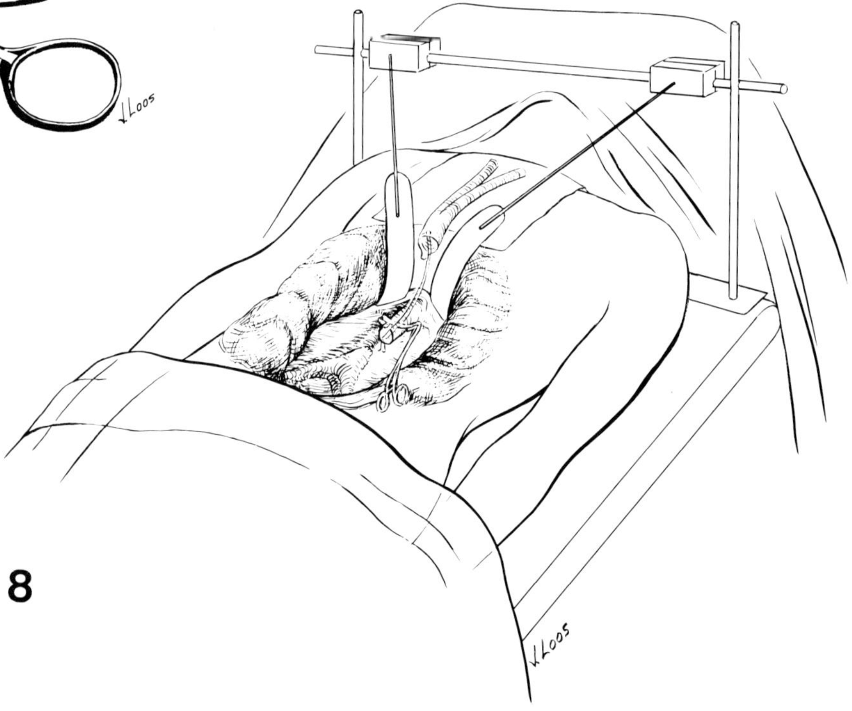

8

Fig. 7. Needles are passed through Dacron graft from outside to inside, through corresponding points on aortic wall, and through a pledget of Teflon felt.

Fig. 8. Placing the aortic graft on patient's chest wall with the distal limbs pointing towards the head facilitates suturing of the posterior row.

Figure 9 illustrates the completed posterior row and the first suture being placed at the apex of the anterior aortotomy. Beginning the anterior row in this manner lines up the graft and host aorta and facilitates the placement of the remaining sutures in a manner identical to that employed posteriorly. When all the anterior sutures have been placed, they are tied and the excess suture cut. Figure 10 illustrates the completed anastomosis.

The time required to perform an aortic anastomosis with this technique will vary depending on the amount of endarterectomy of the aortic wall that must be performed. However, in our experience, the mean operating time for this technique is 35 minutes. Following temporary release of the aortic clamp, the anastomosis will usually be found secure. However, if a bleeding point is identified, the everting nature of this anastomosis simplifies rapid hemostasis by the placement of an additional mattress suture as necessary. If additional preclotting of the Dacron graft is instead required, 100 to 200 cc of blood are allowed to pool in the abdomen. The aortic clamp is then reapplied and, using the Toomey syringes, blood from the abdomen is repeatedly forced through the graft until preclotting is complete. This maneuver will rarely be necessary if the clotting technique described above is precisely followed. Once hemostasis of both the suture line and the Dacron graft has been achieved, the distal limbs of the graft are clamped and the proximal aortic clamp is temporarily released. This will confirm adequate hemostasis under conditions of full aortic pressure. At least 50 cc of blood are flushed through the graft to clear it of any debris or atheromatous material that may have accumulated above the anastomosis. Following completion of this maneuver, we usually reapply the clamp to the aortic wall, although the body of the graft itself may be clamped if a suitable instrument, such as the Fogarty Hydra-grip clamp, is available. Standard aortic clamps should not be applied to a Dacron graft, if possible, since fiber damage may result.

The lumen of the graft must be carefully evacuated of any blood to prevent the formation of luminal thrombi. It is carefully inspected following this maneuver and, if necessary, flushed with saline to remove any residual debris.

The retroperitoneum is irrigated with saline to remove any blood or atheromatous debris. Careful inspection for any bleeding is best performed at this stage, since distal anastomosis will make inspection of the posterior aortic wall subsequently difficult. Both limbs of the graft are then carried through their retroperitoneal tunnels to the site chosen for distal anastomosis, which is performed end-to-side with running sutures of 4–0 braided Dacron in a manner similar to that described in the previous chapter.

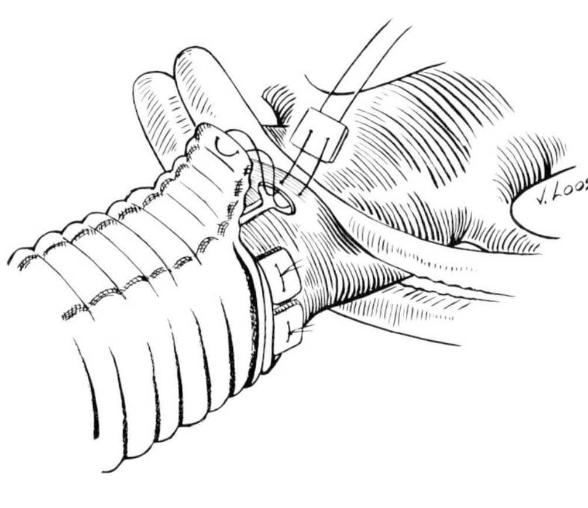

Fig. 9. Completed posterior row and the first suture at apex of anterior aortotomy.

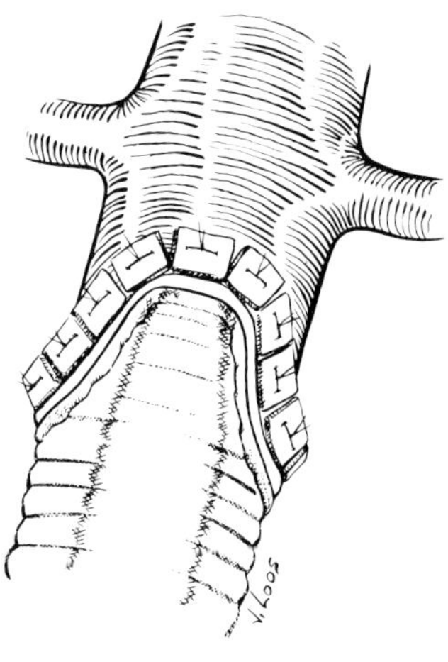

Fig. 10. Completed anastomosis.

CONCLUSION

We have described a technique for end-to-end anastomosis of a Dacron prosthesis to the infrarenal aorta using interrupted horizontal mattress sutures with individual Teflon felt pledgets as a buttress for the aortic wall. Our reported experience with this technique[6] has shown it to be a durable means of ensuring a secure anastomosis with even the most difficult aortas. We have never seen anastomotic bleeding, false aneurysm formation, or an aortoduodenal fistula from an aortic anastomosis performed in this manner. Although we employ it routinely, we would certainly recommend it to other vascular surgeons when aortic anastomosis is difficult or the aortic wall appears unduly fragile.

REFERENCES

1. Malone JM, Moore WS, Goldstone J: The natural history of bilateral aortofemoral bypass grafts for ischemia of the lower extremities. Arch Surg 110:1300, 1975
2. Kempczinski RF: Lower-extremity arterial emboli from ulcerating atherosclerotic plaques. JAMA 241:807, 1979
3. Brewster DC, Darling RC: Optimal methods of aortoiliac reconstruction. Surgery 84:739, 1978
4. Yates SG, Barros D'Sa AAB, Berger K, et al: The preclotting of porous arterial prostheses. Ann Surg 188:611, 1978
5. Linton RR: Atlas of Vascular Surgery. Philadelphia, WB Saunders Company, 1973
6. Jones AF, Kempczinski, RF: Operative therapy for aortoiliac arterial occlusive disease (submitted for publication)

Thoracoabdominal Aortic Aneurysm: Surgical Techniques

E. Stanley Crawford, Salwa A. Saleh

Thoracoabdominal aortic aneurysms and aneurysms involving the upper or entire abdominal aorta are relatively rare and were first treated by excision and graft replacement using homografts.[1–3] The visceral vessels were reattached to corresponding branches of the homograft or by separate grafts sutured end-to-end to vessel and end-to-side to homograft. Hypothermia and temporary shunts were employed to minimize organ ischemia during operation. With the advent of prosthetic grafts and to simplify operation, a technique was devised in which a permanent bypass with appropriate side arm branches to be attached to visceral vessels was first inserted and then the visceral vessels were attached sequentially to the side-arm grafts starting with the left renal artery as the aneurysm was excised reducing renal occlusion time for periods ranging from 15 to 30 minutes.[4] These operations were extensive, time consuming, and frequently associated with excessive bleeding both during and after operation. Moreover, the mortality rate from this form of treatment was 26 percent. Both to further simplify operation and to avoid complications, the senior author introduced the technique of graft inclusion and direct visceral artery reattachment to graft without temporary bypass or hypothermia approximately 15 years ago. A small series of cases treated in this manner was first reported in 1974, and a larger series in 1978.[2,5] To date, this operation has been employed in 145 patients, with survival in 92 percent of cases.

The duration of the operation varies from 2.5 to 3.5 hours, depending upon extent of lesion and size of patients. Hemorrhage has been eliminated as a significant complication and the incidence of paraplegia in patients with extensive aneurysms has been reduced by reattaching or preserving intercostal and lumbar arteries.[5–8] Renal insufficiency, being a problem of failure to anatomically restore renal circulation, has been almost eliminated through increased experience in surgical techniques, and judgment in their application. Moreover, improvement in results has been achieved by better evaluation and preparation of patients through study of the aortic and associated arterial lesions, improvements in anesthesia, monitoring, and blood volume replacement. The purpose of this report is to briefly identify the important aspects of these adjuncts and to present in more detail the technical aspects of the operation.

PATIENT SELECTION AND PREOPERATIVE PREPARATION

All patients are considered for operation, regardless of age, associated disease, and extent of aneurysm. Final selection for operation is based upon thorough hospital evaluation, including cardiac, pulmonary, and renal function and the presence of associated untreatable disease. Good-risk patients without evidence of associated disease are well hydrated and then submitted to aortography visualizing the entire aorta and its major branches to determine the extent of aneurysm, the anatomic arrangement of branches, and associated disease of these branches. Good hydration is continued and renal function studied at 24 and 48 hours to determine the occurrence of transient renal dysfunction resulting from aortography. Operation is usually performed electively within 48 hours but is delayed in those rare instances in which there is a rise in BUN and creatinine until these values are normal. CT scanning may be employed as a secondary procedure to evaluate the abdominal aortic segment but is never employed alone as the primary method of study for planning of operation.

Patients with heart disease are evaluated by the usual battery of diagnostic procedures to determine the etiology and severity of disease and the best method of treatment. Elective patients best managed by operation, ie, those requiring coronary artery bypass or valve replacement, are treated by cardiac operation and are later readmitted for aneurysm operation. Those best treated medically are placed on a medical program and observed in the hospital for 5 to 10 days. Those who show good response are then submitted to aneurysm operation, and those who do not are rejected. Patients with pulmonary disease, blood dyscrasia, diabetes, and gastrointestinal disorders are managed in a similar manner.

The great vessels arising from the aortic arch including thoracic, cervical, and cranial segments are visualized at the time of aortography in patients with either neck murmurs or symptoms of cerebrovascular disease. Occlusive lesions of these vessels, which may produce stroke, are either treated at the time of aneurysm operation or a week to 10 days earlier. Iliac and femoral arteries are also visualized at the time of aortography in patients with pulse changes to determine location and extent of distal occlusive disease. Iliac occlusive disease is usually treated by bypass operation at the time of aneurysm operation by extending the aortic graft as external iliac or common femoral bypass, using a bifurcation aortic graft attached to the end of the main graft used to replace the aneurysm.

With this approach, the majority of patients are eventually treated by operation. Those with advanced cardiac, pulmonary, renal, and neoplastic disease, and those with lesser manifestations who do not respond to treatment are advised not to have graft replacement. As best as can be determined, less than 10 patients have been turned down for operation in the past 15 years.

ANESTHESIA, MONITORING, AND BLOOD REPLACEMENT

Patients arrive in the anesthesia area well hydrated, on digitalis, with normal electrolytes and blood gases from careful preparation. The following lines are inserted: bilateral radial intra-arterial catheters, a central venous line, a Swan-Ganz catheter, and four peripheral venous catheters. All lines are inserted percutaneously. Intra-arterial blood pressure, central venous pressure, pulmonary artery pressure, capillary wedge pressure, cardiac output, and electrocardiogram are monitored continuously or intermittently, dependent upon method. Blood gases and electrolytes are also monitored every 30 minutes. Developing abnormalities are corrected by appropriate therapy as they occur.

Anesthesia is obtained using drugs (narcotics) that do not depress the myocardium, and muscle relaxation is achieved by using muscle relaxants. A double-lumen bifurcation endotracheal tube is used to deflate the left lung during operation upon the thoracic segment of aneurysm to protect the lung from injury, to avoid cardiac compression during lung retraction, and to increase the exposure of the operative site. Electrolyte solutions begun before operation are continued during operation. The first liter is given as 5 percent dextrose and Ringer's lactate solution, and the remainder as plain Ringer's lactate solution, maintaining the central venous pressure between 7 and 10 mm of water and pulmonary wedge pressure and cardiac output at normal levels. Mannitol solution, 25 gm, is given intravenously after induction of anesthesia. Blood replacement is by component technique using packed red cells, fresh frozen plasma, platelets, and albumin. A unit of albumin and two units of fresh frozen plasma are given at the onset of operation; as blood replacement becomes necessary, 250 cc of packed red blood cells to which 100 cc of sodium chloride, U.S.P., have been added, are given and continued as necessary. A unit of fresh frozen plasma is given after the third transfusion and then alternated with two units of red cells. Fresh platelets, 10 to 16 units, are given rapidly when flow is restored through the graft. Operation is delayed in patients taking coumarin until prothrombin time is normal. If operation is urgent, Aquamephytin and 2 to 4 units of fresh frozen plasma are given before operation, and plasma administration is continued until prothrombin time is within normal range. Disturbances of fibrinolysis have been corrected by giving Cryoprecipitate (4 to 6 units).

Temporary shunts, bypasses, and heparin are not employed in the operation. Normal cardiac hemodynamics are maintained during aortic clamping by the administration of drugs including nitroprusside. The proximal aorta is clamped slowly, as this drug is administered at a rate such that aortic clamping does not significantly elevate blood pressure or pulmonary capillary wedge pressure. Blood-volume replacement and intravenous fluid administration during aortic clamping are coordinated with nitroprusside to maintain normal blood pressure and cardiac hemodynamics. When the graft has been inserted and before removal of the aortic clamps, the vasodilator drugs are discontinued. The rate of blood replacement and electrolyte administration is increased, maintaining normal blood pressure as the proximal aortic clamp is slowly removed.

SURGICAL TECHNIQUES

The techniques of graft inclusion and direct arterial reattachment to graft are illustrated by line drawings of actual cases showing positioning on operating table, placement of incision, exposure of lesion, and method of graft insertion and vessel reattachment, with variations according to extent and nature of disease, presence of associated arterial branch disease, and anatomic variations.

Positioning and Incision

The operation is performed with the patient lying on the right side with the left elevated 60 degrees (Fig. 1C). This position is maintained by cradling the patient in a "bean bag" molded to the thighs, hips, and dependent part of the trunk. A thoracoabdominal incision is made, the location of which is dependent upon the location and extent of aneurysm. In patients with extensive aneurysms involving most of the descending thoracic aorta and all of the abdominal aorta in whom the upper thoracic aorta and iliac arteries must be exposed for cross-clamping or reconstruction, the incision is started as a full midline abdominal incision which enters the abdomen and is completed by extension across the costal arch into sixth or seventh intercostal space (Fig. 1A). The incision in patients with more limited involvement to distal thoracic aorta and upper abdominal aorta is made obliquely across the upper abdomen just above the umbilicus and extended across the costal arch into eighth or ninth intercostal space (Fig. 1B). With more extensive abdominal involvement, the oblique abdominal incision is made about 3 cm below the umbilicus.

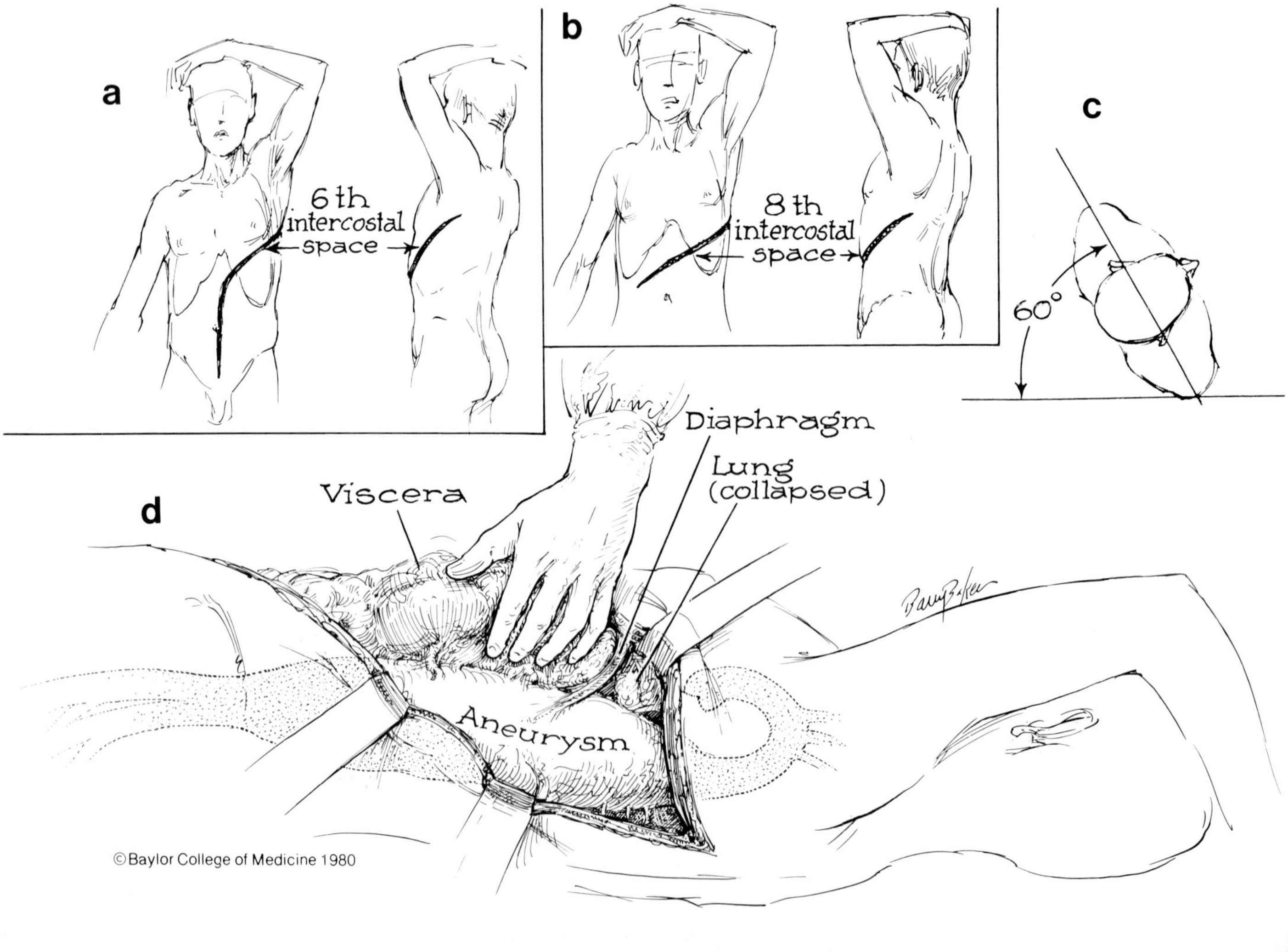

Exposure of Operative Field

The diaphragm is cut radically from the costal arch incision directly to the aortic hiatus. The left lung is collapsed using the double lumen endotracheal tube and gently retracted medially, exposing the chest cavity and posterior mediastinum containing the upper segment of aneurysm. Aortic dissection in the chest is limited to mobilization of enough uninvolved proximal aorta to apply the proximal clamp, which is accomplished by incising the mediastinal pleura. This step of the operation is completed by blunt digital dissection, which permits the necessary palpation to avoid injury to aorta, adjacent structures, and intercostal arteries. The abdominal segment of aneurysm is next exposed extraperitoneally from the left (Fig. 1D). This is accomplished by making an incision in the peritoneum lateral to the left colon. The relatively avascular retroperitoneal tissue plane is entered and the left colon, including mesentery and ureter, are mobilized down to the aorta. Dissection in this plane is continued upward to the aortic hiatus behind the kidney, lateral to and behind the spleen, tail of the pancreas, and the stomach down to the posteriolateral aspect of the aortic aneurysm. The mobilized organs are retracted upward and to the right, exposing the area for reconstruction (Fig. 1D). Either the uninvolved distal aorta or the iliac arteries are exposed for temporary clamping during operation. The left iliac artery is exposed by extension of the above incision. The right may be exposed through the same incision; however, a separate peritoneal incision may be required in some cases. When the iliac system is involved by extensive dissection or associated atherosclerotic occlusive disease, the common femoral arteries are exposed in the groins.

Reconstruction Techniques

Working with the anesthesiologist, the surgeon slowly clamps the aorta proximally to avoid significant elevation of proximal blood pressure and disturbances in cardiac hemodynamics as previously described. The uninvolved segment or segments are then clamped distally. The aneurysm is entered, making a longitudinal incision using electrocautery to control bleeding from the cut edges of the aneurysmal wall, which are retracted using heavy sutures. This maneuver opens the aneurysm and gently retracts the lung and abdominal viscera, providing good exposure of the inside of the aneurysm. The incision is made posteriolaterally in the chest and extended in the same position in the abdomen posterior to origin of left renal artery, so that by retracting the upper aneurysmal wall, all visceral vessel origins come into view on the medial wall of the aneurysm, with the left renal artery being at the top (Figs. 2–5). Bleeding from visceral arteries is controlled by No. 4 Fogerty catheters (Figs. 2,5). Bleeding from intercostal and lumbar arteries is controlled by suture, except where these are to be reattached to the graft (those involving most descending thoracic and abdominal aortas). Bleeding in the latter cases is controlled by No. 3 Fogerty catheters placed in the vessels to be reattached. Those not reattached are sutured. To avoid excessive bleeding, the aneurysm is opened gradually from above down as intercostal bleeding is controlled. The method of reconstruction is dependent upon extent and nature of aneurysm and associated aortic-branch lesions.

Fig. 1. (A,B) Diagrams showing location of incisions made according to extent of disease. (C) Position of patient on the operating table. (D) Exposure of the aneurysm.

Extensive Fusiform Arteriosclerotic Aneurysms

A transverse incision is made in the anterior half of the aortic circumference at each end of the longitudinal aortic incision, exposing the site for graft anastomosis (Fig. 2A). One end of a woven Dacron graft of appropriate size is sutured to the uninvolved aorta proximally using either No. 00 or No. 000 prolene suture. Hemostasis at the suture line is tested by occluding the graft just distal to the suture line and temporarily removing the proximal aortic clamp. Suture line bleeding is controlled with interrupted sutures. The graft is placed under tension, and an opening is made in it opposite the intercostal arteries to be attached, which usually are a pair of arteries arising from the mid or low descending thoracic aorta. This opening in the graft is sutured circumferentially around the orifices of these vessels (Fig. 2B). The graft is again placed under tension and openings made in it opposite the origins of the visceral vessels. The number of openings is dependent upon the distance between the orifices. When closely approximated, all four vessels may be reattached to one opening. When widely separated as in large fusiform aneurysm, each vessel may be attached to a separate opening. In still other cases the celiac, superior mesenteric, and right renal arteries may be attached to one opening and the left renal artery to a second opening.[5-8] In any case, the appropriate attachment is made by suturing the graft opening circumferentially around the origin or origins of vessels. After completion of these anastomoses, the aortic graft is flushed by temporarily removing the proximal aortic clamp. The Fogarty catheters are removed by deflating and withdrawing them through the suture line. The head of the operating table is lowered, the graft is allowed to fill with blood to expel air, the graft is clamped distal to the renal arteries, and the proximal aortic clamp is slowly removed, restoring circulation into intercostal and visceral arteries. The clamp is removed synchronously with the previously described activities of the anesthesiologist. A pair of lumbar arteries may next be reattached using a technique just described for reattachment of intercostal arteries or they may be reattached by graft (Fig. 2B). When these vessels are reattached, the largest pair is selected. When graft reattachment is employed, one end of a 10-, 12-, or 16-mm knitted Dacron tube is sutured around the orifices of these vessels and the other end is sutured to an opening made in the graft. The length of this tube is limited to 1 cm or less to avoid kinking. When reattachment is made opposite the visceral vessels, it is made to the aortic graft using partial occlusion clamps. If made distally, it is attached to the open graft, and lumbar artery flow is reestablished by moving the clamp down on the aortic graft distal to the lumbar arterial reattachment. Reconstruction is then made distally either end-to-end to distal uninvolved aorta, end-to-end to uninvolved common iliac arteries, or end-to-side either to external iliac or common femoral arteries, as required. The latter cases require the addition of a bifurcated graft (Fig. 4). After flow is restored in the entire graft, the head of operating table is elevated to neutral position and the aneurysmal wall is sutured tightly around the graft employing imbrication techniques (Fig. 2C). This maneuver tamponades bleeding through the graft and suture lines and separates the graft from adjacent structures. The operation is completed by closure of the wound.

Fig. 2. Diagrams illustrating method of reconstruction employed in a patient with extensive aneurysm involving most of the descending thoracic and abdominal aorta.
(A) Location of incision in the aneurysm, which is made posteriolaterally and behind the origin of the left renal artery.
(B) The wall of the aneurysm is retracted using stay sutures; back bleeding from visceral vessels is controlled using Fogarty catheters; lumbar arteries have been reattached using graft (this sequence of attaching lumbar arteries is out of order and for the convenience of the artist); intercostal arteries are being reattached; and separate openings made in graft for visceral artery reattachment (in practice these openings are made sequentially as the vessels are to be reattached).
(C) Reconstruction has been completed, and aneurysmal wall is being sutured around the graft.

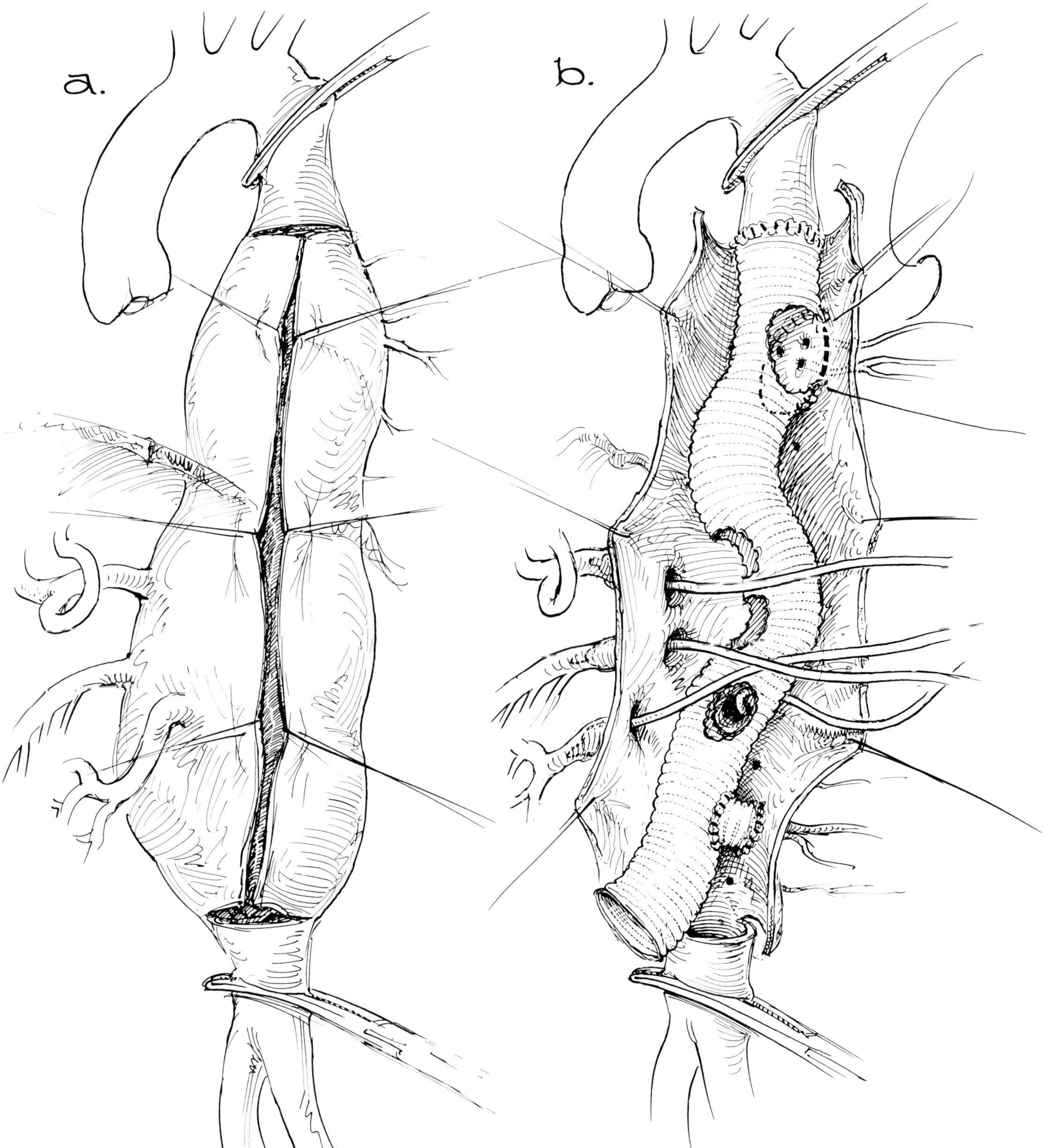
a.
b.

C.

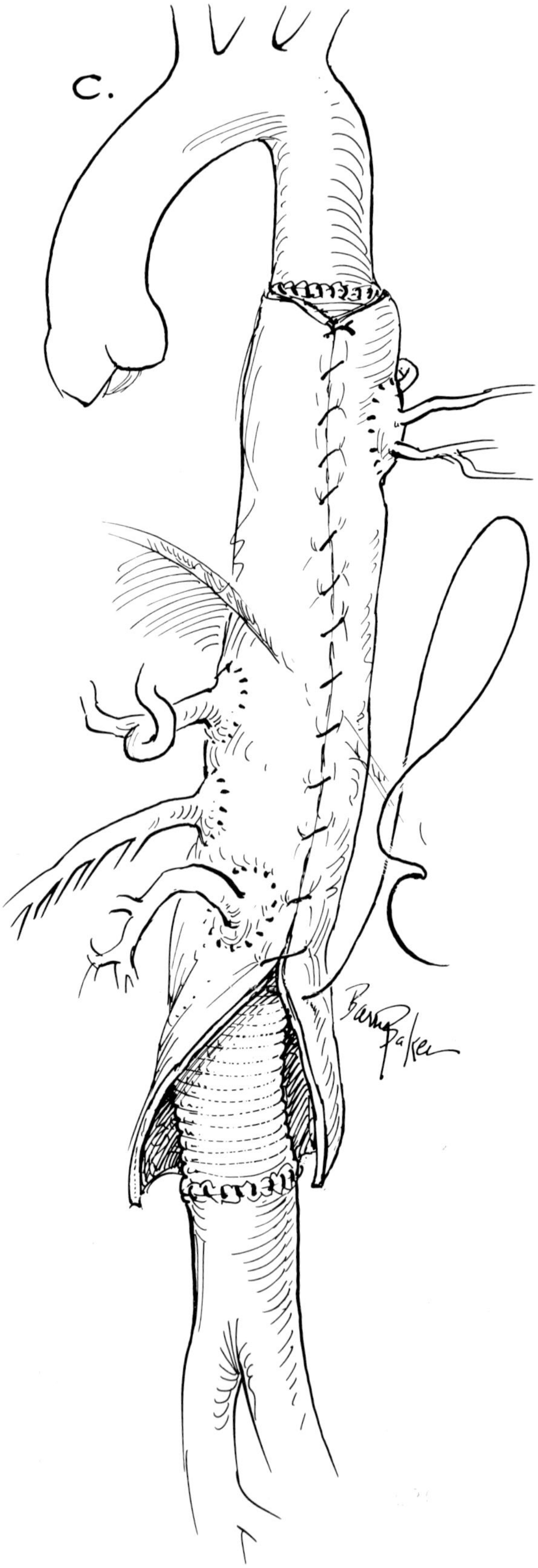

Chronic Dissecting Aneurysms Involving Descending Thoracic and Abdominal Aorta

The aneurysm in such cases results from dilatation of the weakened outer wall of false lumen. The thoracic aortic segment from which the intercostal arteries arise is usually not involved in the dissecting process, and the dilated false lumen is therefore located anteriorly and laterally. In the abdomen, the false lumen is located on the left in 85 percent of cases and on the right in 15 percent. The left renal artery arises from the false lumen in the former cases, and the right renal artery arises from the false lumen in the latter cases. The origin of the celiac and mesenteric vessels in these chronic cases may be involved to some extent; however, they usually arise from the true lumen. Regardless of location of the false lumen, the vessel origins are frequently located near each other. In any case, after clamping the aorta proximally, the aneurysm or false lumen is entered by a longitudinal incision as described above.[3] The septum between false and true lumens is excised, and reconstruction preserving intercostal arteries or intercostal and lumbar arteries is performed using a bevelled end of a woven tubular Dacron graft, the edges of which are sutured to the uninvolved aorta proximally and to the edges of undissected aorta distally (Figs. 3,4). The visceral arteries are reattached singly or in combinations as previously described. Distal reconstruction of circulation to pelvis and legs is also performed as described above.

The authors have not seen it necessary to perform such extensive operations in patients with acute dissections. Moreover, due to the friability of tissues, limited application of this patch technique to relatively short segments of thoracic aorta has not always controlled the dissecting process. We find tubular grafting more appropriate in the control of acute dissections.

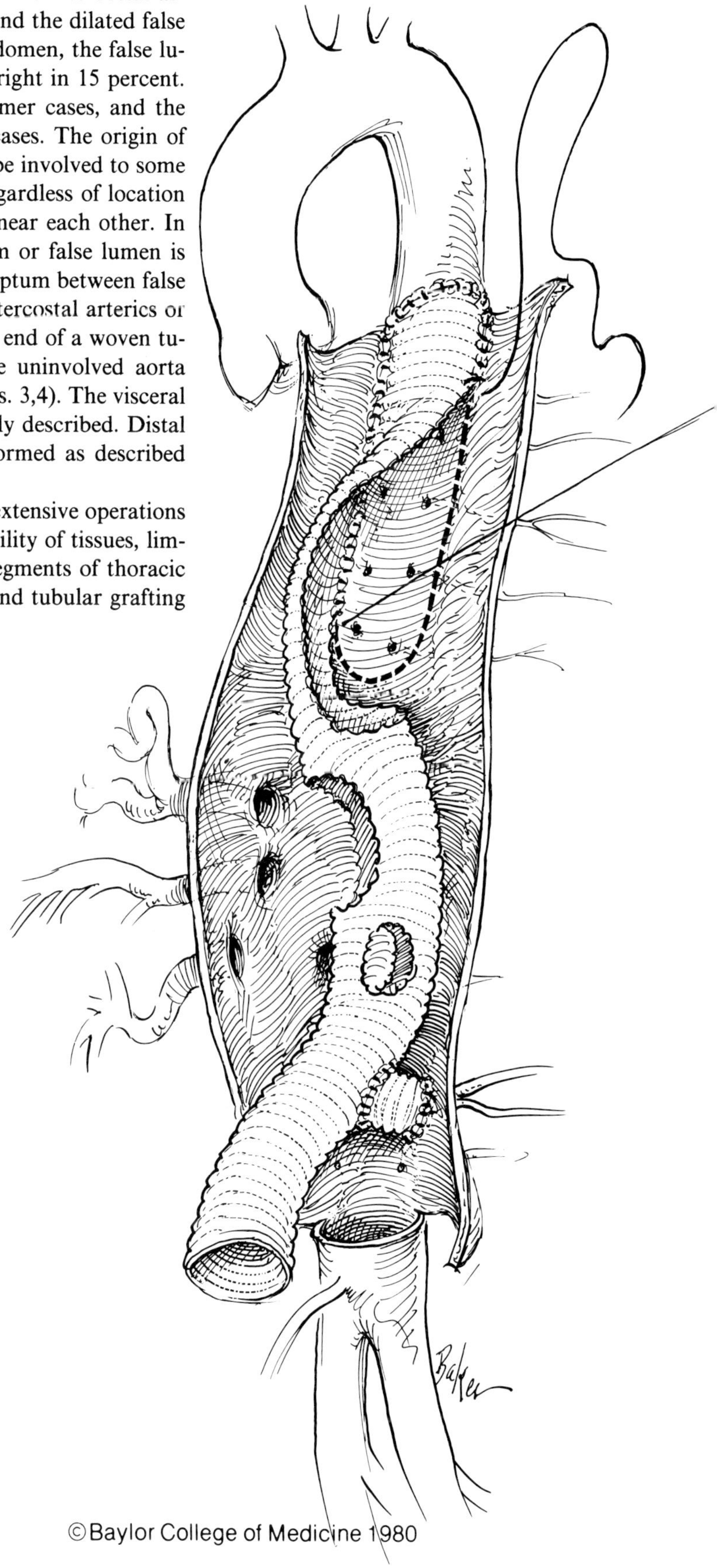

Fig. 3. Illustrations of technique employed in a patient with extensive chronic dissecting aneurysm involving both the descending thoracic and abdominal aorta. Intercostal arterial circulation is preserved by replacing the dissected portion of aortic circumference by a corresponding portion of woven Dacron tube. Lumbar arteries are reattached by graft, the celiac axis and superior mesenteric arteries are reattached to one opening in the aortic graft, and each renal artery is reattached to a separate opening in the graft.

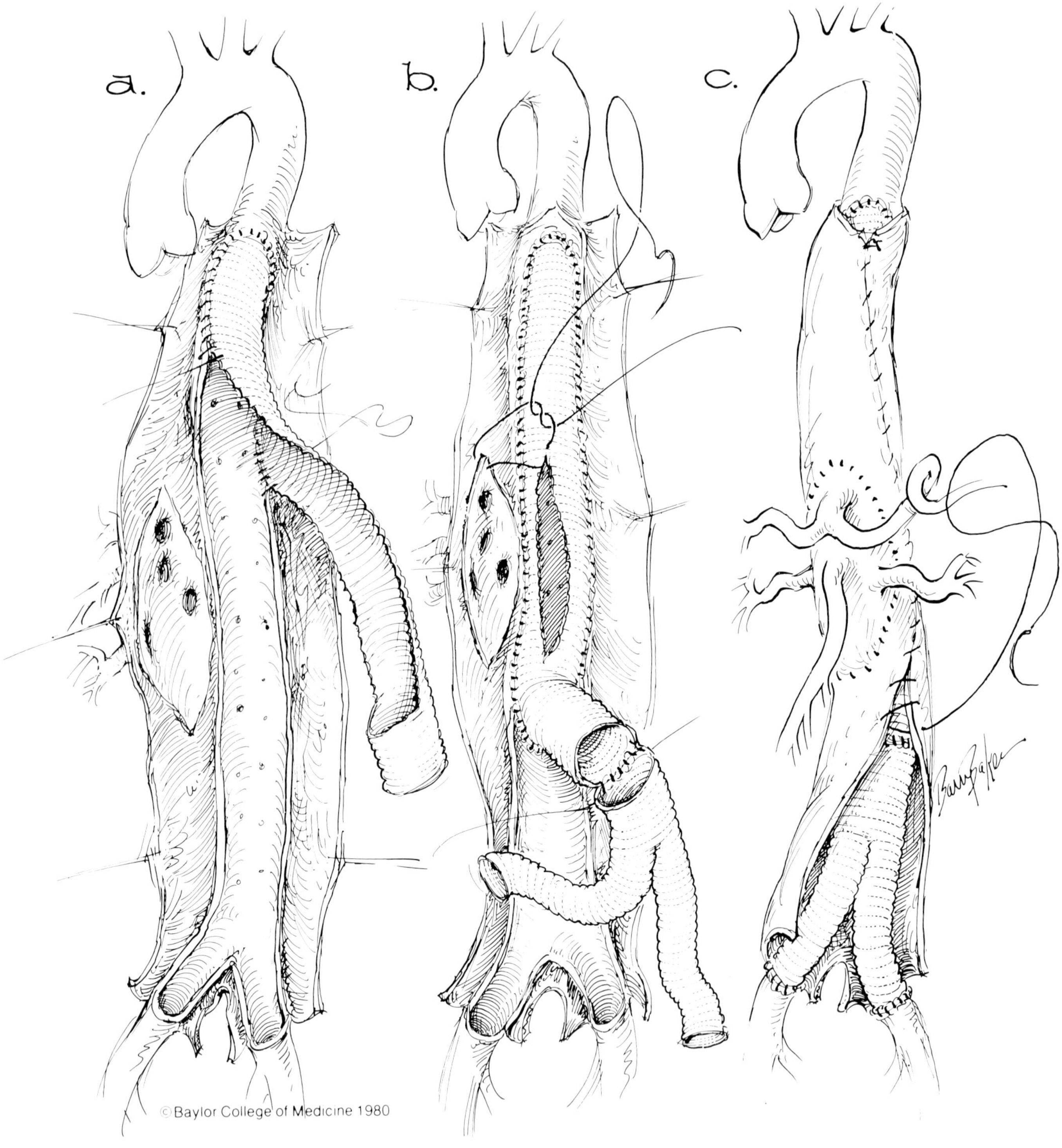

Fig. 4. Illustrations of patient with extensive chornic dissection of the descending thoracic and abdominal segments of aorta and iliac arteries reconstructed as in Figure 3, except that all visceral vessels are attached to one opening made in the aortic graft and distal circulation is restored using bifurcation graft, the iliac limbs of which were attached to distal uninvolved segments of iliac arteries.

TREATMENT OF ASSOCIATED VISCERAL ARTERY DISEASE

The most common associated disease of the visceral arteries is atherosclerotic occlusive disease involving the celiac axis, superior mesenteric, or renal arteries. Involvement of one or more of these vessels has been present in 20 percent of our cases. Occlusive lesions involving the celiac axis and superior mesenteric arteries are located at the origins of these vessels. When both are involved, they are treated by endarterectomy. When only one of these vessels has been involved, collateral circulation has been excellent, either from the other vessel or from the inferior mesenteric artery. Treatment in the latter cases has been preservation or reattachment of the collateral source of circulation.[4] Occlusive lesions of the renal arteries are usually located at the origin of these vessels; however, in some cases the lesions may be distal in location. The former are treated by endarterectomy and the latter by graft technique.[3,4] When grafts have been necessary, 8-mm knitted Dacron tubes have usually been employed. The distal end of the splenic artery, after splenectomy, has been employed in some cases to bypass distal lesions of the left renal artery.[4] Lesions producing renal infarction manifested by nonfunctioning atrophic kidneys are treated by nephrectomy.

Fig. 5. Illustrations of technique employed in patient with aneurysm involving the entire abdominal aorta associated with atherosclerotic occlusion of both celiac axis and superior mesenteric arteries.
(A) Extent of aneurysm.
(B) Method of reconstruction and endarterectomy. The lesion has been removed from the celiac axis, and endarterectomy of superior mesenteric artery is in progress.
(C) Reattachment is being completed by reattaching the left renal artery.

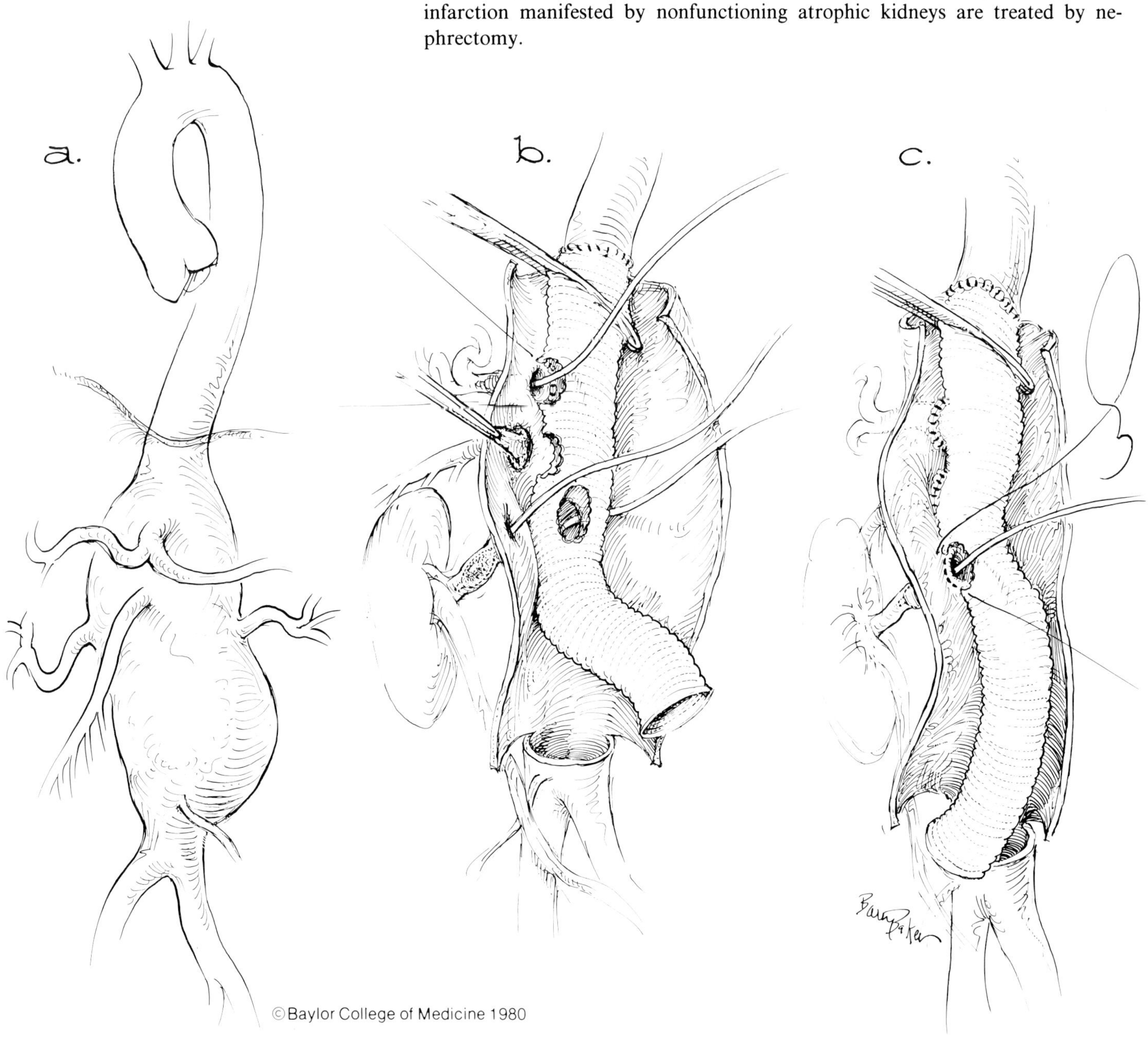

Endarterectomy is performed from inside the opened aneurysm (Fig. 5). A circular incision is made around the involved vessel orifice in the diseased aortic intima. The cleavage plane between the diseased inner layer and the normal outer layer of aortic wall is entered and dissected circumferentially to vessel origin (Fig. 5B). This plane of dissection is then continued distally into the involved vessel until the obstructing atheroma is removed. Back bleeding is controlled as described when all lesions have been removed. Reattachment of vessels to graft is performed as previously described (Fig. 5C).

Grafts are employed for reconstruction in the rare cases in which endarterectomy cannot be successfully performed and when the lesion is either extensive or located distally.[4] On the left, one end of the graft is attached to the side of the aortic graft at about the level of the diaphragm, and the other end of graft is attached end-to-end to the splayed distal uninvolved renal artery (Fig. 6). The proximal attachment of the graft and its length allows inclusion within aneurysmal wall without kinking. On the right, the distal end of the graft is attached end-to-end or end-to-side to the distal uninvolved renal artery, and the proximal end of the graft is attached to the side of the right iliac limb of the aortic graft or to the side of the uninvolved right iliac artery. This method of proximal attachment is necessary due to the fact that the aortic graft is not accessible for proximal anastomosis, since the aortic aneurysmal wall is intact and covered by retroperitoneal tissues on the right.[3,4]

Associated aneurysms of the superior mesenteric, celiac axis, and renal arteries are rare, occurring in 2 percent of cases. Sacciform aneurysms are treated by excision and patch graft repair. Fusiform aneurysms are treated by excision and graft replacement, using 8-mm knitted Dacron tubes.

Fig. 6. Patient with thoracoabdominal aortic aneurysm and diffuse renal artery occlusion requiring grafts for renal artery reconstruction.
(A) Diagram showing extent of lesions in renal arteries.
(B,C) Aortogram and diagram showing renal artery bypass grafts in place and functioning.

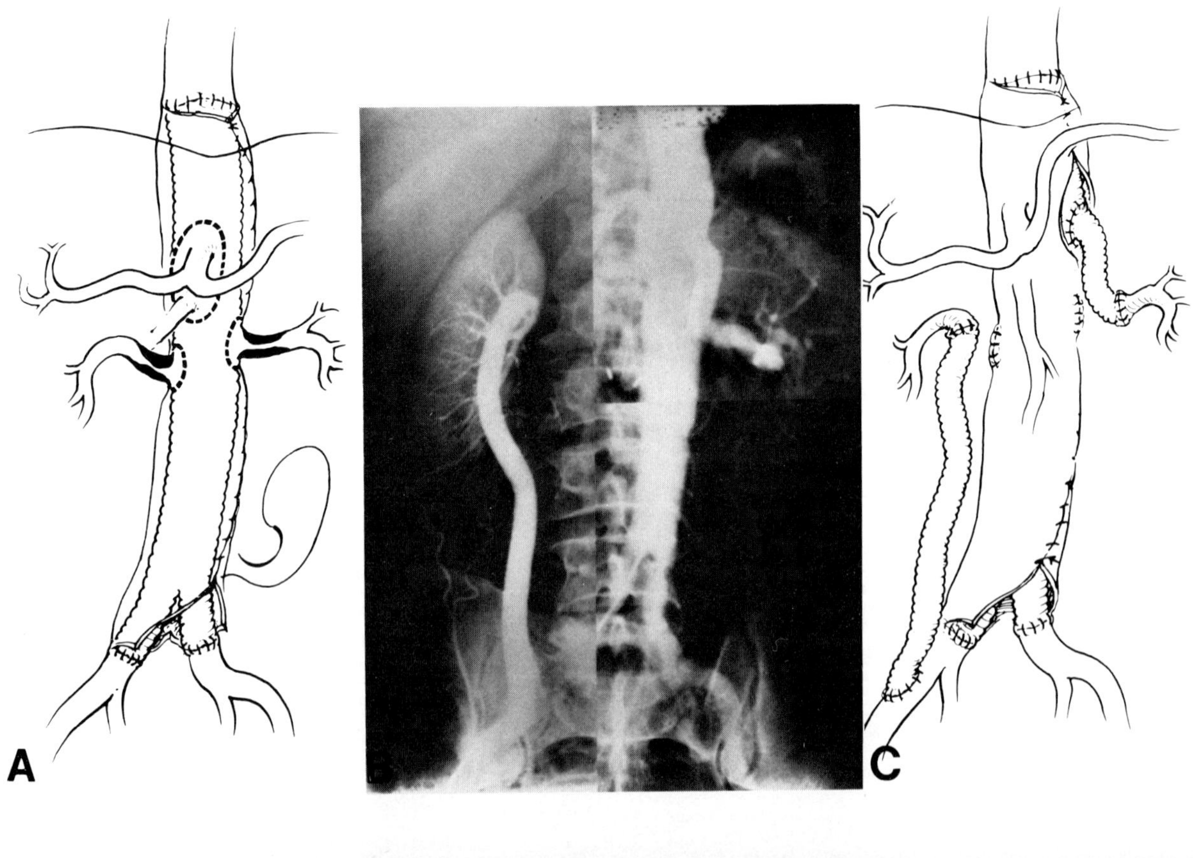

REFERENCES

1. DeBakey ME, Creech O Jr, Morris GC Jr: Aneurysms of thoraco-abdominal aorta involving the celiac, superior mesenteric, and renal arteries: Report of four cases treated by resection and homograft replacement. Ann Surg 144:459, 1956
2. Ellis FH, Helden RA, Hines EA Jr: Aneurysm of the abdominal aorta involving the right renal artery: Report of case with preservation of renal function after resection and grafting. Ann Surg 142:992, 1055
3. Etheredge SN, Yee J, Smith JV, Schonberger S, Goldman MJ: Successful resection of a large aneurysm of the upper abdominal aorta and replacement with homograft. Surgery 38:1071, 1955
4. DeBakey ME, Crawford ES, Garrett HE, Beall AC Jr, Howell JF: Surgical considerations in the treatment of aneurysms of the thoraco-abdominal aorta. Ann Surg 162:650, 1965
5. Crawford ES: Thoraco-abdominal and abdominal aortic aneurysms involving renal, superior mesenteric, and celiac arteries. Ann Surg 179:763, 1974
6. Crawford ES, Cho GC, Roehm JOF Jr: Thoraco-abdominal and abdominal aortic aneurysms involving celiac axis, superior mesenteric, and renal arteries. Bergan JJ, Yao JST (eds): Surgery of the Aorta and Its Body Branches. New York, Grune & Stratton, 1979, pp 145–169
7. Crawford ES, Schuessler JS: Thoraco-abdominal and abdominal aortic aneurysms involving celiac, superior mesenteric, renal arteries. Surgery Rounds 2:14, 1978
8. Crawford ES, Snyder DM, Cho GC, Roehm JOF Jr: Progress in treatment of thoracoabdominal and abdominal aortic aneurysms involving celiac, superior mesenteric, and renal arteries. Ann Surg 188:404, 1978

Special Problems Associated with Aortic Aneurysm Surgery

Jesse E. Thompson

A number of unusual manifestations associated with abdominal aortic aneurysms have been observed and recorded. Table 1 lists the more common ones. Awareness of these problems, recognition at the time of operation, and proper handling are imperative if such catastrophic complications as massive hemorrhage, loss of a kidney, or intestinal gangrene are to be averted. Appropriate methods of managing all these special problems have been reported and have undoubtedly resulted in reduced morbidity and mortality.[1]

Renal artery problems are best recognized from preoperative aortograms, allowing appropriate surgical plans to be made. Aberrant vessels may be implanted into the graft, or bypass grafts to the renal artery may be constructed to relieve occlusive lesions. Shunts may be used to perfuse the kidney in complicated resections.[2]

Figure 1A depicts the problem when a renal artery arises from the aneurysm. In this situation, following systemic heparinization the proximal aorta, distal iliac arteries, and right renal artery are clamped. The aneurysm is opened, and a button of aortic wall approximately 2 cm in diameter including the orifice of the renal artery, is excised. A preclotted knitted Dacron graft is then sutured end-to-end to the upper aortic stump with 3–0 polyester sutures. The aorta is flushed and the graft cleaned of clots. A hole of appropriate size is then made on the right side of the tubular portion of the graft. The button of aortic wall containing the renal artery orifice is then sutured to this orifice with a continuous suture of 4–0 polyester (Fig. 1B). Flow is then restored to the right kidney and the graft clamped below the renal artery suture line. The iliac anastomoses are then completed.

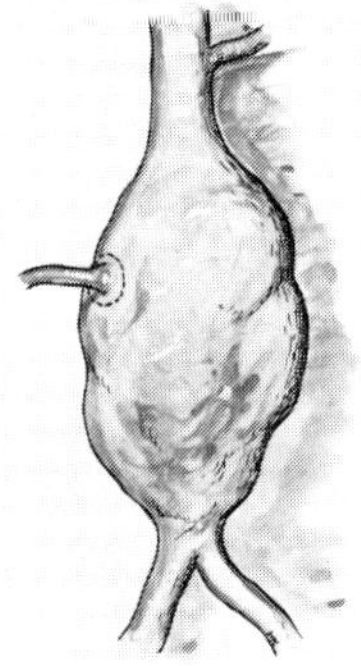

A

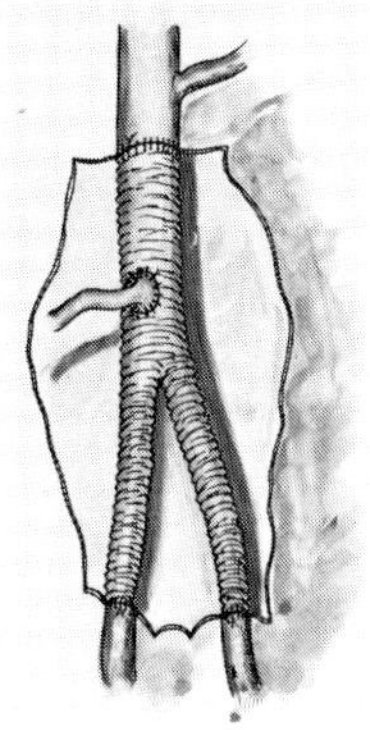

B

Fig. 1. Method of reimplanting an aberrant renal artery into an aortic graft.

I am indebted to Manoutch Kazemzadeh for his skill in executing the drawings to illustrate the text.

Figure 2A shows the problem of severe renal artery stenosis associated with aortic aneurysm. Reconstruction of the aneurysm is carried out in the usual fashion with a knitted Dacron graft. The renal artery is then freed up and prepared for anastomosis. A graft of autologous saphenous vein or 6-mm knitted preclotted Dacron is then sutured to the side of the aortic graft using a partial occlusion clamp for control. The left renal artery is ligated, transfixed, and divided, after instillation of heparinized saline into the kidney. The distal end of the renal artery is then sutured end-to-end to the previously placed graft with 5–0 polyester sutures (Fig. 2B). End-to-end anastomosis done in this fashion is more satisfactory and expeditious than the formerly used method of suturing the distal end of the renal graft to the side of the in situ renal artery.

Retroaortic left renal vein is the most common venous variant seen, but one does encounter occasionally a left-sided or double vena cava.[3] Careful dissection is necessary for definition of the particular problem and avoidance of massive hemorrhage.

Aortic aneurysms occasionally rupture into the vena cava, producing aortocaval fistulas. These lesions must be repaired promptly to prevent acute congestive heart failure. Another major problem is pulmonary embolism of debris from the aneurysm lumen.[4,5]

Table 1.
Unusual Manifestations of Aortic Aneurysms

Renal artery problems
Multiple, arising from aneurysm
Stenosis at origin
Renal vein variations
Retroaortic left renal vein
Low-lying left vein
Circumaortic collar
Vena cava problems
Double vena cava
Left-sided vena cava
Aortocaval fistula
Horseshoe kidney
Mesenteric artery problems
"Meandering mesenteric"
Inflammatory aneurysm

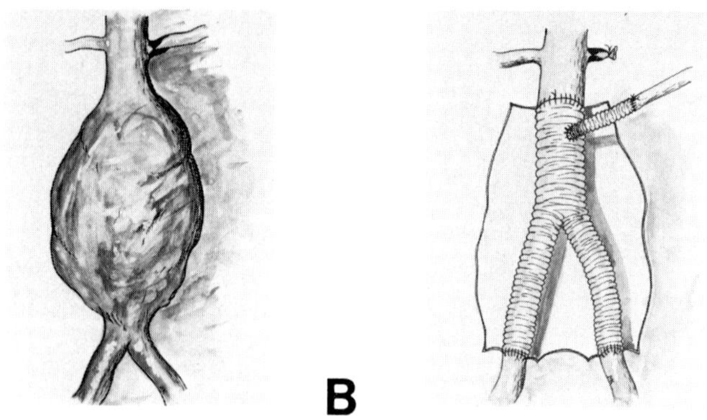
A B

Fig. 2. Technique of aortorenal bypass graft.

Figure 3 outlines the steps in repair of an aortocaval fistula. Control of both the aorta and vena cava are first obtained. The aneurysm is then incised and the fistula closed from within the aneurysm sac with running sutures of 3–0 or 4–0 polyester (Fig. 3B). Following closure, flow is then restored in the vena cava. A preclotted knitted Dacron graft is then employed to replace the aneurysm in the usual manner (Fig. 3C). Some surgeons interrupt the vena cava with a partially occluding clip, but this step is not necessary in all cases.

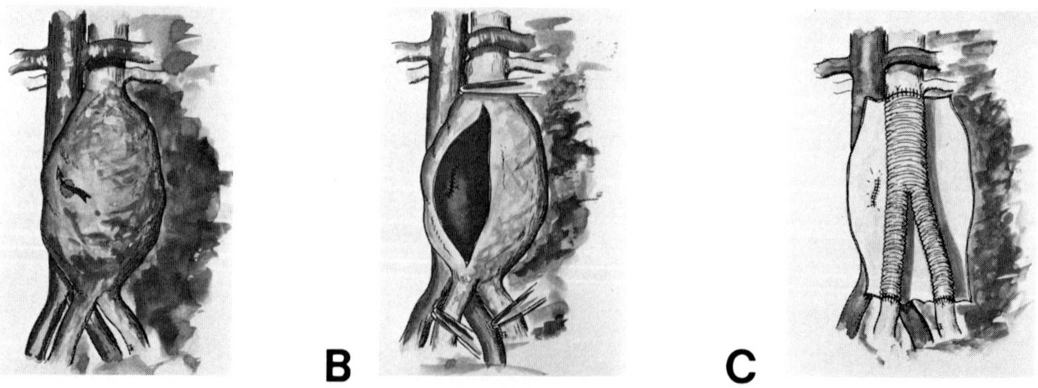
A B C

Fig. 3. Steps in the repair of an aortocaval fistula.

The management of horseshoe kidney is variable and depends on the origin of the blood supply to the kidney.[6] Preoperative aortograms and careful delineation of the vessels at operation are necessary prerequisites for successful surgical repair. Figure 4A depicts the situation in which two renal arteries arising in the normal location supply the right and left sides of the kidney mass, but, in addition, a single trunk with two large branches arises from the aneurysm to supply the isthmic region. As with the aberrant renal artery in Figure 1A, here the origin of the vessel from the aneurysm is excised with a surrounding cuff of aneurysm wall. The Dacron graft is first sutured to the proximal aortic stump, and the cuff of aneurysm wall containing the aberrant renal artery is then sutured to the anterior wall of the graft with 4–0 polyester sutures. Flow can then be restored to the lower renal arteries (Fig. 4B). The graft is then passed under the mass of horseshoe renal tissue, and the iliac anastomoses are completed in routine fashion with 4–0 sutures.

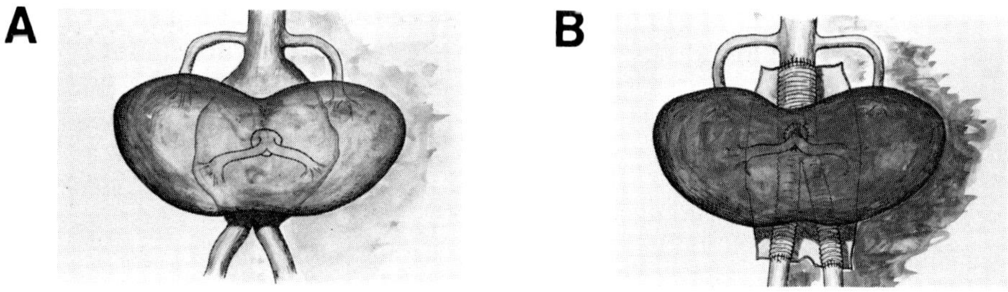

Fig. 4. A method of handling horseshoe kidney associated with abdominal aortic aneurysm.

In the usual case of aneurysm repair, the inferior mesenteric artery (IMA) is either occluded with old thrombus or it can be ligated with impunity. In some cases, however, the IMA is quite large and carries the major blood supply to the intestines, especially if the superior mesenteric and/or coeliac arteries are compromised[7] (Fig. 5A). Under these circumstances it is obligatory to resuture the IMA into the aortic graft to avoid intestinal gangrene. Following aortic clamping, a button of aortic wall including the origin of the IMA is excised, with particular care to preserve the left colic branch, which arises near the IMA source. After the aortic graft has been sutured into place proximally and one iliac anastomosis has been completed, the button containing the IMA is then reimplanted into the left side of the graft and flow restored to the bowel (Fig. 5B). The other iliac anastomosis is then completed.

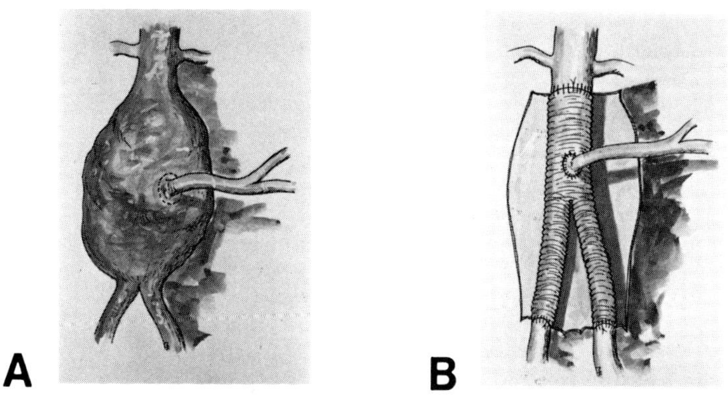

Fig. 5. Reimplantation of a large inferior mesenteric artery into an aortic graft.

Inflammatory aneurysm repair may be a very difficult technical problem because of the fibrosis and inflammation, making proximal control extremely difficult.[8] Intra-aortic balloon tamponade may be required. This may be accomplished from below, as depicted in Figure 6, or from above via the transaxillary approach, using a specially designed Fogarty catheter. The distal end of the graft may be sutured to the distal aorta in tubular fashion, to the internal iliacs, to the external iliacs in the abdomen, or to the femoral arteries in the groin, depending upon the situation with regard to the extent of the inflammatory process.

Figure 6 shows one method of repair. Distal control of the iliacs is first obtained, and the proximal aorta is then compressed manually or with a special depressor in the suprarenal area at the diaphragm. The aneurysm sac is then incised and a large (24 or 26 French with 30-ml bag) Foley catheter is then inserted into the aortic lumen for proximal control (Fig. 6A). A Dacron graft is then directed over the catheter and the proximal anastomosis completed from within the aneurysm sac using 3–0 running polyester sutures (Fig. 6B). The aorta is then again controlled manually from above as the Foley catheter is deflated and removed. The graft is then clamped with a vascular clamp below the proximal suture line and flow restored to the renal and mesenteric arteries (Fig. 6C). The distal anastomosis is completed at whatever level is feasible, and flow is restored to the lower extremities. In Figure 6D the distal suture line is within the aneurysmal sac, the completed reconstruction being a tubular graft in this instance.

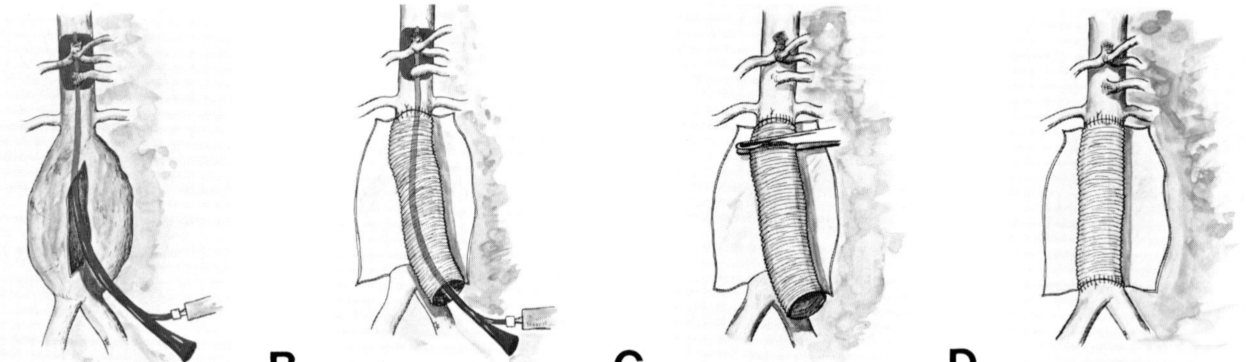

A B C D

Fig. 6. Method of handling inflammatory aortic aneurysm when proximal control in the usual fashion is not possible.

In all cases of aortic surgery, systemic as well as local heparin is employed during vascular occlusion, with reversal by protamine at the close of the procedure. Prophylactic antibiotics are used routinely both systemically and topically. The fluid regimen employed is one we have previously reported, its basis being 5% dextrose in lactated Ringer's solution, with blood replaced as it is lost.[9]

REFERENCES

1. Hardy JD, Timmis HH: Abdominal aortic aneurysms: Special Problems. Ann Surg 173:945, 1971
2. Cox JL, Sabiston DC Jr: The use of heparin bonded shunts for perfusion of the renal artery during resection of complex abdominal aortic aneurysms. Surg Gynecol Obstet 147:859, 1978
3. Brener BJ, Darling RC, Frederick PL, Linton RR: Major venous anomalies complicating abdominal aortic surgery. Arch Surg 108:159, 1974
4. Doty DB, Wright CB, Lamberth WC, Spoto G III, Garrett WV, Cram AE.: Aortocaval fistula associated with aneurysm of the abdominal aorta: Current management using autotransfusion techniques. Surgery 84:250, 1978
5. Hollier LH, Thompson JE, Patman RD, Persson AV: Ruptured aortic aneurysm with aorto-caval fistula. Rev Surg 32:444, 1975
6. Bietz DS, Merendino KA: Abdominal aneurysm and horseshoe kidney. Ann Surg 181: 333, 1975
7. Ernst CB, Hagihara PF, Daugherty ME, et al: Inferior meseneric artery stump pressure: A reliable index for safe IMA ligation during abdominal aortic aneurysmectomy. Ann Surg 187:641, 1978
8. Goldstone J, Malone JM, Moore WS: Inflammatory aneurysms of the abdominal aorta. Surgery 83:425, 1978
9. Thompson JE, Hollier LH, Patman RD, Persson AV: Surgical management of abdominal aortic aneurysms: Factors influencing mortality and morbidity: A 20-year experience. Ann Surg 181:654, 1975

CEREBRAL REVASCULARIZATION

Carotid Endarterectomy

Jesse E. Thompson

The most common operation used in the treatment of cerebrovascular insufficiency is carotid endarterectomy. Technical considerations are of the utmost importance in this operation, since the limits of tolerance to temporary occlusion of the blood supply to the brain may be quite narrow. Safety factors must be employed, which will eliminate in most instances the occurrence or aggravation of neurologic deficits. Any method of carotid endarterectomy should carry low mortality, few complications, satisfactory immediate and long-term anatomical results, and good functional results relative to cerebrovascular insufficiency. The technique to be described has evolved over a period of 20 years and has proved safe and reliable.[1]

The operation is performed under light general anesthesia. The head is turned away from the side to be operated upon and placed on a rubber ring. The shoulders are elevated slightly using a folded sheet, but no undue extension of the neck is allowed. An oblique incision is made along the anterior border of the sternocleidomastoid muscle, curving medially at its lower end, centered over the bifurcation of the common carotid artery, and curved slightly inferiorly to the lobe of the ear at the upper end. Adequate exposure of the common carotid and of the internal and external carotid divisions is essential. The carotid sinus area is infiltrated with 1% lidocaine. The artery is freed completely, including division of the carotid sinus plexus if necessary. One must avoid injury to the mandibular branch of the facial nerve and the vagus, hypoglossal, and superior laryngeal nerves. A small branch of the external carotid artery, passing to the sternocleidomastoid muscle, usually passes over the hypoglossal nerve, holding it down as a sling. This small artery should be ligated and divided to free the hypoglossal nerve off the external and internal carotid divisions. Though rarely necessary, the superior thyroid artery may be ligated and divided to facilitate dissection and exposure. An umbilical tape is first placed around the external carotid artery. Umbilical tapes are then placed around the common and internal carotid arteries and segments of No. 16 French rubber catheters are threaded over the tapes to act as tourniquets.

The occluding plaque is usually located at the bifurcation of the common carotid and extends only a short distance into the internal carotid. The distal internal carotid is ordinarily soft and thin-walled and is freed up for at least 1 cm beyond the palpable distal end of the plaque. Utmost gentleness is used throughout manipulation and the artery is simply palpated, never squeezed, since platelets, thrombi, or atherosclerotic debris may break off and embolize intracranially.

When satisfactory exposure is obtained, systemic heparinization is effected with 3500 units of heparin. The external carotid is occluded with a bulldog clamp and heparinized locally with 10 ml of a solution containing 100 units of heparin per ml. The common carotid is then clamped proximally with an angled vascular clamp. The distal internal carotid is occluded with a soft bulldog clamp, and a linear arteriotomy is made from the common carotid into the internal carotid beyond the distal extend of the plaque (Fig. 1A). It is important that the internal carotid be opened beyond the plaque and that the entire extent of plaque be visualized, in order to facilitate the succeeding steps of the operation. A plastic catheter shunt is then inserted into the distal internal carotid and the artery allowed to backflow. The proximal end of the plastic shunt is then placed into the common carotid lumen and the umbilical tapes with rubber tourniquets are made snug (Fig. 1B). Cerebral blood flow is thus restored through the shunt. This step of the operation requires from 45 to 90 seconds. The average size shunt that fits the distal internal carotid is a No. 10 French plastic catheter about 9 cm in length. A No. 8 or No. 12 catheter may be used as a shunt if the artery is smaller or larger than usual. The internal diameter of the No. 10 catheter used is 2.5 mm. With normal levels of blood pressure, this shunt carries approximately 125 ml of blood per minute. Experience has shown that this is adequate flow during the period required for endarterectomy.

A

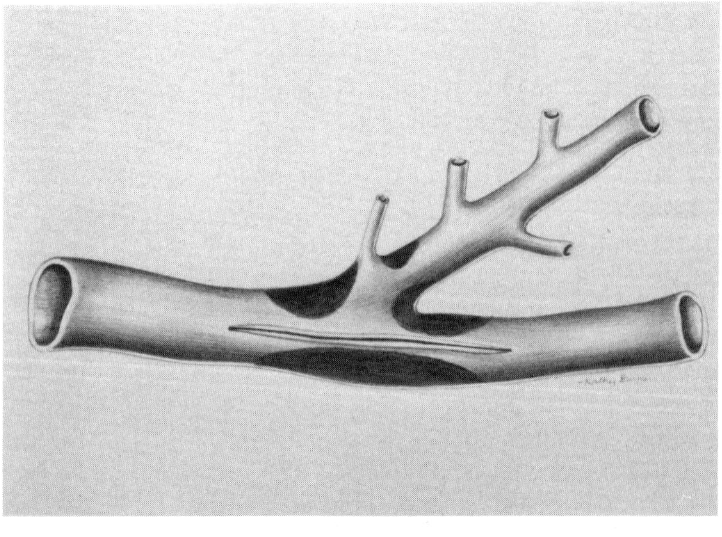

Fig. 1. Steps in the technique of carotid endarterectomy using a temporary inlying shunt. (Used by permission from Thompson JE: Internal carotid and vertebral artery occlusive disease, in Hardy JD (ed): Rhoads Textbook of Surgery. Philadelphia; JB Lippincott Co, 1977.)

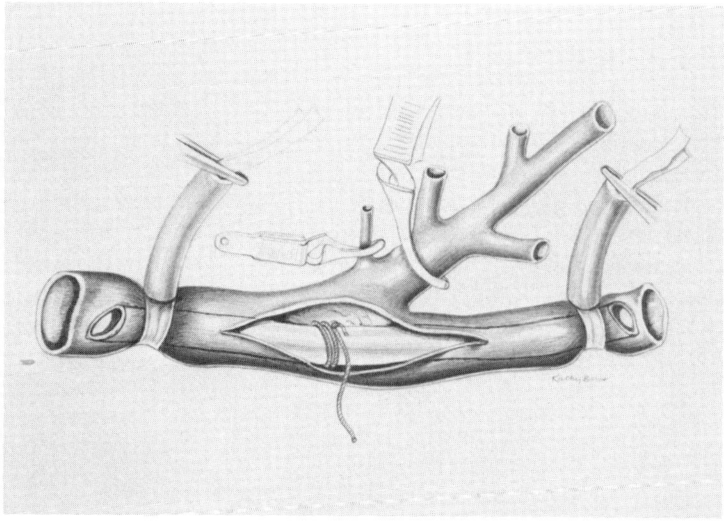

B

With the intraluminal shunt in place, one may endarterectomize the vessel without undue haste (Fig. 1C). The appropriate plane is entered with a fine-pointed clamp and the plaque is dissected from the common carotid, the bifurcation, the first portion of the external carotid, and that portion of the internal carotid containing the plaque. The distal end of the plaque in the internal carotid usually feathers off quite smoothly, leaving only thin intima above, which should not be disturbed. Small bits of debris may be lifted out with forceps or flushed out with saline. It is of the utmost importance that the distal extent of the endarterectomy be visualized so that no large pieces of intima be left to dissect distalward and produce a postoperative occlusion. Occasionally it is advisable to secure the distal intima with a few interrupted stitches to prevent dissection. 6–0 polyester sutures serve well to tack down the intima as well as to close the arteriotomy. It is also important to endarterectomize carefully the origin of the external carotid, since this artery is an important source of blood supply to the brain.

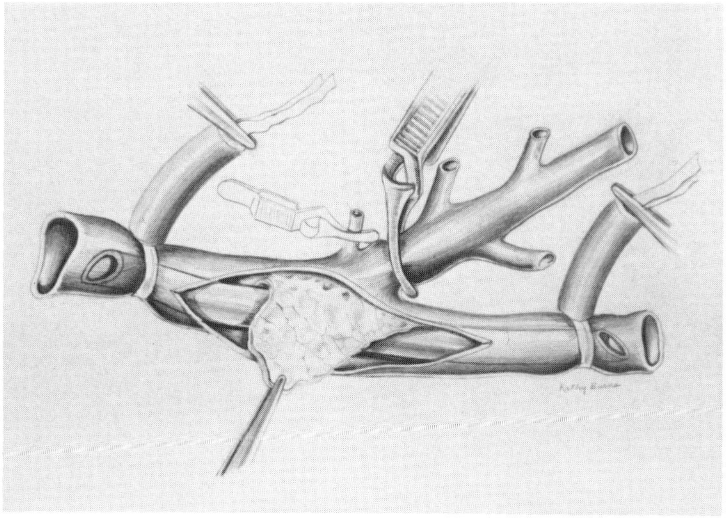

C

The arteriotomy is then closed with running sutures of 6–0 polyester beginning at each end (Fig. 1D). Immediately prior to placing the final three or four sutures, the common carotid and internal carotid are clamped and the shunt removed. The vessels are then flushed. The final sutures are quickly placed and tied. At this point the internal carotid is allowed to backflow and is then reclamped.

Clamps are removed from the external carotid and common carotid arteries, and flow is restored into the external carotid, allowing any debris or air to be flushed into it rather than into the internal carotid. The clamp is then removed from the internal carotid and flow restored to the brain. The occlusion time during this final step is from one to two minutes. The heparin is then reversed with protamine.

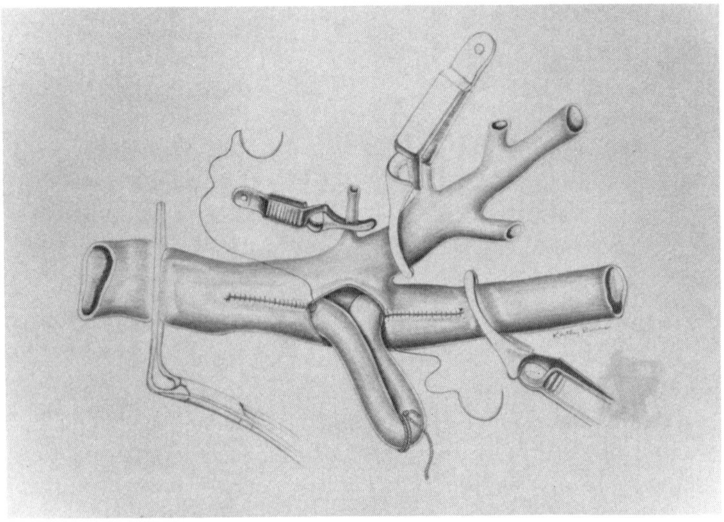

D

One may vary the technique of arteriotomy closure by using a fine partially occluding clamp to include the unfinished portion of the suture line after the shunt is removed. In this way cerebral flow is quickly reestablished and the suture line is then completed (Fig. 1E).

If one is concerned about the completeness of endarterectomy or the quality of pulsation in the internal carotid following restoration of flow, arteriograms may be performed on the operating table. Some surgeons perform this step routinely,[2] but the author has not found its routine use necessary. Towne and Bernhard[3] have utilized the technique of vascular endoscopy to examine the endarterectomized area for any residual debris or unattached intimae prior to closure of the arteriotomy.

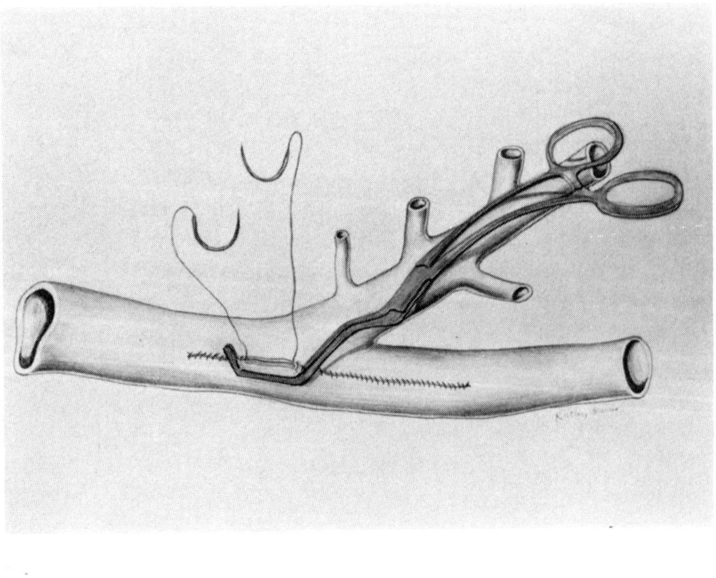

E

It is rarely necessary to use a patch graft for closure of the arteriotomy (Fig. 1F), but if the artery is quite small a patch graft of autologous vein or Dacron may be used. The wound in the neck is then closed anatomically in two layers with interrupted sutures of fine cotton and a small rubber drain brought out the lower end of the wound, to be removed 24 hours postoperatively. The operation as described requires from one to two hours to perform. Bilateral operations, when necessary, are done in separate stages about a week apart to avoid complications of laryngeal edema, transient hypoglossal paresis, and cerebral edema.

For totally occlusive lesions in contrast to stenotic ones, a shunt is not necessary during endarterectomy. When a thrombus is present in the distal internal carotid, thrombectomy is performed with endarterectomy forceps or small balloon catheters.

F

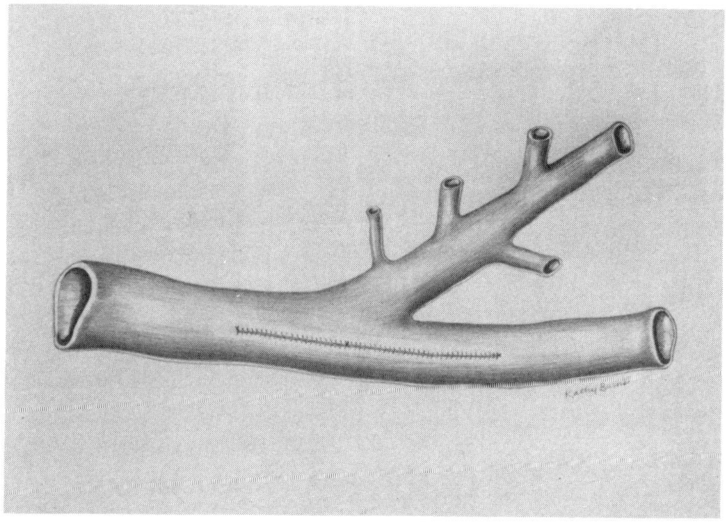

It is important that adequate levels of blood pressure be maintained during operation and in the immediate postoperative period. The most satisfactory way to achieve this is to administer 500 to 1000 ml of lactated Ringer's solution during the operation and postoperatively. Vasopressors are occasionally necessary even when adequate fluids have been given. Routine postoperative heparinization is not used.

The technique may vary depending upon pathology. If the plaque is long and extends quite far distally, a longer arteriotomy is necessary, as is a longer shunt. At times it is prudent to close the distal portion of the arteriotomy and move the shunt proximally before completing the endarterectomy at the common carotid bifurcation. Occasionally one finds a plaque in the common carotid a centimeter or so proximal to the bifurcation. In this case the arteriotomy may be extended proximally, as it is important to remove this plaque as well.

Only rarely does one encounter a patient with bilaterally occluded internal carotid arteries that cannot be opened by operation. Under such circumstances it is important that patency of the external carotid arteries be maintained. Endarterectomy of the orifices of these arteries may be necessary to improve collateral cerebral blood flow. The shunt technique is easily adapted to endarterectomy of the external carotid arteries.

The technique as described depicts carotid endarterectomy with the aid of a temporary inlying bypass shunt, which is the most reliable method for cerebral support. Some surgeons use the shunt routinely in all partially occlusive lesions,[4,5] some use it selectively based on an assessment of cerebral collateral circulation, and a few rarely if ever use it. Those who advocate selective shunting rely on the criterion of inadequacy of cerebral collateral circulation. Some test the patient under local anesthesia and use a shunt if temporary clamping cannot be tolerated. Others, using general anesthesia, insert a shunt if internal carotid artery stump pressure is below 50 to 55 mm Hg or if EEG changes occur upon carotid clamping.[1] In the hands of experienced operators, results comparable to routine shunting may be obtained using selective shunting.

REFERENCES

1. Thompson JE, Patman RD, Talkington CM: Carotid surgery for cerebrovascular insufficiency, in Current Problems in Surgery, Ravitch MM, (ed): Chicago, Yearbook Medical Publishers Inc, vol 15, December, 1978
2. Rosental JJ, Gaspar MR, Movius HJ: Intraoperative arteriography in carotid thromboendarterectomy. Arch Surg 106:806, 1973
3. Towne JB, Bernhard VM: Vascular endoscopy: Useful tool or interesting toy? Surgery 82:415, 1977
4. Javid H, Julian OC, Dye WS, et al: Seventeen-year experience with routine shunting in carotid artery surgery. World J Surg 3:167, 1979
5. Thompson JE, Talkington CM: Carotid endarterectomy: Surgical progress. Ann Surg 184:1, 1976

Technical Advances in Carotid Surgery

William H. Baker

A symptomatic patient with an ulcerated, stenotic, atherosclerotic lesion in the proximal internal carotid artery is a stroke-prone patient. Thus various treatment regimens have as their goal long-term stroke prevention. Nonoperative treatment with warfarin sodium and acetylsalicylic acid are directed against embolizing blood clots but do not arrest the growth of the underlying atheroma. Although the results of nonoperative therapy are impressive, they cannot compare with the best results obtained by carotid endarterectomy.[1–3] However, carotid endarterectomy is not universally free of operative risk, and an operation that is associated with a double-digit morbidity/mortality rate cannot compete successfully in today's medical marketplace. Many factors, such as patient selection, timing of the operation, safe anesthesia avoiding extremes of hypertension and hypotension, and close postoperative monitoring are all important in reducing operative complications. Nonetheless, the single most important factor in achieving good results remains technical perfection.

Stroke associated with carotid endarterectomy is most often due to either intraoperative embolization or carotid occlusion, both of which are the result of a technical misadventure. The emphasis of this chapter will be on avoidance of these complications as well as on pointing out other pitfalls, so that a safe operation with an anticipated excellent result will result.

OPERATIVE TECHNIQUE

Carotid endarterectomy at Loyola University Medical Center is performed under general anesthesia. An indwelling radial artery catheter is inserted prior to induction to help avoid extremes in blood pressure. The patient is supine, with the head turned away from the operative side and the neck extended.

A transverse incision is made approximately two fingerbreadths below the angle of the mandible or lower, depending upon the position of the carotid bifurcation (Fig. 1). A transverse incision is cosmetically superior to one placed along the anterior border of the sternocleidomastoid, but this is a moot point. The incision is placed at this level, not higher, to avoid possible trauma to a low-lying mandibular branch of the seventh cranial nerve, which may traverse the neck inferior to the mandible underneath the platysma muscle. The platysma is sharply incised, and the subplatysmal flaps are created cephalad and caudad. At the lateral aspect of the wound, the external jugular vein and greater auricular nerve are encountered (Fig. 1). The external jugular vein is an excellent source for a vein patch, should angioplasty be performed. The greater auricular nerve is a cutaneous branch of the cervical plexus supplying sensation to the ear. Whereas nerve severance does not cause major disability, the patient will have a permanently numb and uncomfortable ear.

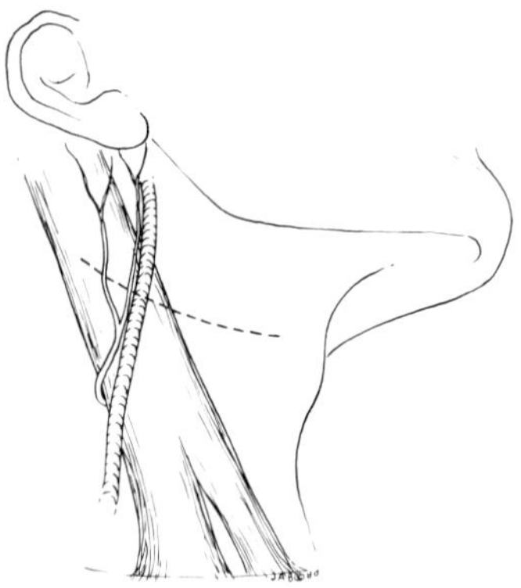

Fig. 1. A cosmetic transverse incision is made two fingerbreadths below the angle of the mandible. The greater auricular nerve and external jugular vein are shown crossing the sternocleidomastoid.

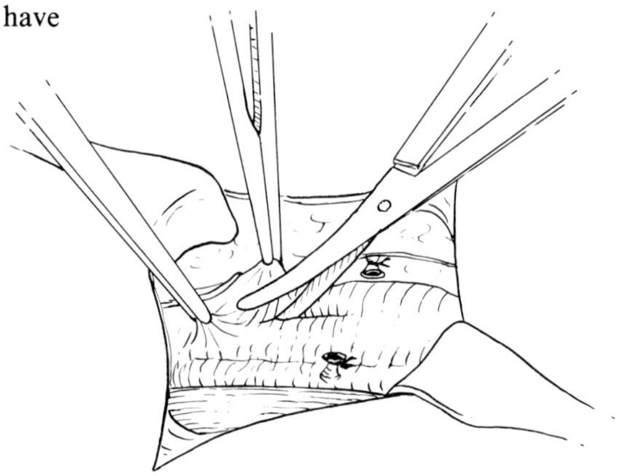

Fig. 2. The lymph nodes lying anteriorly over the carotid sheath are cleaned from lateral to medial, preserving the ansa hypoglossi nerve. Division of the facial vein exposes the carotid bifurcation. The pickups are shown splaying the tissue out away from the carotid, thus avoiding trauma to the carotid. (Reproduced by permission.[7])

The sternocleidomastoid muscle is dissected along its anterior border until the carotid sheath is encountered. The dissection is kept directly on the anterior border of the sternocleidomastoid in a relatively avascular plane to avoid disturbing the rather bloody lymph nodes lying directly over the carotid sheath. This dissection is carried posteriorly until the lateral aspect of the internal jugular vein is identified. Then, going from lateral to medial, the lymph nodes and adipose tissue are swept anterior-medially off the vein. By using this approach to the carotid sheath, the ansa hypoglossi nerve, which comes anteriorly and supples the strap muscles, should not be injured (Fig. 2). Occasionally branches of this nerve cross directly in front of the surgical field, and they may be severed without untoward effect. Next the facial vein or veins entering the internal jugular vein are divided and ligated, exposing the carotid bifurcation.

During any dissection near the carotid, the artery is minimally manipulated. This technique is based on the premise that each and every carotid artery contains a potentially stroke-producing thrombus and that any manipulation increases the odds of embolization. The tissue surrounding the vessel is splayed out between pickups and sharply incised (Fig. 2), avoiding trauma to the artery. In other words, the artery is *not* dissected away from the patient, but rather the patient is dissected away from the artery.

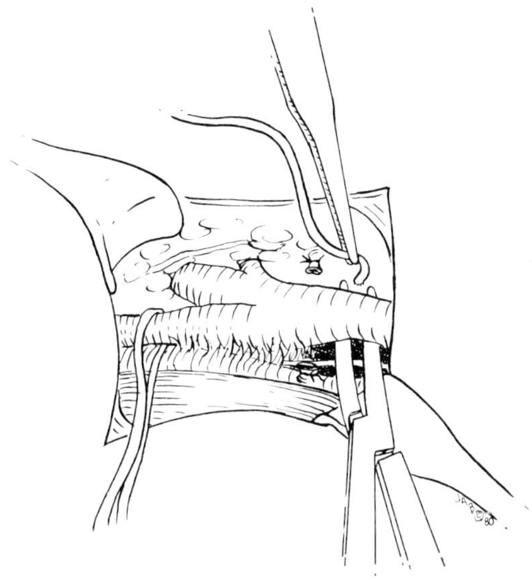

Fig. 3. The common and internal carotid artery are encircled away from the carotid bifurcation. The hypoglossal nerve can be seen coursing across the external carotid artery. (Reproduced by permission.[7])

The common carotid artery is encircled at a point as far caudad in the wound as possible (Fig. 3). This maneuver, which is necessary to gain proximal arterial control, should be performed in an area that is relatively free of atherosclerosis. The carotid bifurcation is not dissected free at this time but is merely cleaned anteriorly to help identify both the internal and external carotid arteries. Distal arterial control is achieved by encircling the internal carotid artery at the most craniad extent of the wound. Whereas the atherosclerotic carotid bulb has a yellowish tinge, the distal internal carotid artery should have the normal bluish color of a nonatherosclerotic vessel. If the internal carotid is obviously atherosclerotic, then the dissection must be carried distally until a normal artery is identified. This distal dissection of the internal carotid artery again emphasizes avoiding the atherosclerotic carotid bifurcation, thereby reducing the chance of embolization.

Finally, the external carotid artery is dissected free. This aspect of the dissection is carried along the medial common carotid artery until the superior thyroid artery is cleared. The undersurface of the external carotid artery is next identified, and this plane is developed, taking care not to traumatize the atherosclerotic internal carotid artery. When the surrounding tissue has been dissected away from the carotid, the external carotid is carefully palpated to insure that this portion of the artery is normal. If the external carotid artery is normal at this location, no further dissection is carried out. The lateral aspect of the external carotid artery between the external carotid and internal carotid artery containing the carotid body is not dissected, thus avoiding a potentially bloody dissection and destruction of the carotid body. This latter point is esepcially important in patients undergoing bilateral operations.[4]

During dissection of the carotid sheath, one must be aware at all times of the cranial nerves contained therein. The vagus nerve descends from the jugular foramen posteriorly between the internal jugular vein and the internal carotid artery. The vagus then continues down into the chest, sending a recurrent laryngeal nerve back up along the trachea to supply the vocal cords. Developmentally, this nerve ducks under the sixth embryologic arch. On the left side, this corresponds to the ligamentum arteriosum, and on the right side, because the fifth and sixth arches disappear, it corresponds to the subclavian artery. If the patient has abnormalities of the great vessels as they come off the arch, the recurrent laryngeal nerve might not be recurrent. Instead, it may leave the carotid sheath in the neck.

The vagus nerve, in addition, gives rise to the superior laryngeal nerve. This nerve arises from the lower part of the inferior ganglion and passes obliquely downward and medially towards the larynx behind both the internal and external carotid arteries. The internal branch of the superior laryngeal nerve swings forward and pierces the thyrohyoid membrane. The external branch of the superior laryngeal nerve (motor to the cricothyroid muscle) descends medially and posteriorly with the superior thyroid artery. If the superior thyroid artery or the external carotid artery is not cleanly dissected on its undersurface, this nerve can be injured by the vascular clamps. The resultant lack of tension on the vocal cord may lead to a weakened voice that is more monotonous and lower in pitch.

The hypoglossal nerve descends from the jugular foramen in the carotid sheath traveling over the internal carotid artery and anterior to the external carotid artery towards the tongue (Fig. 3). In most instances, it crosses craniad to the common carotid bifurcation, but when the carotid bifurcation is located high in the neck, this nerve is sometimes uncommonly low. The nerve may be partially entrapped by a branch of the external carotid artery, which supplies the sternocleidomastoid muscle. Division of this artery and the accompanying vein frees the hypoglossal nerve and allows more distal dissection of the internal carotid artery. The spinal accessory nerve leaves the carotid sheath laterally to supply the sternocleidomastoid muscle quite high in the neck and is infrequently seen. Nerves may be damaged directly during the dissection by an improperly placed retractor (Fig. 4) or vascular clamp.

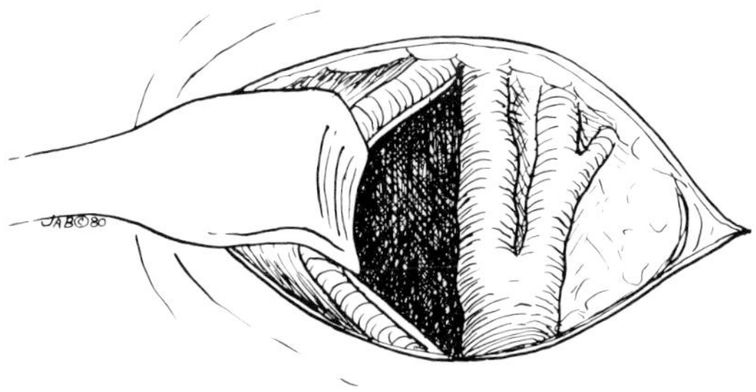

Fig. 4. Improper retraction upon the nerves will result in nerve dysfunction.

It should be emphasized that up until this time the carotid bifurcation itself has been cleaned only anteriorly and medially, not laterally or posteriorly. The purpose of this technique is to avoid trauma to the atherosclerotic area that is the most common site of intraoperative thromboembolism.

The patient is given approximately 5000 units of heparin (depending on the patient's size). We have made no attempt to completely heparinize the patient, as this dosage of drug works empirically. If the surgeon desires to measure an internal carotid back pressure or stump pressure, a 19-gauge needle is inserted into the distal common carotid artery after the common and external carotid arteries have been controlled. Although many different clamps may be used, we employ a multipurpose clamp on the common carotid and external carotid artery and a small curved pediatric clamp on the distal internal carotid artery. The superior thyroid artery is controlled by the loose application of a metallic clip, which is removed at the end of the procedure.

Only after all the clamps are in place is the carotid bifurcation directly palpated and dissected (Fig. 5). This dissection can be done fairly expeditiously, as there is no threat of embolism with the clamps in place. The lateral and posterior dissection allows the carotid artery to be rotated anterior-medially closer to the skin surface, making the remainder of the endarterectomy much easier. A lateral arteriotomy is performed from the distal common carotid artery to the end of the enlarged carotid bulb at the origin of the internal carotid artery (Fig. 6). A plane is developed both medially and laterally between the atheroma and the remaining normal arterial wall (Fig. 7). The endarterectomy proceeds caudally in the common carotid artery, and when the atheroma thins it is sharply divided (Fig. 8). This shelf of atheroma will be pinned to the arterial wall by the cranial flow of blood, and tacking sutures are not necessary. The atheroma is next teased from the external carotid artery using an endarterectomy spatula or a fine hemostat. Admittedly a blind end-point is sometimes obtained. Others are more meticulous concerning the external carotid and ensure its patency with operative arteriography.[5]

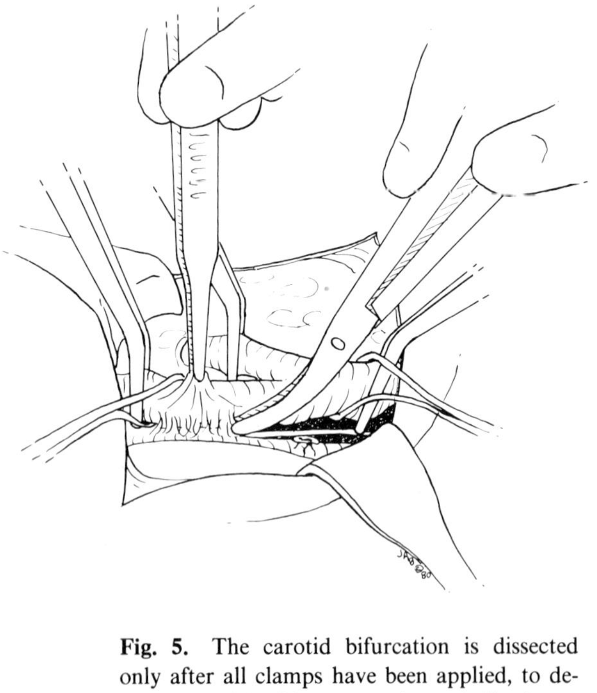

Fig. 5. The carotid bifurcation is dissected only after all clamps have been applied, to decrease the risk of intraoperative embolization.

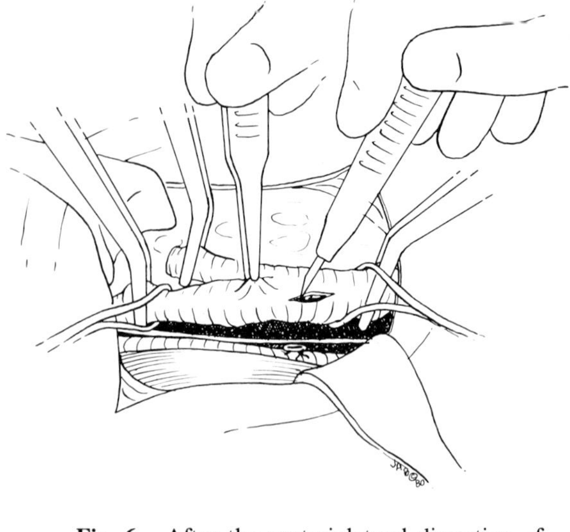

Fig. 6. After the posteriolateral dissection of the carotid has been completed, the carotid bifurcation is rolled up into the wound and a lateral arteriotomy is performed. The vagus nerve can be seen along the jugular vein.

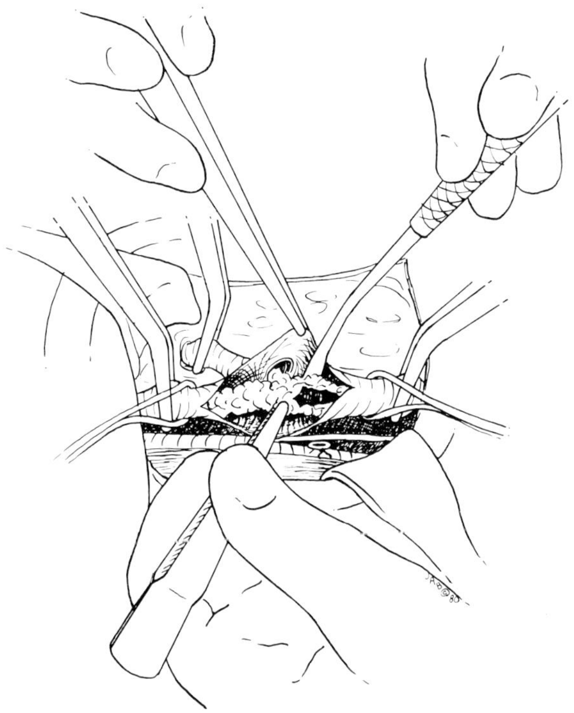

Fig. 7. The endarterectomy is begun using a small flat spatula.

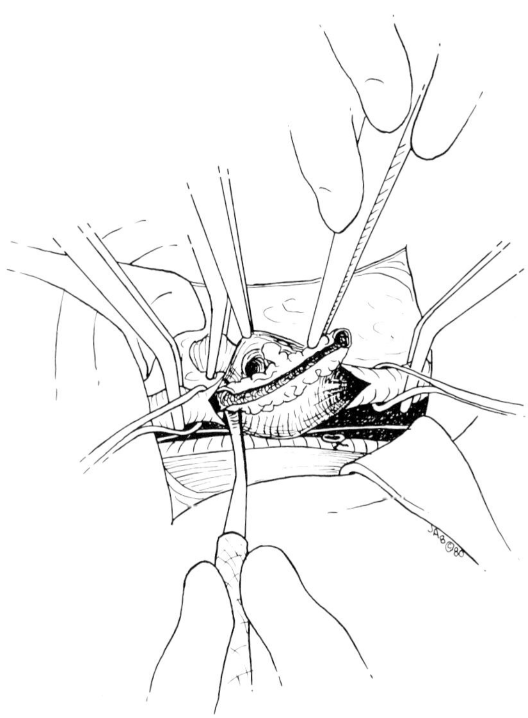

Fig. 8. The common carotid end of the atheroma is sharply divided and the atheroma is teased from the external carotid artery before completing the most important internal carotid dissection.

The completion of the endarterectomy in the internal carotid artery so that an excellent end-point is obtained requires some practice. The plane of dissection, at the origin of the carotid bulb where the atheroma is thickest, frees not only the intima but also the superficial portion of the media. However, as the atheroma thins out distally, it usually tapers and becomes very superficial, lying on top of a relatively normal intima (Figs. 9 and 10). The surgeon must recognize this transition, and must seek a more superficial plane as the atheroma thins by maintaining the pressure of the spatula upon the atheroma. It is to be remembered that the surgeon can always take off more atheroma if a too-superficial plane is entered, but it is not possible to replace the normal intima. When this more superficial plane between the atheroma and normal intima is entered, the dissection is carried distally until the tapering atheroma thins and breaks cleanly away.

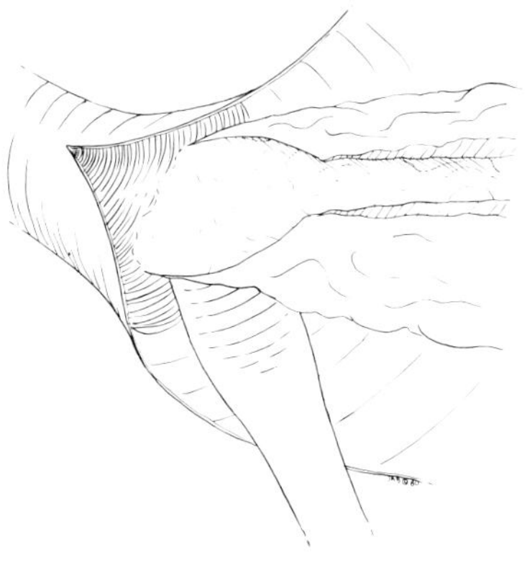

Fig. 9. As the atheroma thins distally, there is a transition to a more superficial plane of dissection. The spatula is shown between the atheroma and this superficial plane. Proximally, a transition between the deep and superficial layers of dissection can be seen.

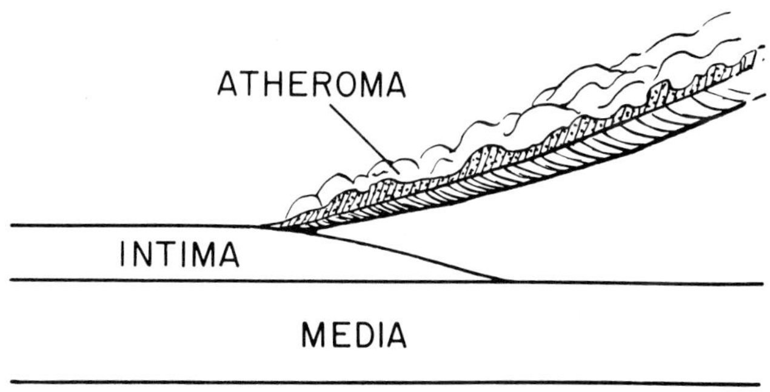

Fig. 10. Diagrammatic visualization of the distal dissection of the internal carotid endpoints. (Reproduced by permission.[7])

This leaves two different and distinct end-points, each of which must be adherent to the arterial wall so that postoperative craniad blood flow will not dissect them loose and cause a carotid occlusion. The first end-point is the transition zone between the deep and superficial planes of the endarterectomy. The second is where the most distal portion of the atheroma breaks from the very thin normal intima. The inside of the artery is flushed with heparinized saline, and the end-points are inspected. If the arteriotomy is inadequate to visualize these end-points, it is lengthened. If the end-points are not adherent to the arterial wall and require tacking, simple sutures oriented longitudinally are used at the edge of the end-point to make the intima adherent. Flushing with heparinized saline, in addition, will detect loose tags of circumferentially oriented media (Fig. 11). These are then grasped with a fine hemostat and removed.

The arteriotomy is closed with a running continuous layer of 6–0 fine monofilament suture (Fig. 12). As mentioned earlier, the arteriotomy is ordinarily carried only to the distal bulb so that closure does not result in any constriction of the artery. If the patient has a small internal carotid, necessitating an extended arteriotomy, the closure may compromise the lumen. Although in practice angioplasty is done infrequently, in these circumstances a vein patch angioplasty is always performed. Prior to completing the closure, the artery is vented so that clot, atheromatous debris, and air all escape completely. The arteriotomy closure is completed and the internal carotid clamp is released temporarily to force any remaining air at the internal carotid artery orifice more caudad. This clamp is reapplied and flow is restored into the external carotid system for a few seconds before internal carotid flow is allowed. In this way, intracranial embolization is minimized.

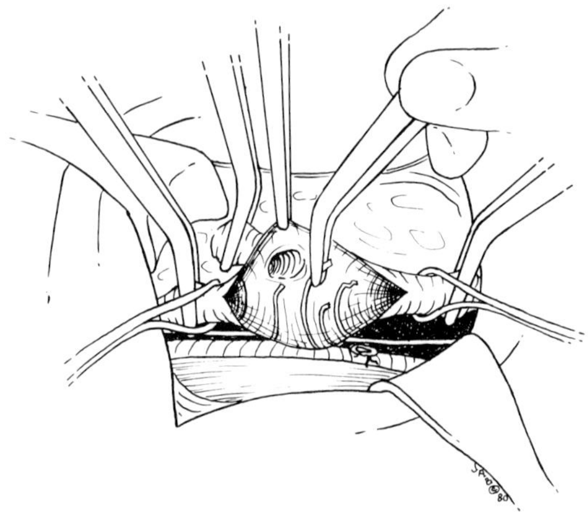

Fig. 11. Loose circumferential fibers are pulled from the endarterectomy site.

COMMENT

Carotid endarterectomy, while not a difficult operation, requires exacting attention to detail to insure low morbidity (stroke) rates. Any deviations from the basic principle of avoidance of intraoperative embolization and careful completion of the internal carotid end-point cannot be tolerated. Protection of the other vital structures in this area is also important.[6]

Cerebral protection utilizing a temporary indwelling shunt is not used. Rarely will a patient suffer neurologically because of its absence, and no patients will suffer because of improper insertion or air emboli. Furthermore, the absence of a shunt allows better visualization of the critical internal carotid end-point. Our series[7] as well as another[8] attest to the safety of this technique as measured by a combined morbidity/mortality rate of less than 2 percent. The fact that carotid endarterectomy can be performed safely with a shunt[9] is a tribute not to the shunt but to the surgeon.

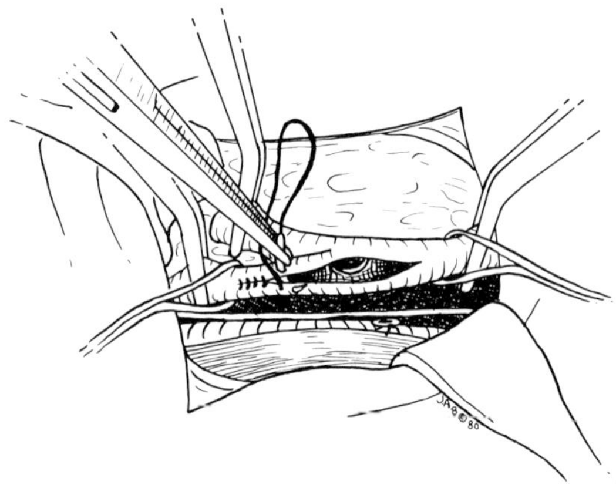

Fig. 12. The closure is performed by a running monofilament suture.

REFERENCES

1. Whisnant JP: Indications for medical and surgical therapy for ischemic stroke, in Thompson RA, Green JR (eds): Advances in Neurology. New York, Raven Press, vol 16, 1977, pp 133–144
2. The Canadian Study Group: A randomized trial of aspirin and sulfinpyrazone in threatened stroke. N Engl J Med 299:53, 1978
3. Wylie EJ, Ehrenfeld WK: Extracranial Occlusive Cerebrovascular Disease, Diagnosis and Management. Philadelphia, WB Saunders Co, 1970
4. Wade JG, Larson CP, Hickey RF, Ehrenfeld WK, Severinghaus JW: Effect of carotid endarterectomy on carotid chemoreceptor and baroreceptor function in man. N Engl J Med 282:823, 1970
5. Rosenthal JJ, Gaspar MR, Movius HJ: Intraoperative arteriography in carotid thromboendarterectomy. Arch Surg 106:806, 1973
6. Verta MJ, Applebaum EL, McClusky DA, et al: Cranial nerve injury during carotid endarterectomy. Ann Surg 185:192, 1977
7. Baker WH; Carotid endarterectomy. in Baker WH (ed): Diagnosis and Treatment of Carotid Artery Disease. Mount Kisco, NY, Futura Publishing Co, 1979, pp 161–192
8. Whitney DG, Kahn EM, Estes JW, Jones CE: Carotid artery surgery. Presented at the North American Chapter of the International Cardiovascular Society, Chicago, Illinois, June, 1980
9. Thompson JE, Talkington CM: Carotid endarterectomy. Ann Surg 184:1, 1976

Carotid-Subclavian Bypass

D. Preston Flanigan, James S. T. Yao

Carotid-subclavian bypass may be employed to improve blood flow to the upper extremity and to the posteriocerebral circulation via the vertebral artery when proximal subclavian artery disease is present, by using the common carotid artery as the donor vessel. Alternatively, the technique may be used to restore blood flow to the anterior cerebral circulation when proximal common carotid disease is present, using the subclavian artery as the donor vessel.

The patient is positioned supine on the operating table. Intra-arterial pressure monitoring is usually not necessary, but, if used, the catheter should be placed in the arm opposite the operated side. Although regional cervical block is an acceptable method of anesthesia, general anesthesia is preferred, as it allows for better patient control and cerebral protection during carotid clamping, through reduction of cerebral metabolism. The neck is extended and the head is turned toward the side opposite the planned procedure, stablized by a ring support (Fig. 1A).

The entire anterior thorax, shoulders, and neck are antiseptically scrubbed with providone iodine; the thorax is prepared as a precautionary step should more proximal vascular control be required. One leg may additionally be prepared if the use of autogenous saphenous vein is intended.

The skin incision is made 1 cm above and parallel to the clavicle, beginning medially at the sternal head of the sternocleidomastoid muscle and extending laterally to the midpoint of the clavicle (Fig. 1A). The incision is carried through the subcutaneous tissue and platysma muscle to expose the clavicular head of the sternocleidomastoid muscle (Fig. 1B). The muscle is then divided parallel to the clavicle using the coagulation mode of the electrocautery, exposing the scalene fat pad (Fig. 1C).

At this point the dissection may proceed along either of two different lines of approach. The standard technique, as described by Diethrich,[1] involves exposure of the proximal portion of the subclavian artery. Dissection medially in the scalene fat should identify the anterior scalene muscle and its attachment to the first rib (Fig. 1C). Particular care must be given to this dissection, as the phrenic nerve courses along the anterior border of the anterior scalene muscle and is to be preserved. The phrenic nerve is dissected from the anterior scalene muscle and retracted gently with a silastic sling (Fig. 1D). The anterior scalene muscle may then be divided close to its junction with the first rib, thus exposing the more proximal portion of the subclavian artery (Fig. 1D). It must be remembered that the subclavian vein lies just anterior to the anterior scalene muscle and should be protected during division of the muscle. Also, the thoracic duct, which enters the junction of the left internal jugular vein and the left subclavian vein, can easily be inadvertently injured at this point in the dissection.

Fig. 1. Exposure of the subclavian artery.
(A) The skin incision is made one cm above and parallel to the clavicle.
(B)The incision is carried through the subcutaneous tissue and platysma muscle to expose the clavicular head of the sternocleidomastoid muscle.
(C) The muscle is divided parallel to the clavicle using the coagulation mode of the electrocautery, exposing the scalene fat pad.
(D) The phrenic nerve is dissected from the anterior scalene muscle and retracted gently with a silastic sling.
(E) For lateral exposure of the artery the dissection is carried laterally along the artery as it proceeds beneath the clavicle.

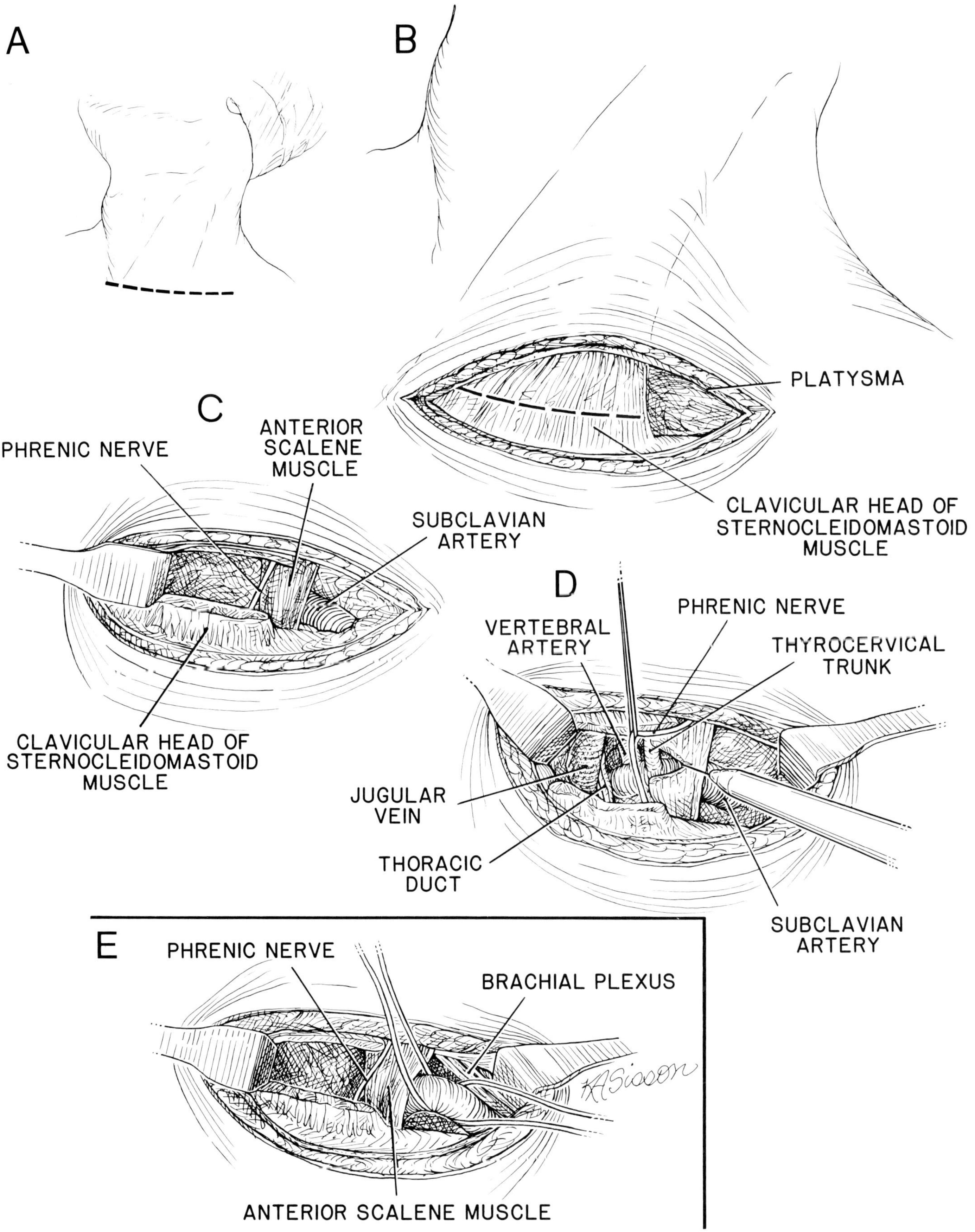
A
B
PLATYSMA
CLAVICULAR HEAD OF STERNOCLEIDOMASTOID MUSCLE
C
PHRENIC NERVE
ANTERIOR SCALENE MUSCLE
SUBCLAVIAN ARTERY
CLAVICULAR HEAD OF STERNOCLEIDOMASTOID MUSCLE
D
VERTEBRAL ARTERY
PHRENIC NERVE
THYROCERVICAL TRUNK
JUGULAR VEIN
THORACIC DUCT
SUBCLAVIAN ARTERY
E
PHRENIC NERVE
BRACHIAL PLEXUS
ANTERIOR SCALENE MUSCLE

At this time, the subclavian artery is dissected. (Remember that the pleura lies just deep to the vessel.) The vertebral artery should be preserved unless occluded by atherosclerotic disease. The internal mammary artery and thyrocervical trunk should be preserved. Vascular control is obtained through the use of silastic slings on the proximal and distal extent of the subclavian artery, proximal control being obtained as early as possible in the dissection. Branch vessels are controlled by the double-looping of silastic slings that are placed on mild tension prior to arteriotomy (Fig. 2A).

An alternative approach to the standard proximal dissection is that of lateral supraclavicular exposure of the subclavian artery. Using this approach, division of the anterior scalene muscle and retraction of the phrenic nerve are not required. Dissection through the scalene fat is begun by first localizing the position of the subclavian artery by finger palpation. Proximal control is obtained first where the artery courses over the first rib. The dissection is then carried laterally along the artery as it proceeds beneath the clavicle. The artery at this location is very mobile and easily can be pulled up into the wound (Fig. 1E). Inferior displacement of the shoulder often facilitates this part of the dissection. At this level, cords of the brachial plexus are adjacent to the subclavian artery and should be avoided. Distal control of the subclavian artery and any branch vessels is then obtained.

Although the lateral approach to the subclavian artery involves dissection near the brachial plexus, it avoids the need to divide the anterior scalene muscle and retract the phrenic nerve. Likewise, injury to the thoracic duct is obviated. Lateral dissection of the artery near the brachial plexus is not difficult, as the tissue planes are easily entered and retraction of the nerves is not required. Occasionally, in small, particularly stock patients, the lateral approach does not afford an adequate length of exposure of the subclavian artery.

Attention is next turned to the dissection of the common carotid artery. The sternal head of the sternocleidomastoid muscle is retracted medially, exposing the carotid sheath. The artery can be localized by gentle palpation and will be found medial to the jugular vein. The carotid sheath is opened longitudinally over the artery and the artery dissected free for a distance of 4 to 5 cm (Fig. 2A). No arterial branches are generally encountered at this level. The vagus nerve, which is located deep to the vessels, should be avoided. Proximal and distal control of the artery is obtained with silastic slings as described previously.

Because Dacron has had excellent success as a bypass material in this location, it is often preferred to saphenous vein, which may be small in caliber and requires a separate incision for procurement. An 8-mm knitted Dacron graft is usually employed. However, if desired, adequate-caliber saphenous vein or polytetrafluoroethylene grafts may be used, as they have also been used quite successfully in the carotid-subclavian location. Blood is drawn from the jugular vein for preclotting of the graft. Five-thousand units of heparin are then administered intravenously. Appropriate atraumatic vascular clamps are placed proximally and distally on the common carotid artery, and a longitudinal arteriotomy is made (Fig. 2B). An end-to-side anastomosis is then performed using 6–0 monofilament polypropylene suture in a continuous fashion (Fig. 2C). Following completion of the carotid anastomosis, the distal carotid clamp is removed, thus flushing any air and debris through the graft. The distal clamp is reapplied and the proximal clamp is loosened in the same manner. When the surgeon is sure that all potential embolic material has been flushed from the carotid artery, the graft is clamped close to the anastomosis and both carotid clamps are then removed, thus reestablishing cerebral perfusion. The graft lateral to the clamp should next be cleansed of blood to avoid thrombus formation. Use of an indwelling carotid artery shunt is not recommended. Carotid clamp time is routinely less than 10 minutes; thus, reduction in clamp time through the use of a shunt is minimal. We have encountered no strokes in patients undergoing this procedure.

Fig. 2. Subclavian arteriotomy.
(A) Branch vessels are controlled by the double-looping of silastic slings placed on mild tension prior to arteriotomy.
(B) Appropriate atraumatic vascular clamps are placed proximally and distally on the common carotid artery, and a longitudinal arteriotomy is made.
(C) An end-to-side anastomosis is performed using 6–0 monofilament polyproplyene suture in a continuous fashion.
(D) A longitudinal arteriotomy is made in the subclavian artery and the anasotmosis is completed as shown.
(E) An end-to-side anastomosis as end of carotid artery to side of subclavian artery is fashioned when treatment is for proximal common carotid disease.
(F) An end-to-side anastomosis as end of subclavian artery to side of carotid artery is fashioned when proximal subclavian artery disease is present.

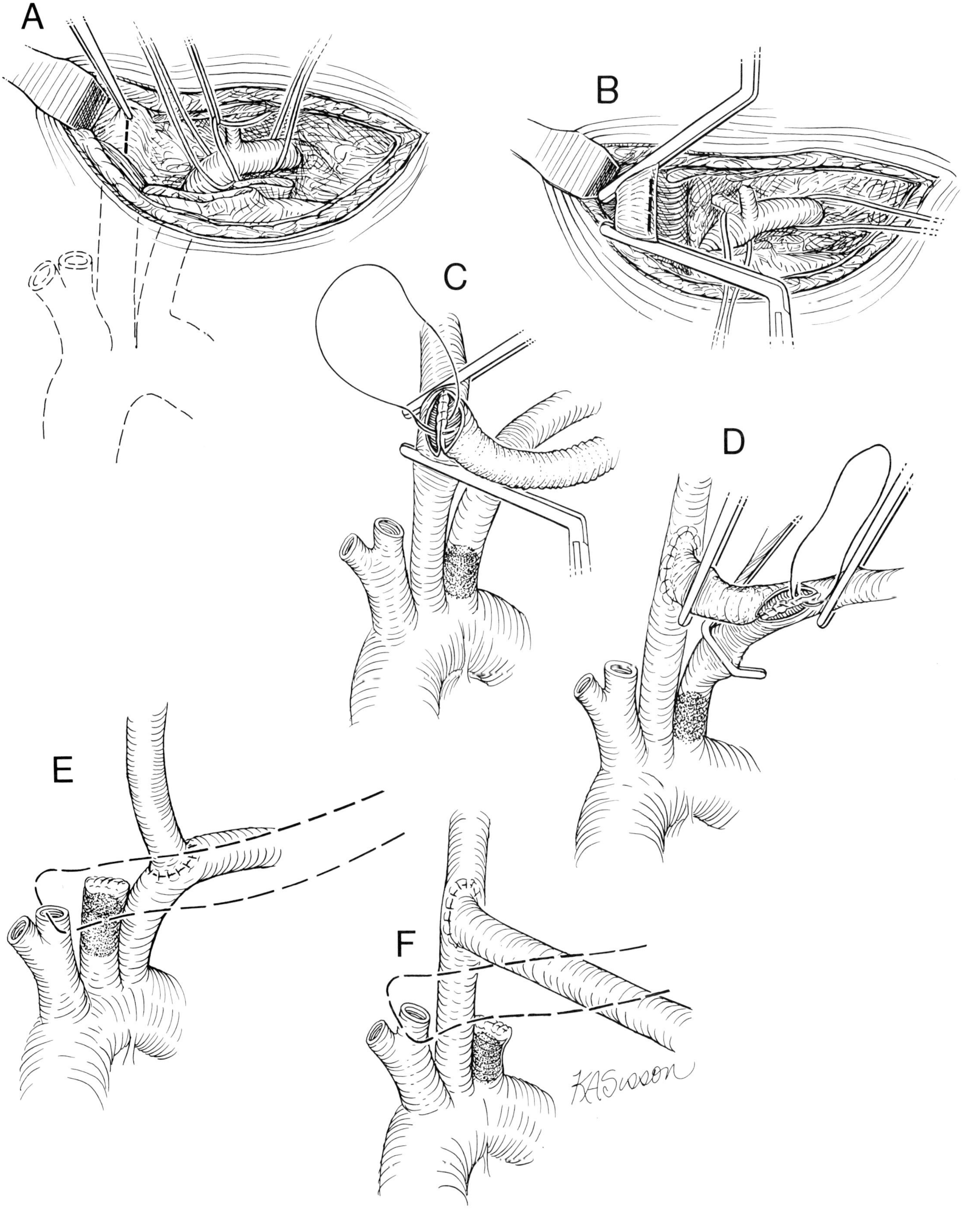
A
B
C
D
E
F
KASwisson

Atraumatic vascular clamps are next placed on the subclavian artery, and a longitudinal arteriotomy is made. An end-to-side anastomosis is fashioned using a 6–0 monofilament polypropylene suture (Fig. 2D). Prior to completion of the anastomosis, air and residual debris are flushed from the graft. Following completion of the anastomosis, the clamps on the graft and the distal subclavian artery are removed, thus re-establishing blood flow to the arm. Subsequent to this, the proximal subclavian clamp (or the silastic loop controlling the vertebral artery) is removed, thus re-establishing vertebral artery flow. In this manner, any inadvertently missed embolic material is not likely to enter the vertebral circulation.

Occasionally, individual anatomy may allow the construction of a carotid subclavian anastomosis using only autogenous artery. This requires the proximal dissection of the subclavian artery as described above with division of the anterior scalene muscle, and is possible when the carotid and subclavian arteries are in close proximity at the clavicular level. Three variations exist: (1) Rarely, a side-to-side anastomosis is possible, as it requires very close proximity of the vessels; More commonly, end-to-side anastomoses are fashioned as (2) end of carotid artery to side of subclavian artery when treatment is for proximal common carotid disease (Fig. 2E), or as (3) end of subclavian artery to side of carotid artery when proximal subclavian artery disease is present (Fig. 2F). This type of autogenous approach has also proved to be very useful in treating proximal great vessel trauma using such approaches as medial clavicular resection, thoracic trapdoor exposure, and standard thoracotomy or sternotomy.

It is not uncommon to find disease of the carotid bifurcation in association with proximal disease of the common carotid or subclavian arteries. In this situation, it is often necessary to combine cartoid bifurcation endarterectomy with carotid-subclavian bypass.

The positioning of the patient is the same as for standard carotid-subclavian bypass (Fig. 3A). In addition to the supraclavicular incision already described for carotid-subclavian bypass, an additional incision is made over the carotid bifurcation. This incision is curvilinear, following Langer's lines, and extends from 1 cm lateral of the midline near the thyroid cartilage laterally, posterially, and superiorally toward the ear, extending approximately 2 cm over the sternocleidomastoid muscle. The incision is through the skin, subcutaneous tissue, and platysma muscle only. At this point, superior and inferior subplatysmal flaps are created using the knife and a gentle wiping motion with a gauze sponge.

A detailed description of the technique of carotid endarterectomy is covered elsewhere in this volume and will not be repeated here. Suffice it to say that the dissection of the carotid arteries and performance of a standard bifurcation endarterectomy (Fig. 3B and C) are carried out. The longitudinal carotid arteriotomy is not closed but rather is used for the end-to-side anastomosis of the carotid-subclavian bypass graft. This anastomosis is performed as described above using a continuous 6–0 monofilament polypropylene suture. If an indwelling carotid shunt is employed, it is removed before completing the last half of the anterior suture line. The internal carotid clamp is always removed first to provide flushing of the internal carotid artery and the bypass graft. The internal carotid clamp is then reapplied and the proximal clamp loosened for additional flushing. A clamp is then placed on the graft close to the carotid anastomosis and the common and external carotid clamps are removed, followed by removal of the internal carotid clamp.

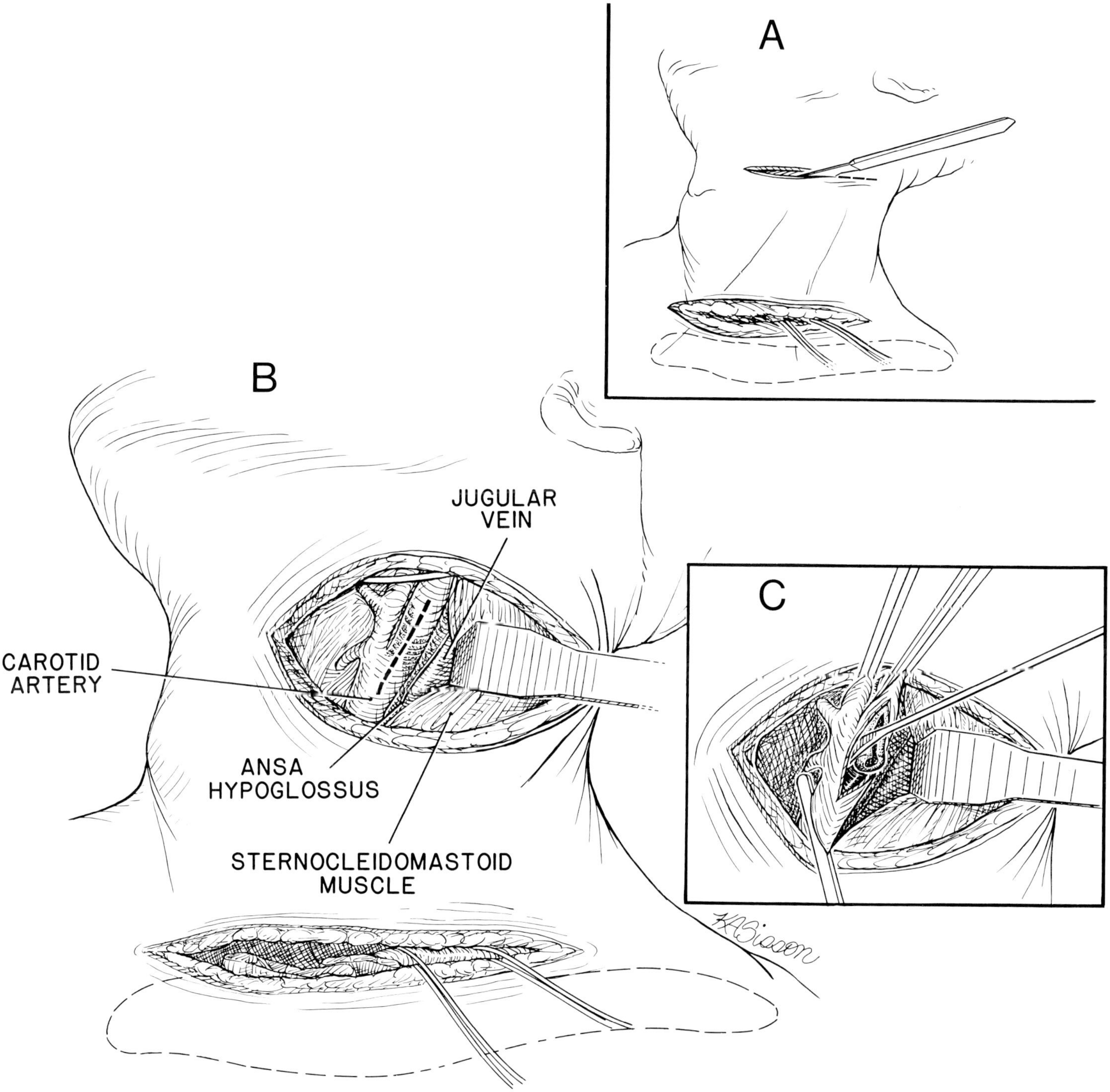

Fig. 3. Combined carotid bifurcation endarterectomy with carotid-subclavian bypass.
(A) In addition to the supraclavicular incision already described for carotid-subclavian bypass, an additional incision is made over the carotid bifurcation.
(B) The carotid arteries are skeletonized.
(C) Standard bifurcation endarterectomy is performed.

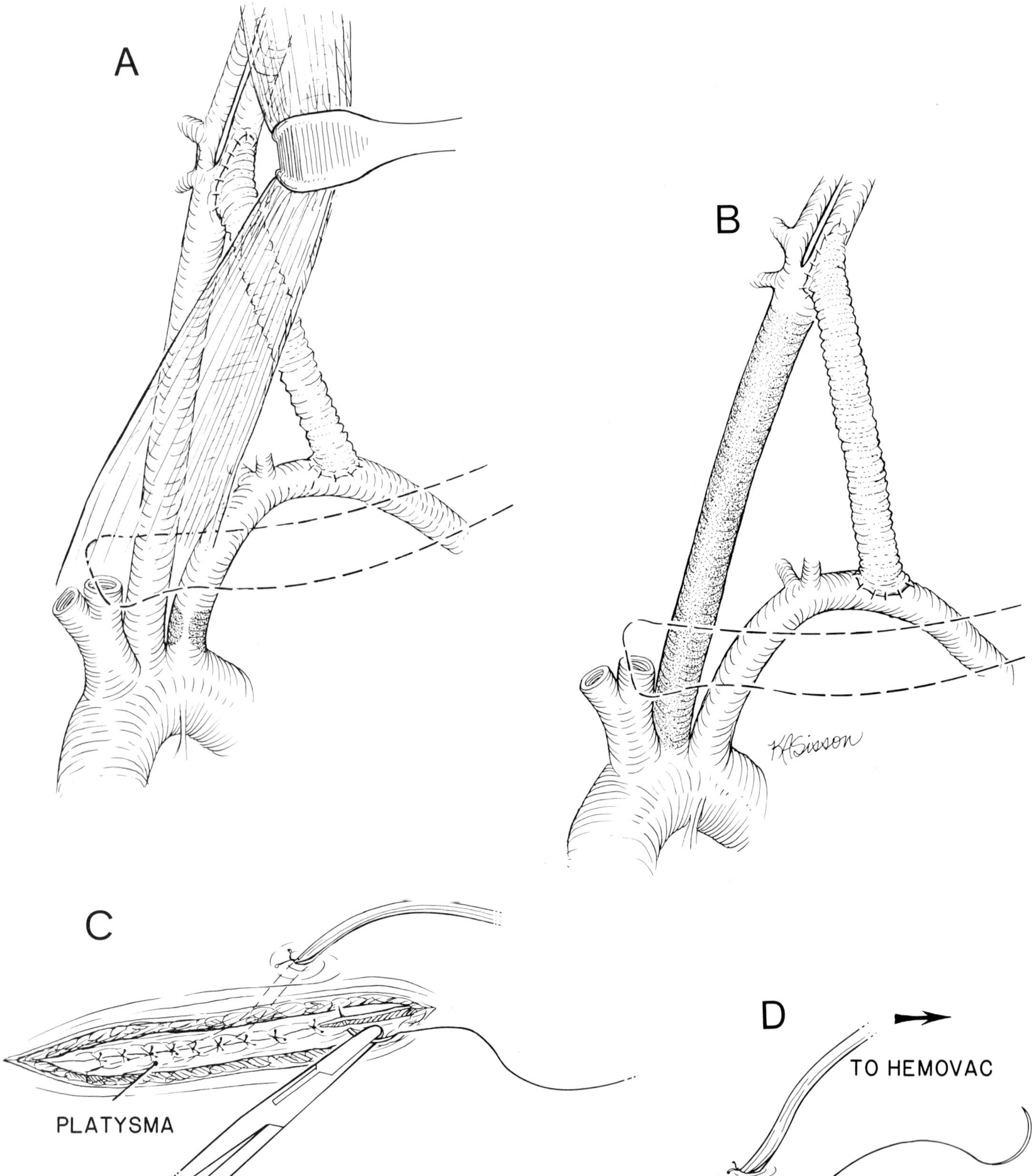

Fig. 4. Use of prosthetic material in carotid subclavian bypass. Subclavian anastomosis (A) in the subclavian artery, and (B) in the proximal common carotid artery. Wound closure is in two layers: (C) The deep layer approximates platysma muscle using interrupted sutures of 3–0 synthetic absorbable sutures. (D) The skin closure employs a running 4–0 subcuticular suture of the same type.

Using blunt dissection, a tunnel between the two incisions is then created deep to the sternocleidomastoid muscle, and the graft is passed through it. The subclavian anastomosis is then performed as described above. Like the standard carotid-subclavian bypass, this procedure may be used when it is thought necessary to bypass disease in either the proximal subclavian artery (Fig. 4A) or the proximal common carotid artery (Fig 4B).

Following removal of all vascular clamps and restoration of flow, an appropriate dosage of protamine sulphate is given to reverse the heparin effect. Both the carotid and supraclavicular wounds are closed in similar fashion. At times, hematoma formation in the supraclavicular wound is a problem. This problem can generally be avoided by institution of closed-suction drainage of the wound for 24 hours. The drain is brought through a separate stab incision and placed deep to the platysma muscle but not adjacent to the graft. The drain is secured at the skin level with a 2–0 silk suture.

Wound closure is in two layers. The deep layer approximates platysma muscle using interrupted sutures of 3–0 synthetic absorbable sutures (Fig. 4C). The skin closure employs a running 4–0 subcuticular suture of the same type (Fig. 4D). The wounds are dressed with occlusive dressings.

REFERENCES

1. Diethrich EB, Garrett HE, Ameoriso J, Crawford ES, El-Bayer M, DeBakey ME: Occlusive disease of the common carotid and subclavian arteries treated by carotid subclavian bypass. Am J Surg 114:800, 1967

Proximal Vertebral Artery Stenosis: Surgical Relief

William H. Edwards, Joseph L. Mulherin, Jr.

The first successful correction of vertebral artery stenosis was performed by Cate and Scott[1] in 1957. Crawford, DeBakey, and Fields,[2] however, were the first to report such a surgical procedure, in 1958. Surgical principles formulated and utilized then are still applicable, but certain refinements and extensions of techniques have been made possible.

OPERATIONS AVAILABLE

Endarterectomy

The dissection required to perform an endarterectomy of the vertebral artery requires control of the proximal and distal subclavian artery. Distally, this may require division of the scalenus anticus muscle, as well as the internal mammary artery and thyrocervical trunk. It also requires preservation of the phrenic nerve. On the left side, any exposure of the vertebral artery requires careful division of the thoracic duct to prevent lymph drainage. Care must be taken to avoid injury to the vagus and recurrent laryngeal nerve. If possible, the ansa subclavia is preserved.

Removal of the diseased intima in the proximal vertebral artery continues to be the operation utilized by most surgeons when operating for vertebral artery stenosis. Either a trans-subclavian incision (Fig. 1A-C) with dissection and extraction of the intima, or a combined subclavian and vertebral incision (Fig. 1D-F) with more direct visualization of the distal intima can be used. Control of the distal intima at the point of termination of the endarterectomy remains a sound principle of vascular surgery. A patch graft would seem to be ideal in this type of operation to prevent narrowing in what may well be a small vessel. Shunting, although possible, is fraught with technical problems and probably is not necessary. Heparinization can be safely achieved with 5000 units intravenously. Reversal at the termination of the endarterectomy is accomplished with 50 mg of protamine sulfate.

Fig. 1.
(A,B,C) Endarterectomy performed through the subclavian artery; distal control of the intima is not possible.
(D,E,F) Arteriotomy through origin of vertebral with visual control of distal intima following the endarterectomy; vein patch graft applied.

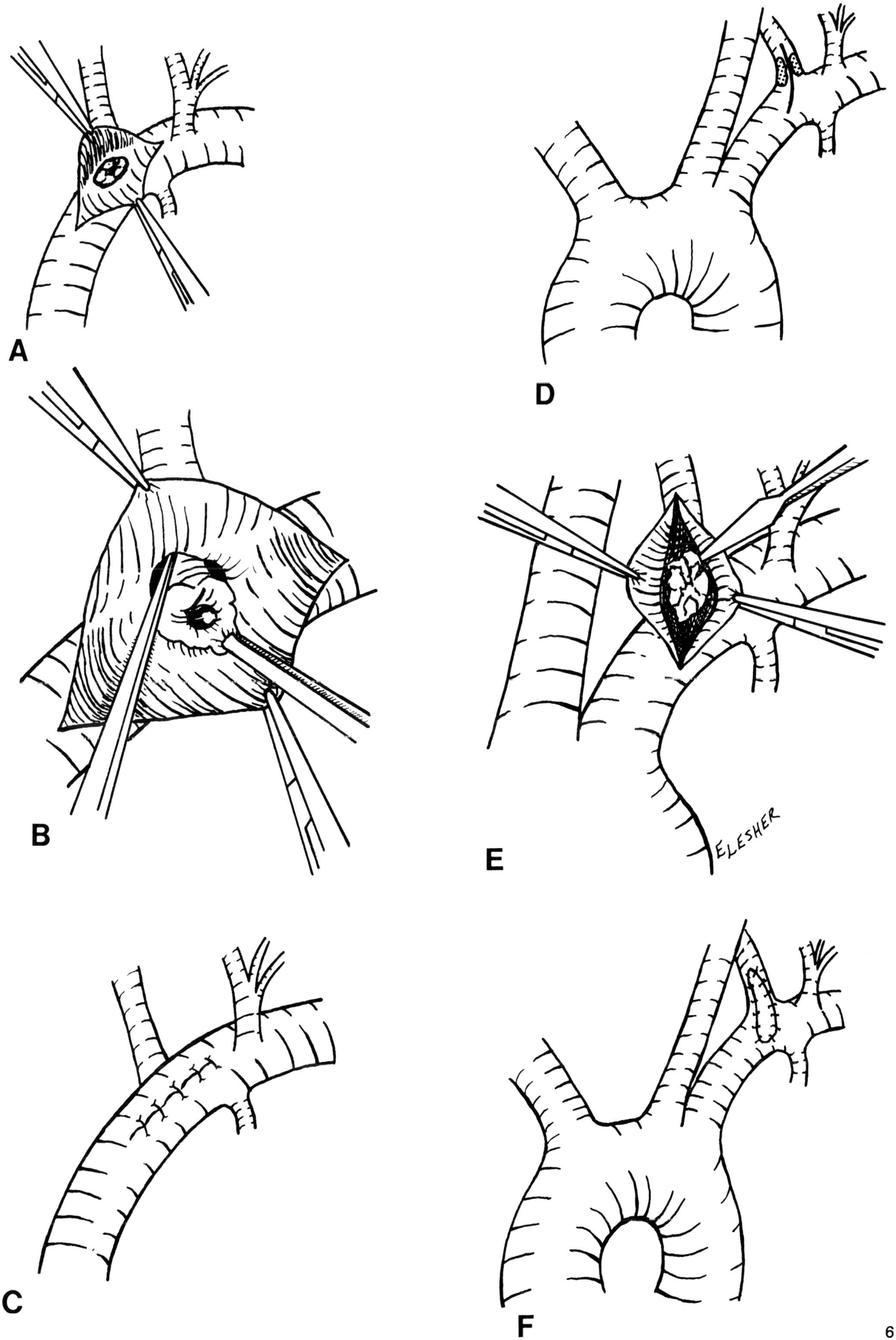
A
D
B
E
ELESHER
C
F

Bypass

The surgical exposure to achieve a subclavian-to-vertebral bypass differs little from that required for endarterectomy. The proximal subclavian must be controlled slightly more distally in order to have a site for the bypass. This is achieved by dividing the scalenus anticus muscle and exposure of a short segment of subclavian artery distally. A sufficient segment of vertebral artery must be exposed to allow the anastomosis. Several centimeters of the artery are usually available before it courses beneath the longus colli muscle to enter the bony canal at C-6.

Autogenous saphenous vein would seem to be the best material for bypass. Polytetrafluoroethylene or Dacron either might well be difficult to work with in the rather limited area exposed.[3]

Following harvesting of a segment of saphenous vein from the thigh or ankle, systemic heparin is again administered (5,000 units). The subclavian anastomosis can be accomplished first, with restoration of flow in the subclavian after completion of the anastomosis. An end-to-side anastomosis with 6–0 or 7–0 polypropylene is performed (Fig. 2).

Care must be taken to avoid buckling of the vein graft. Slight tension will prevent this from occurring. An end-to-side or end-to-end anastomosis of vein to vertebral may then be accomplished.

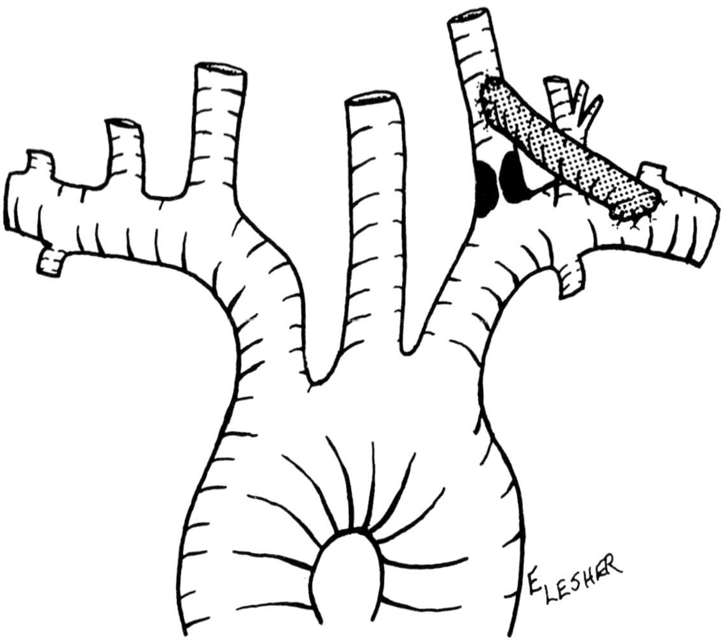

Fig. 2. Subclavian to vertebral bypass with vein.

Vertebral-to-carotid anastomosis

The surgical technique that we have found to be most ideal for proximal vertebral stenosis is amputation at its subclavian origin and a direct anastomosis to the adjacent common carotid artery.[4,5]

OPERATIVE TECHNIQUE

The incision (Fig. 3A) is placed just above the clavicle, extending from the suprasternal notch laterally for 7 to 8 cm. The platysma and sternocleidomastoid muscles are divided. The sternohyoid and sternothyroid muscles are also divided. This exposes the common carotid artery, the internal jugular vein with the vagus nerve between, and deep to the jugular vein. At this point, cephalad and caudad dissection along the course of the jugular vein and carotid artery facilitate the deeper dissection that will follow, as well as preparing a portion of the carotid artery for anastomosis (Fig. 3B). We generally loop the vagus nerve with a Vesseloop (Medgeneral, Minneapolis, Minn.) to remind us of its location. Care is taken not to stretch the nerve. The jugular vein and vagus nerves are retracted laterally and the common carotid medially. The exposure from this point on is beneath the deep cervical fascia and does not require exposure of the scalenus anticus muscle or phrenic nerve. Visualization of these structures alerts the surgeon that the dissection is too far lateral. On the right side, the recurrent laryngeal nerve looping over the subclavian may at times need identification. The ansa subclavia is usually visualized and is preserved if possible. When on the left side, the thoracic duct is identified, ligated, and divided (Fig. 3C). Deep to this lies the vertebral vein, which is also ligated. It is generally not necessary to expose or control the subclavian artery, thus avoiding any dissection beneath the clavicle in the thoracic outlet. The vertebral artery is the first branch of the subclavian artery, arising from its posterior-superior aspect, and has no branches at this level (Fig. 3D). This is important in identification. The thyrocervical trunk arises from the anterior aspect of the subclavian, branches almost immediately, and can be mistaken for the vertebral. In an occasional patient, the vertebral may arise from the aortic arch, but will follow the same course in the neck to enter the bony canal. The vertebral is cleared of tissue from its origin to its disappearance behind the longus colli muscle. At that time, it is necessary to divide some of the sympathetic fibers crossing the vertebral to obtain length of the vertebral artery.

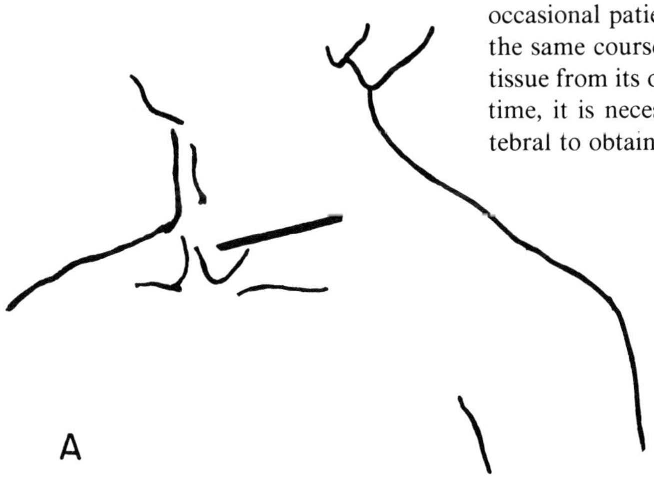

A

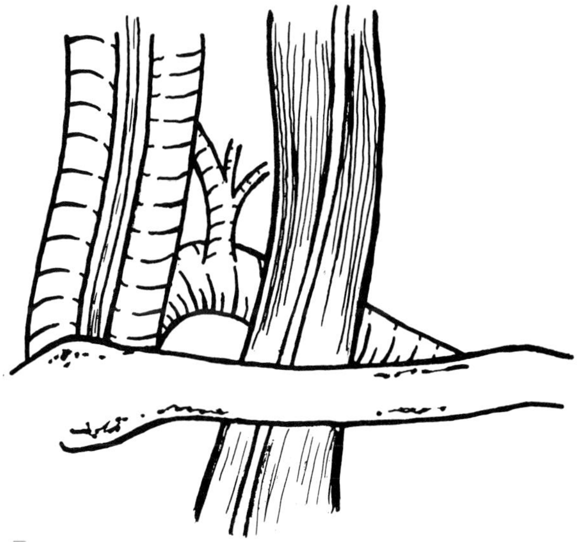

B

Fig. 3.
(A) Supraclavicular incision.
(B) Common carotid artery and jugular vein with vagus nerve lying between.
(C) Common carotid and jugular retracted to demonstrate the ends of the ligated thoracic duct.
(D) Common carotid and jugular vein retracted to show ligated vertebral vein overlying vertebral artery.

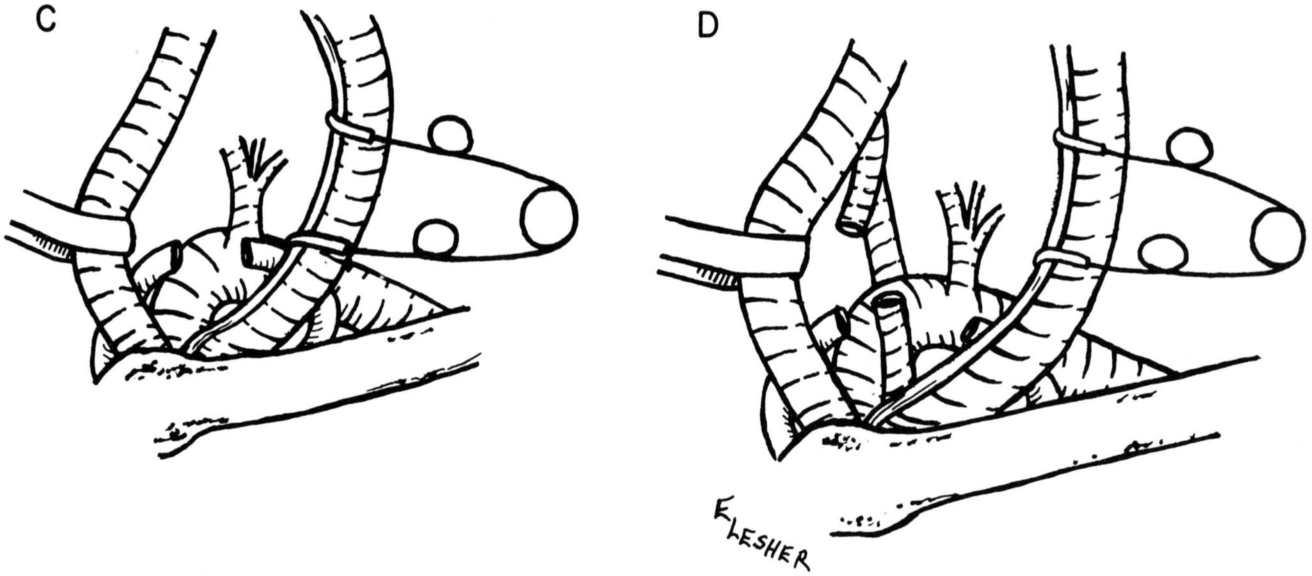

The common carotid artery, having previously been dissected free, is ready for use in the anastomosis. The involved vertebral or subclavian is transected and the stump appropriately occluded. The cut vessel is tailored by incising its medial wall in the case of the vertebral and usually just trimming in the case of the subclavian. The carotid is occluded and opened at the chosen site. We have found that a Goosen punch works well to create an adequate opening in the carotid artery (Fig. 4A). We use an internal shunt only when a combined internal carotid endarterectomy is performed in conjunction with direct anastomosis. The anastomosis is accomplished with 6–0 monofilament nylon on a special small curved needle designed to facilitate the anastomosis in the small vessels. Loop magnification is extremely helpful (Fig. 4B). Following completion of the anastomosis, the wound is closed in layers without drainage (Fig. 4C). Total operative time is about 75 minutes.

A

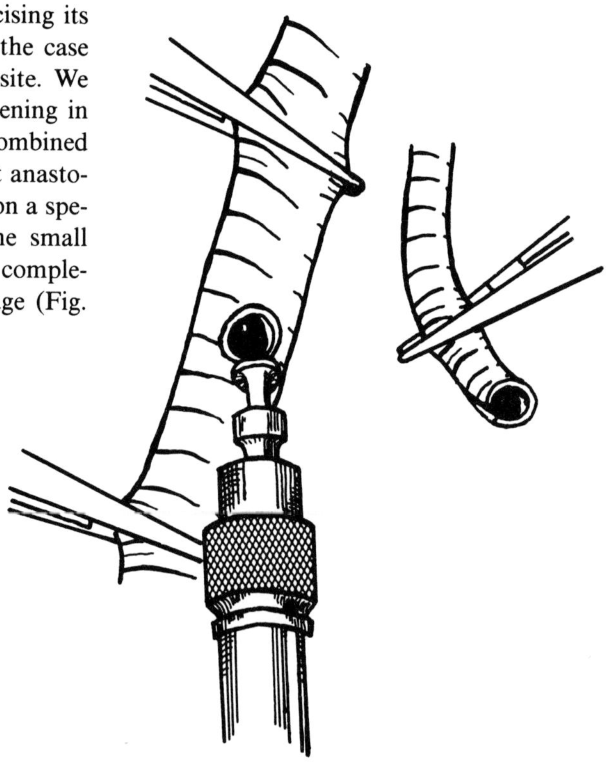

C

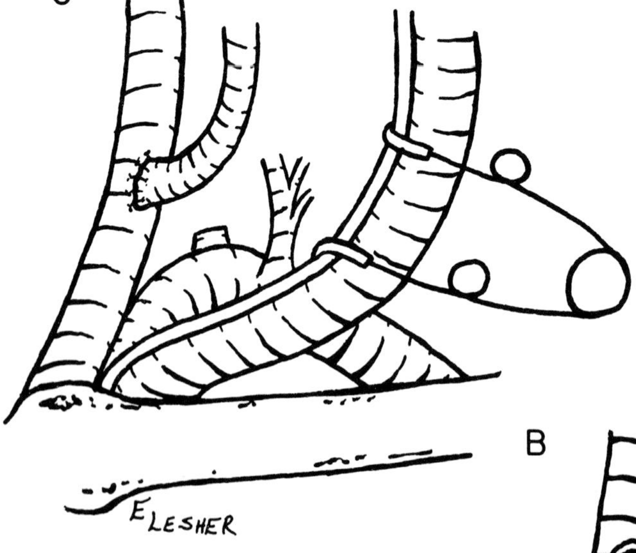

B

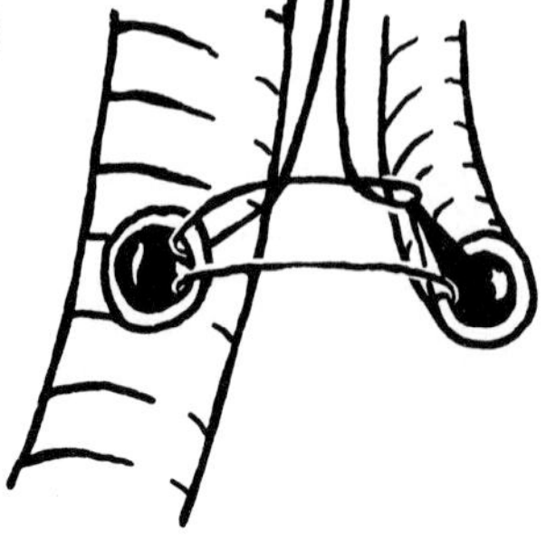

Fig. 4.
(A) The Goosen punch is appropriate for creating a defect in the common carotid to receive the vertebral artery.
(B) The anastomosis.
(C) Completed anastomosis.

COMMENTS

Our experience in the relief of proximal vertebral stenosis for symptomatic brain stem ischemia has been concentrated on a direct vertebral-to-carotid anastomosis. Early in our experience, we utilized endarterectomy but were not entirely satisfied with the technique. We have had very limited experience with the bypass technique. We favor a direct anastomosis.

REFERENCES

1. Cate WR, Scott HW Jr: Cerebral ischemia of central origin: Relief by subclavian-vertebral artery thrombendarterectomy. Surgery 45:19, 1959
2. Crawford ES, DeBakey ME, Fields WS: Roentgenographic diagnosis and surgical treatment of basilar artery insufficiency. JAMA 168:509, 1958
3. Berguer R, Lourdes VA, Bauer RB : Vertebral artery bypass. Arch Surg 111:976, 1976
4. Edwards WH, Mulherin JL Jr: The surgical approach to significant stenosis of vertebral and subclavian arteries. Surgery 87:20, 1980
5. Mehigan JT, Buch WS, Pipkin RD, Fogarty TJ: Subclavian-carotid transposition for the subclavian steal syndrome. Am J Surg 136:15, 1978

External Carotid Endarterectomy

Charles S. O'Mara, James S. T. Yao,
and John J. Bergan

Endarterectomy of the internal carotid artery is widely accepted as an effective method of treatment for cerebral ischemia but is only performed when the vessel is narrow, not occluded. Cerebral ischemia in the presence of total occlusion of the internal carotid artery presents a different therapeutic problem. When the internal carotid artery is occluded, the external carotid artery and its major branches act as collateral channels for perfusion of the brain.[1] Retrograde perfusion of the carotid siphon via the external maxillary-supraorbital anastomosis is often seen on arteriograms which show total occlusion of the internal carotid artery. Emboli may occasionally originate from an external carotid plaque, and emboli to the retina or cerebral hemisphere by way of the external carotid collateral circulation have been reported by Burnbaum et al[2] and Ehrenfeld and Lord[3] when the internal carotid artery is occluded. Therefore, when the internal carotid artery is occluded, cerebral or retinal embolic symptoms caused by an external carotid artery plaque are an indication for external carotid endarterectomy.[4] When bilateral internal carotid artery occlusions are present, an incidental external carotid artery stenosis may compromise the external carotid collateral pathways to the brain to the extent that nonlateralizing symptoms may occur due to diffuse cerebral ischemia. In this situation, external carotid endarterectomy[5,6] may increase total brain perfusion and relieve the ischemia. With the current development of extra-intracranial bypass,[7] external carotid endarterectomy assumes more surgical significance. Endarterectomy of a stenotic external carotid artery may be required to provide satisfactory inflow to the superficial temporal artery in preparation for extra-intracranial bypass.[7]

Supported in part by the Conrad Jobst Foundation and the Northwestern University Vascular Research Fund.

OPERATIVE TECHNIQUE

Under general anesthesia, the patient is positioned supine with the shoulders elevated slightly on a folded sheet and with the head turned away from the side of the operation (Fig. 1A). An oblique neck incision on a natural skin crease at the level of the carotid bifurcation then allows satisfactory exposure and also affords a cosmetically acceptable scar. The incision is deepened through the subcutaneous tissue and then through the platysma muscle.

Flaps are elevated in a plane beneath the platysma muscle for a short distance along the anterior border of the sternocleidomastoid muscle both superiorly and inferiorly (Fig. 1B). This step is important to allow adequate exposure of the carotid artery in subsequent stages of the procedure. Landmarks at this stage of the dissection are the anterior border of the sternocleidomastoid muscle; the external jugular vein, which usually requires ligation and division; and the greater auricular nerve, which is located just deep to the platysma muscle in the lateral aspect of the incision. Retraction of the sternocleidomastoid muscle laterally allows exposure for dissection of the common facial vein as it courses across the neck to join the internal jugular vein (Fig. 1C). The facial vein is a landmark that, along with palpation of the hyoid bone, indicates the position of the carotid bifurcation. The facial vein is ligated and divided, permitting exposure of the underlying carotid sheath (Fig. 1D).

The carotid sheath is entered and the carotid bifurcation is visualized. The carotid sinus area is infiltrated with 1% xylocaine solution to prevent bradycardia and hypotension during its manipulation. The distal common carotid artery and the proximal portion of the occluded internal carotid artery are dissected free. Exposure of the external carotid artery to a point beyond the distal extent of arteriosclerotic disease, which is important, sometimes requires division of the digastric muscle and gentle elevation of the underlying hypoglossal nerve (Fig. 1E). This nerve must, of course, be protected from injury. The distal external carotid and its branches are dissected free and individually encircled with silastic vessel loops. Figure 2A shows in saggital section the typical extent of arteriosclerotic involvement encountered at the carotid bifurcation during this procedure.

Fig. 1. Endarterectomy of stenotic external carotid artery.
(A) An oblique neck incision on a natural skin crease at the level of the carotid bifurcation allows satisfactory exposure and affords a cosmetically acceptable scar.
(B) Flaps are elevated in a plane beneath the platysma muscle for a short distance along the anterior border of the sternocleidomastoid muscle both superiorly and inferiorly.
(C) Retraction of the sternocleidomastoid muscle laterally allows exposure for dissection of the common facial vein as it courses across the neck to join the internal jugular vein.
D) The facial vein is ligated and divided, permitting exposure of the underlying cartoid sheath.
(E) Exposure of the external carotid artery to a point beyond the distal extent of the arteriosclerotic disease sometimes requires division of the digastric muscle and gentle elevation of the underlying hypoglossal nerve.

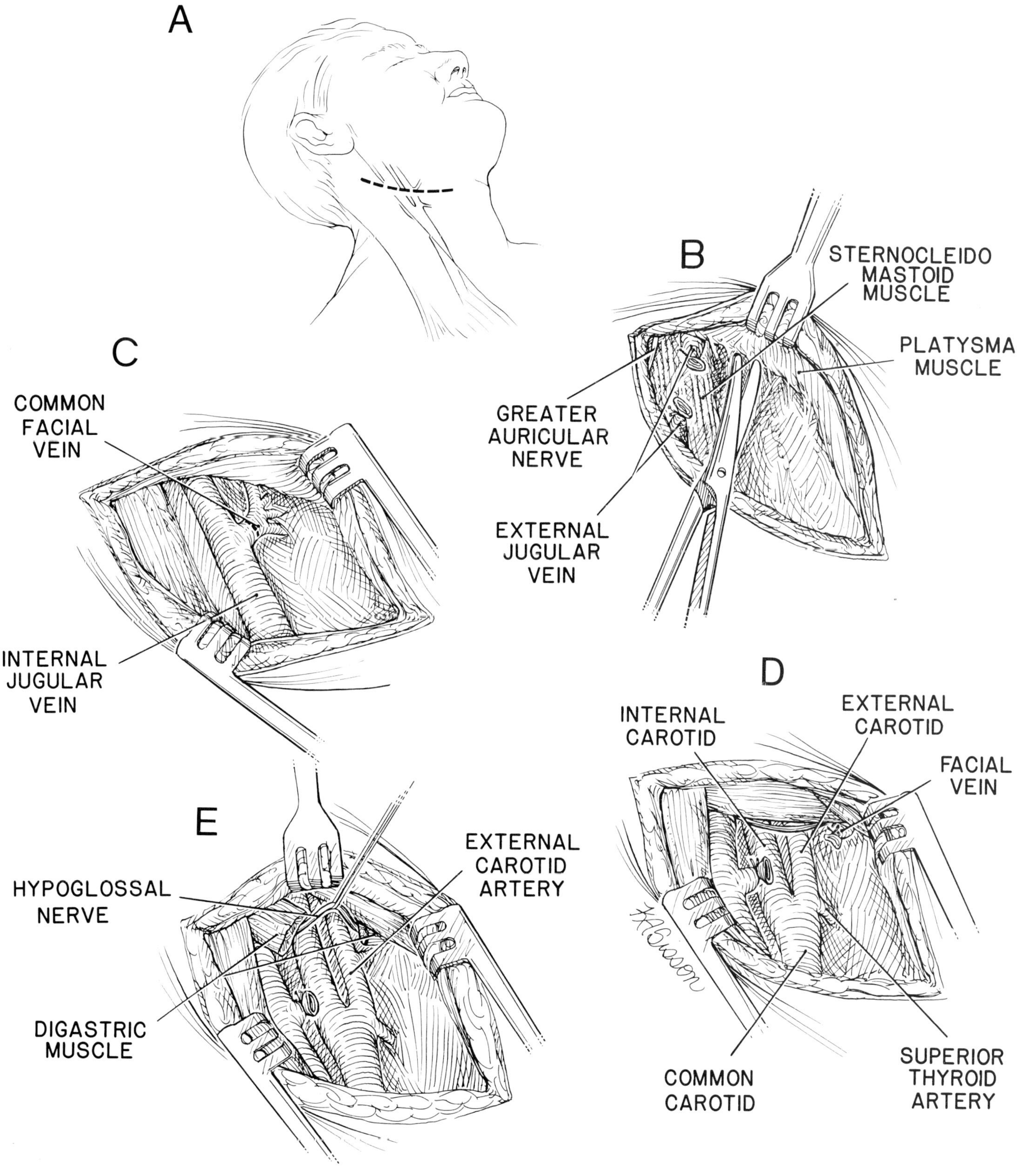
A
B
STERNOCLEIDO MASTOID MUSCLE
PLATYSMA MUSCLE
GREATER AURICULAR NERVE
EXTERNAL JUGULAR VEIN
C
COMMON FACIAL VEIN
INTERNAL JUGULAR VEIN
D
INTERNAL CAROTID
EXTERNAL CAROTID
FACIAL VEIN
COMMON CAROTID
SUPERIOR THYROID ARTERY
E
EXTERNAL CAROTID ARTERY
HYPOGLOSSAL NERVE
DIGASTRIC MUSCLE

Aqueous heparin, 1 mg/kg, is given systemically. The external carotid artery and its branches are doubly encircled with silastic loops for distal control. An angled vascular clamp is used to control the common carotid artery proximally. A longitudinal arteriotomy is begun on the distal common carotid and extended onto the external carotid artery (Fig. 2B). The arteriotomy should extend beyond the distal limit of the arteriosclerotic plaque.

The appropriate cleavage plane for the endarterectomy is established with a curved endarterectomy curette (Fig. 2C).The cleavage plane is created circumferentially in the common carotid artery and the plaque is then transected at this location (Fig. 2D). Interposition of the endarterectomy curette between the plaque and the vessel wall protects the vessel wall as the plaque is being divided. The distal portion of the arteriosclerotic plaque is separated smoothly from the external carotid artery. The plaque is then extracted by eversion technique from the origin of the occluded internal carotid artery (Fig. 2E).

Fig. 2. Endartercotomy of stenotic external carotid artery (continued).
(A) Saggital section shows the typical extent of arterioscelerotic involvement encountered at the carotid bifurcation during this procedure.
(B) A longitudinal arteriotomy is begun on the distal common carotid and extended onto the external carotid artery.
(C) The appropriate cleavage plane for the endarterctomy is etablished with a curved endarterectomy curette.
(D) The cleavage plane is created circumferentially in the common carotid artery and the plaque is then transected at this location.
(E) The plaque is extracted by eversion technique from the origin of the occluded internal carotid artery.

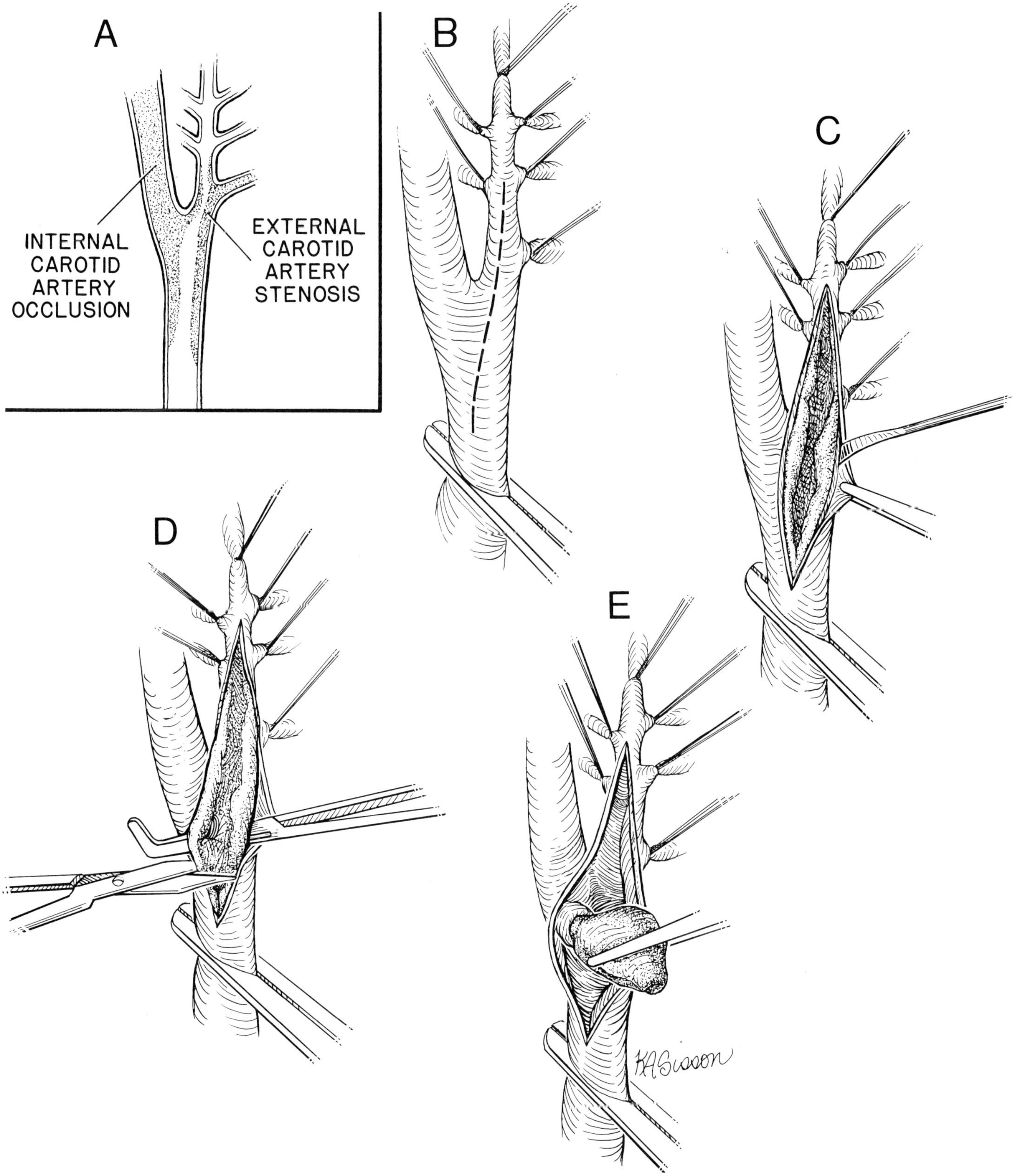
A
INTERNAL CAROTID ARTERY OCCLUSION
EXTERNAL CAROTID ARTERY STENOSIS
B
C
D
E
KASisson

Special care is taken to be certain that there is no distal intimal flap, which will cause postoperative occlusion. If a distal intimal shelf is present, the arteriotomy should be extended distally to a point beyond the arteriosclerotic plaque. If this is done, intimal tacking sutures should seldom be necessary. Atheromatous plugs in branch vessels can be extracted with forceps by eversion (Fig. 3A). Residual debris is meticulously removed using forceps, Kittner dissectors, and local irrigation with heparinized saline (Fig. 3B). The endarterectomized surface should be as smooth as possible. Heparin saline flushes can also be helpful to ascertain that the distal intima is secure.

While a patch is rarely necessary in internal carotid endarterectomy, patch angioplasty closure of the arteriotomy is often needed in external carotid endarterectomy because of the small diameter of the endarterectomized external carotid. Autogenous vein, rather than synthetic material, is preferred for use as a patch. A suitable vein segment can usually be obtained locally from either the common facial, external jugular, or internal jugular vein. The vein segment is tailored to match the arteriotomy. The patch is initially secured with a suture at the distal apex of the arteriotomy (Fig. 3C). The angioplasty is performed with continuous 7–0 monofilament sutures (Fig. 3D). The vein patch is carried down only to the origin of the external carotid artery. The remaining portion of the arteriotomy on the common carotid artery, which is of adequate luminal diameter, is closed without a patch.

Fig. 3. Endarterectomy of stenotic external carotid artery (continued).
(A) Atheromatous plugs in branch vessels can be extracted with forceps by eversion.
(B) Residual debris is meticulously removed using forceps, Kittner dissectors, and local irrigation with heparinized saline.
(C) The patch is initially secured with a suture at the distal apex of the arteriotomy. Autogenous vein, rather than synthetic material, is preferred for use as a patch.
(D) The angioplasty is performed with continuous 7–0 monofilament sutures. The vein patch is carried down only to the origin of the external carotid artery.
(E) Standard flushing techniques are used prior to completion of the arteriotomy closure. The external carotid artery and its branches are opened and flushed retrograde.

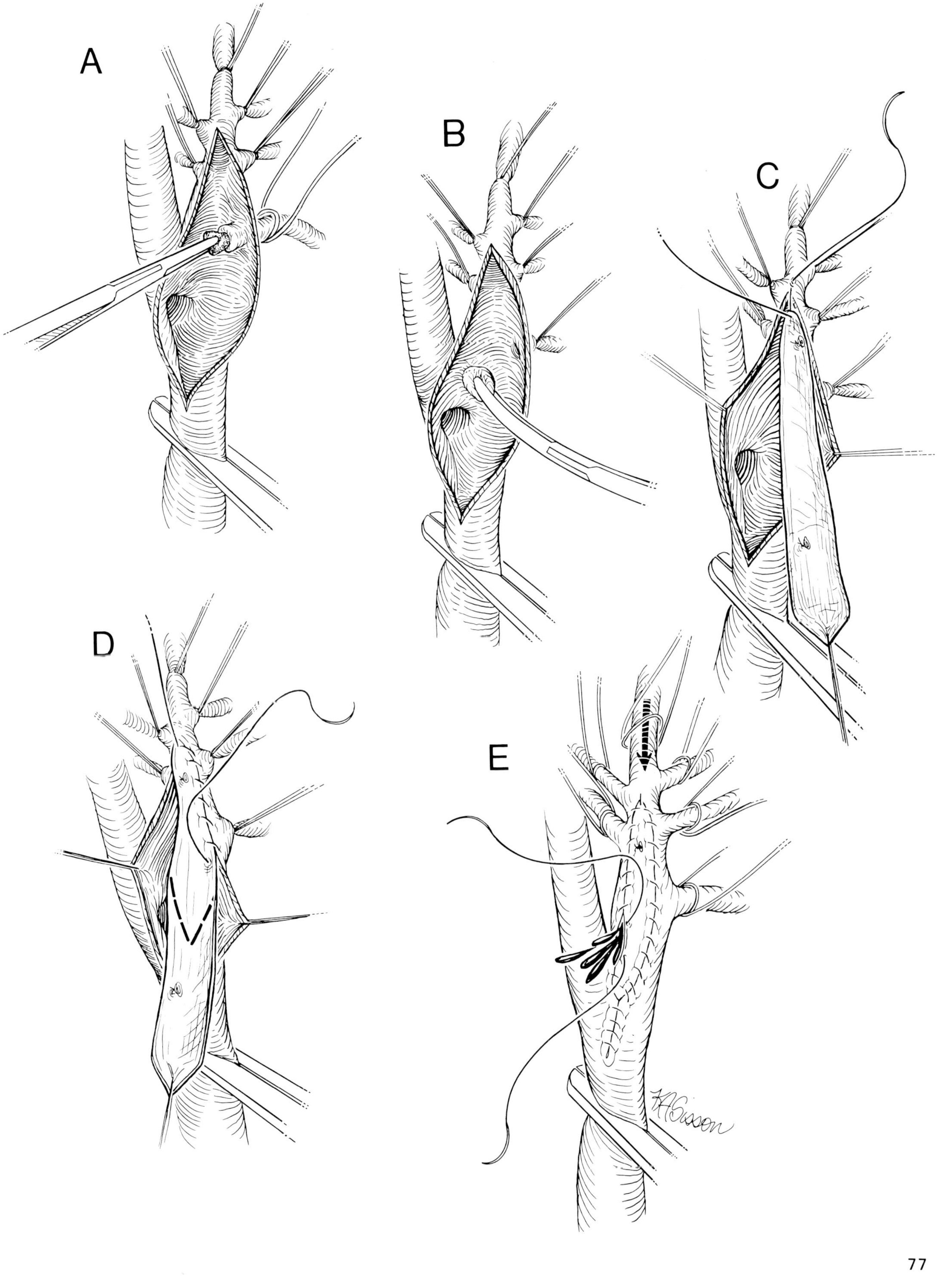
A
B
C
D
E

Standard flushing techniques are used prior to completion of the arteriotomy closure. The external carotid artery and its branches are opened and flushed retrograde (Fig. 3E). Then, the angled vascular clamp is momentarily released and the common cartotd artery is flushed (Fig. 4A). Closure of the arteriotomy is then completed. Flow is restored initially to the superior thyroid artery branch (Fig. 4B) and then to the more important distal branches of the external carotid.

The completed vein patch angioplasty provides a widely patent endarterectomized segment of external carotid artery (Fig. 4C). An alternative method for patch angioplasty is provided by use of the endarterectomized proximal segment of the occluded internal carotid artery,[8] as shown in Fig. 4D and E.

Following complete hemostasis, the platysma muscle and subcutaneous tissue are closed in layers. (Fig. 4F) The skin is approximated with a subcuticular closure of continuous absorbable suture. The reconstruction can be easily monitored in the postoperative period by palpation of the superficial temporal artery pulse.

Fig. 4. Endarterectomy of stenotic external carotid artery (continued).
(A) The angled vascular clamp is momentarily released and the common carotid artery is flushed.
(B) Closure of the arteriotomy is completed. Flow is restored initially to the superior thyroid artery branch.
(C) The completed vein patch angioplasty provides a widely patent endarterectomized segment of external carotid artery.
(D)(E) An alternative method for patch angioplasty is provided by use of the endarterectomized proximal segment of the occluded internal carotid artery.
(F) Following complete hemostasis, the platysma muscle and subcutaneous tissue are closed in layers.

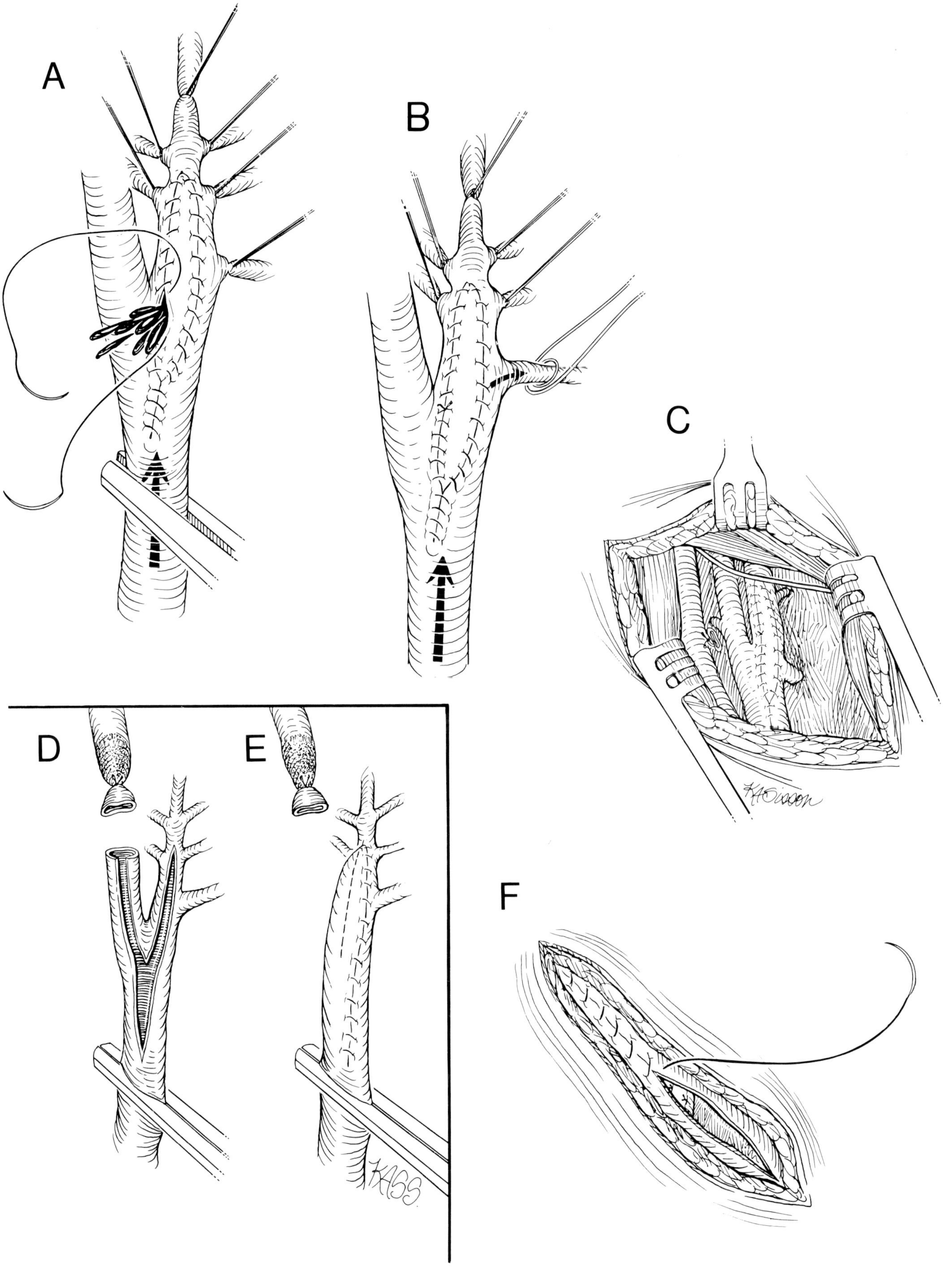
A
B
C
D
E
F

REFERENCES

1. Fields WS, Bruetman ME, Wiebel J: Collateral circulation of the brain. Monographs in Surgical Science 2:183–259, 1965
2. Burnbaum MD, Selhorst JB, Harbison JW, Brush JJ: Amaurosis fugax from disease of the external carotid artery. Arch Neurol 34:532–535, 1977
3. Ehrenfeld WK, Lord RSA: Transient monocular blindness through collateral pathways. Surgery 65:911–915, 1969
4. Countee RW, Vijayanathan T: External carotid artery in internal carotid artery occlusion. Angiographic, therapeutic, and prognostic considerations. Stroke 10:450–460, 1979
5. Clayson KR, Edwards WH: Importance of the external carotid artery in extracranial cerebrovascular occlusive disease. South Med J 70:904–909, 1977
6. Connolly JE, Stemmer EA: Endarterectomy of the external carotid artery: Its importance in the surgical management of extracranial cerebrovascular occlusive disease. Arch Surg 106:799–802, 1973
7. Karmody AM, Shah DM, Monaco VJ, Leather RP: On surgical reconstruction of the external carotid artery. Am J Surg 136:176–180, 1978
8. Javid H, Dye WS, Hunter JA, Najafi H, Goldin MD, Serry C: Surgical treatment of cerebral ischemia. Surg Clin North Am 54:239–255, 1974

SURGERY OF THE AORTIC BRANCHES

Surgery for Renovascular Hypertension

Richard H. Dean

A variety of operative techniques has been used to correct renal artery stenoses in the past twenty years. These techniques include aortorenal bypass using saphenous vein, autogenous hypogastric artery, or synthetic material; endarterectomy; and renal artery reimplantation. Other procedures, such as splenorenal anastomosis and segmental renal artery resection with reanastomosis, have been discarded following their inferior results. Whereas thromboendarterectomy and renal artery reimplantation are only suitable for proximal or orificial lesions, aortorenal bypass can be employed for either atherosclerotic disease or fibromuscular dysplasia of the renal artery.

Although each of these techniques has its proponents, the most important point to be made is that no single method is applicable to all situations and that any one of these techniques may be the superior modality of renal revascularization in any given patient. The indications for operation and the results of the respective procedures are beyond the scope of this chapter. These aspects are outlined elsewhere in detail.[1–3]

PREOPERATIVE PREPARATION

Antihypertensive medications are discontinued two or more weeks before operation if possible. If continued therapy is required, alpha-methyldopa is the drug of choice. There is little effect on hemodynamics when this agent is combined with anesthesia. Occasionally, blood pressure control has required the preoperative use of intravenous nitroprusside. In such instances, continuous monitoring of blood pressure is mandatory. It is also important that the anesthesiologist be aware that the patient has been receiving antihypertensive medications and thereby be prepared to provide appropriate support during the operative and postoperative periods.

Approximately one-third of patients with renovascular hypertension have a deficit in blood volume ranging from 500 to 1500 ml. Such deficits should be replaced preoperatively; failure to do so can lead to intraoperative hypotensive episodes and further embarrassment of an already compromised renal perfusion.

Supported in part by National Heart and Lung Institute Grant No. 5-PD-HL14192.

OPERATIVE TECHNIQUE

Certain measures are applicable in almost all renal arterial operations. Mannitol, 12.5 gm, is administered intravenously at least 10 minutes prior to renal crossclamping and heparin, 75 mg or 7500 units, is given intravenously. Occasionally, protamine is required for reversal of the heparin at the end of the reconstruction. Finally, accurate monitoring of blood loss and fluid replacement during the operation is madatory, for episodes of hypotension are especially detrimental to renal function under these circumstances.

Exposure of the Renal Artery

Adequate exposure is the most difficult but important aspect of renal artery surgery. A midline, xiphoid-to-pubis incision provides excellent access to either renal artery. This incision is carried to the side of the xiphoid process to gain the additional 3 to 4 centimeters of proximal exposure (Fig. 1). To expose the left renal artery, the posterior peritoneum overlying the aorta is incised longitudinally and the duodenum is reflected to the patient's right. By extending the posterior peritoneal incision to the left along the inferior border of the pancreas, an avascular plane behind the pancreas can be entered (Fig. 2A). This allows excellent exposure of the entire renal hilum on the left and is of special significance when distal lesions are to be managed (Fig. 2B). The renal artery lies behind the left renal vein. In some cases, it is easier to retract the vein cephalad in order to expose the artery. In others, caudal retraction of the vein provides better access. Usually, the gonadal and adrenal veins, which enter the left renal vein, have to be ligated and divided to facilitate exposure of the artery (Fig. 2C). Another frequent tributary is a lumbar vein that enters the posterior wall of the left renal vein and is easily avulsed unless special care is taken in mobilizing the renal vein. Similarly, the proximal right renal artery can be exposed through the base of the mesentery by ligating two or more pairs of lumbar veins and retracting the vena cava to the patient's right and the left renal vein cephalad. The distal right renal artery is best exposed, however, by mobilizing the duodenum and right colon medially (Fig. 3A). The right renal vein is mobilized and usually retracted cephalad in order to expose the artery (Fig. 3B). In some patients, there is an accessory right renal artery, which arises from the anterior wall of the aorta about 1 inch above the origin of the inferior mesenteric artery. This artery is unusual in that it courses anterior to the vena cava and then over to the lower pole of the right kidney, as opposed to the retrocaval course of the right renal artery. It can be easily injured if one is unaware of its presence.

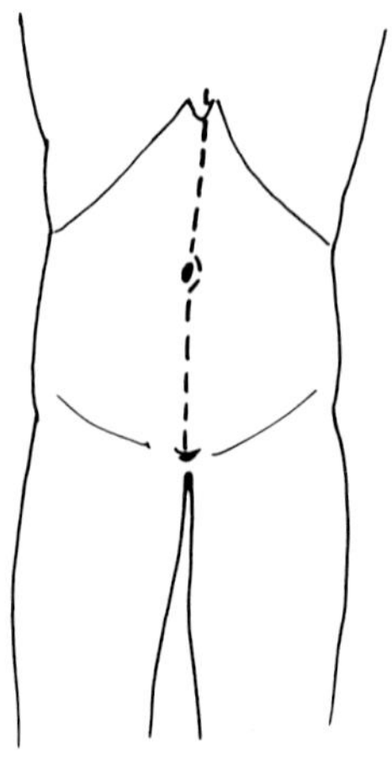

Fig. 1. Drawing of the preferable incision for renal artery exposure. The proximal end of the fascial incision is extended superiorly to the side of the xiphoid process. This allows improved visualization of the proximal aorta and juxtarenal area.

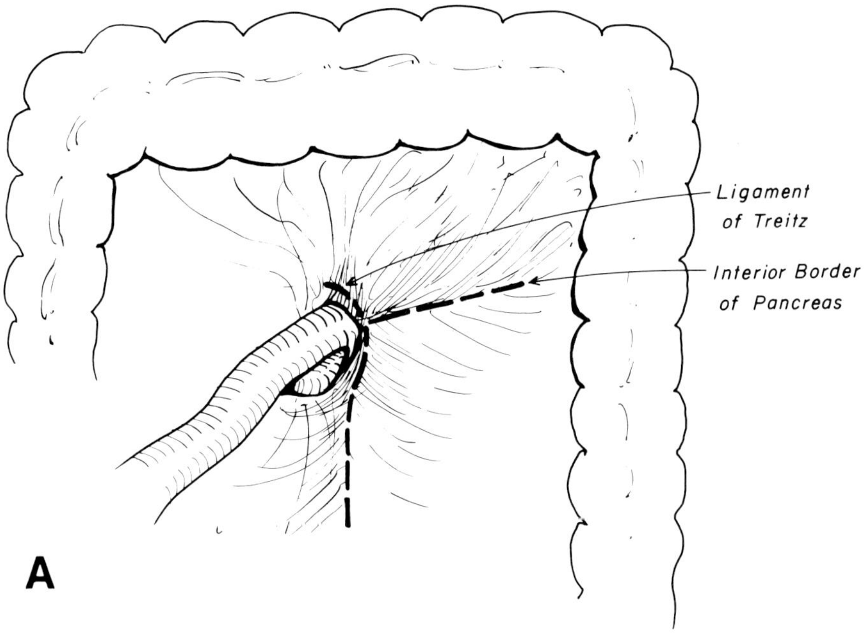

Fig. 2. Exposure of the left renal artery or proximal right renal artery is best obtained through an incision in the posterior peritoneum overlying the aorta. Proximally, the ligament of Treitz is divided with complete mobilization of the duodenum.
(B) The incision is also extended to the left along the inferior border of the pancreas. Dividing the inferior mesenteric vein exposes the entire left upper quadrant and renal hilum. After dividing the left adrenal and gonadal veins, the entire length of the left renal artery can be visualized behind the renal vein.
(C) Similarly, by dividing one or two sets of lumbar veins, the proximal right renal artery can be widely visualized.

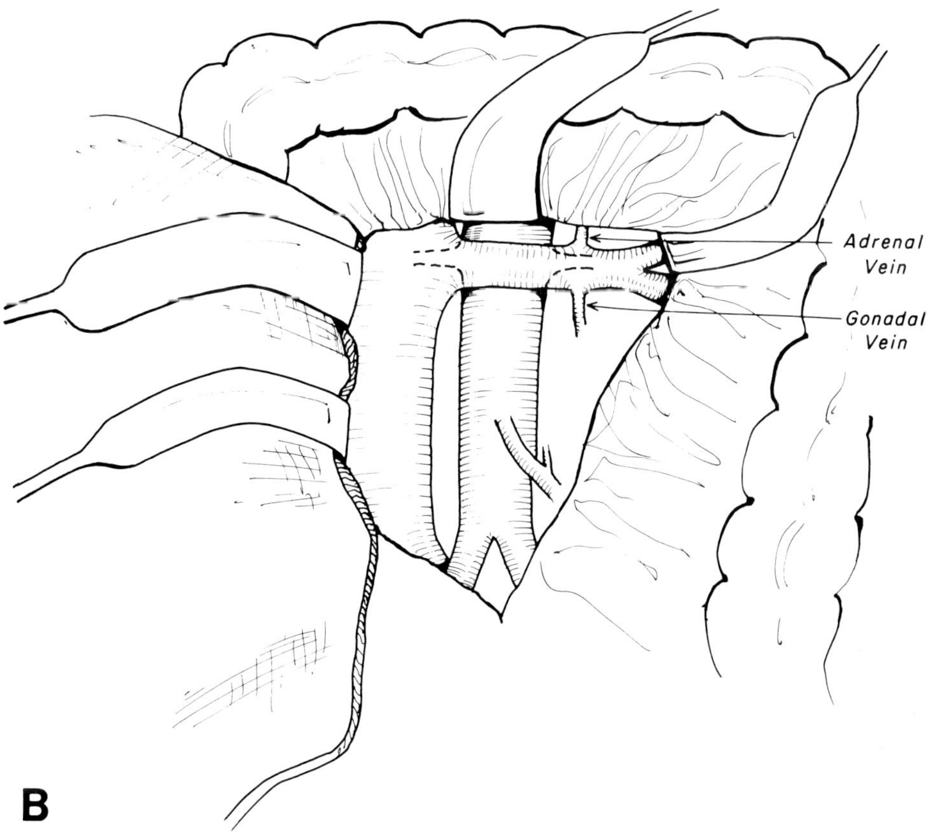

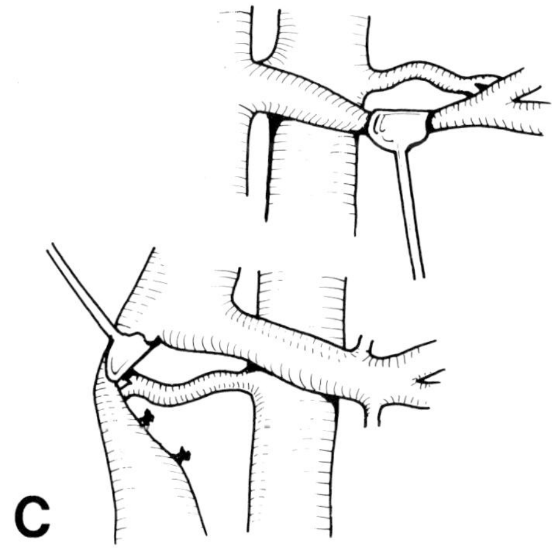

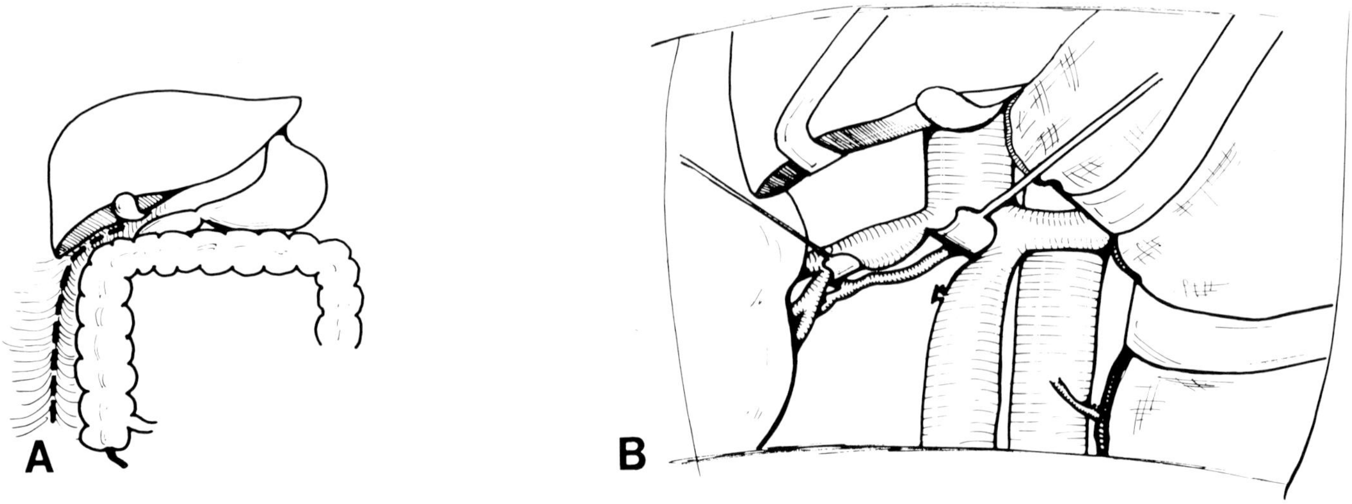

Fig. 3. Most right renal artery lesions are approached through a lateral approach (A) by mobilizing the right colon and duodenum. By retracting the vena cava and right renal vein, the entire length of the right renal artery can be visualized (B).

AortoRenal Bypass

Three types of graft are usually available for aortorenal bypass: These are autogenous saphenous vein, autogenous hypogastric artery, and synthetic prosthesis. Wylie, Perloff, and Stoney[4] have recommended the preferential use of autogenous hypogastric artery for aortorenal bypass. Such arterial autografting has great theoretical appeal, in that autogenous tissue is utilized, which matches in size and consistency the affected renal arteries. Despite these advantages, however, the added risk of pelvic dissection and the fact that the hypogastric artery itself may be atherosclerotic or the source of important collateral flow to the intestines seem to mitigate against its widespread use.

Dacron grafts have been extensively used by Kauffman, Maxwell, and Maloney.[5] They may be useful in atherosclerotic patients when the distal renal artery is large and the saphenous vein is small. Nevertheless, the distal renal artery is often small in atherosclerotic cases as well as in most patients with fibromuscular disease. The technical difficulties of anastomosing Dacron to small vessels with the ensuing high risk of suture-line stenosis and subsequent thrombosis limit its application in many circumstances.

Recently, however, expanded polytetrafluoroethylene has been introduced for use as a vascular prosthesis. We have found it to be technically superior to Dacron in regard to the ease of suturing to small vessels. Although long-term studies are not available to assess its durability, we currently prefer it (in 6-mm diameter) to Dacron when synthetic material is used for aortorenal grafting.

Although circumstances may require the use of these other graft materials, autogenous saphenous vein has emerged as the preferred donor of graft material in most centers. It can be used for bypass in atherosclerotic disease and fibromuscular dysplasia. The advantages of autogenicity and flexibility allow the use of very fine suture for direct anastomosis to branch vessels, if necessary. Further, the procurement of a short segment of saphenous vein through a separate groin incision adds little to either operative time or postoperative morbidity. Nevertheless, if the saphenous vein is small (less than 4-mm in diameter) or if it has been previously sacrificed, other sources of graft material must be used. Although gonadal and iliac veins have been suggested as alternative sources, these intra-abdominal veins withstand aortic pressure poorly and should not be employed as arterial substitutes.

After the renal artery and infrarenal aorta are mobilized, the vein graft is prepared. Mild distention with heparinized saline allows identification of adventitial bands, which should be divided. Extensive removal of the adventitia, or distention under high pressure, however, is unnecessary and potentially detrimental to the long-term function of the vein graft. In "end-to-side" renal artery bypass, the renal artery–vein graft anastomosis should be performed first. Since this is generally the most difficult anastomosis, it is much easier if the graft is completely mobile (Fig. 4).

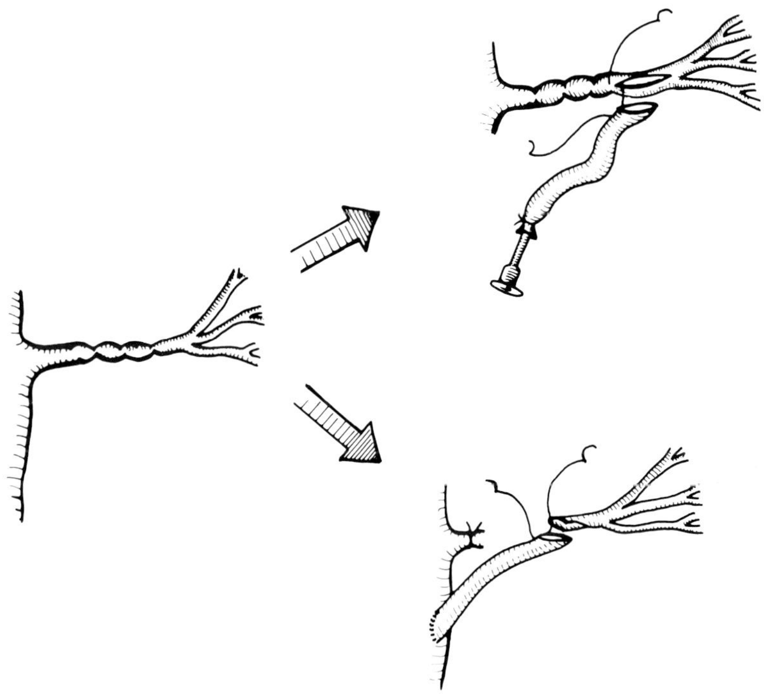

Fig. 4. The renal artery bypass can be constructed with an end-to-side or end-to-end graft renal artery anastomosis. The distal anastomosis is performed first when performing the end-to-side technique. In contrast, the aortic anastomosis is performed first when employing the end-to-end technique.

After an adequate exposure is obtained, small silastic slings can be used to occlude the renal artery distally. This method of vessel occlusion is especially applicable to this procedure. In contrast to vascular clamps, these slings are essentially atraumatic to the delicate renal artery. The absence of clamps in the operative field is also advantageous. Further, when tension is applied to the slings, they lift the vessel out of the retroperitoneal soft tissue for a more accurate visualization.

The length of the arteriotomy should be at least three times the diameter of the renal artery to guard against late suture-line stenosis. Before the anastomosis is created, each of the branches of the renal artery is gauged with renal artery dilators. Since branch stenosis in patients with fibromuscular dysplasia may be missed on angiography, this maneuver may be diagnostic as well as therapeutic. A 6–0 or 7–0 monofilament polypropylene (Prolene) suture material is employed with loop magnification. A continuous suture line is employed to allow the greatest exposure for the placement of sutures at the distal end of the arteriotomy. Greatest emphasis is placed on the placement of these four or five sutures. If these are placed deeply or with an inappropriate advancement, one will create a stenotic outflow for the graft and risk later graft thrombosis (Fig. 5).

Following completion of the renal artery anastomosis, heparinized saline is injected and the suture line is checked for leaks. The occluding clamps and slings are then removed from the renal artery and an atraumatic, small bulldog clamp is placed across the vein graft adjacent to the anastomosis. The aortic anastomosis is then performed (Fig. 6).

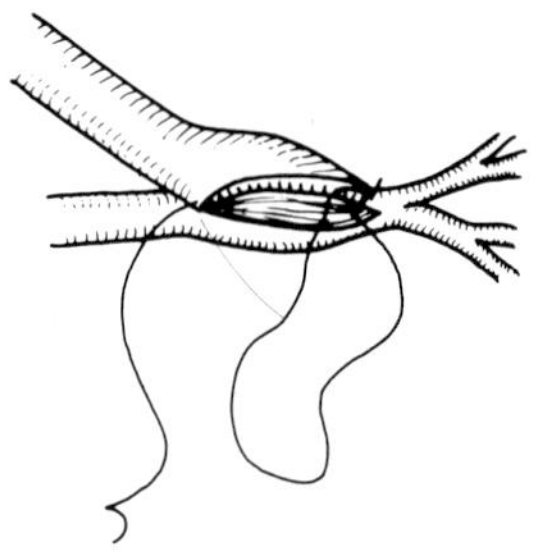

Fig. 5. The renal artery anastomosis is performed with a continuous suture line of 6–0 or 7–0 monofilament polypropylene suture. This allows the best visualization for placement of the sutures around the distal end of the arteriotomy.

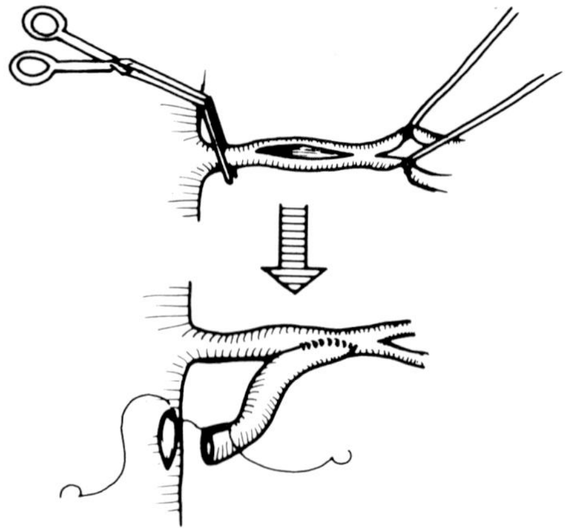

Fig. 6. To perform the aortic anastomosis, a wide button of aorta is excised to create a large orifice for the origin of the renal artery graft.

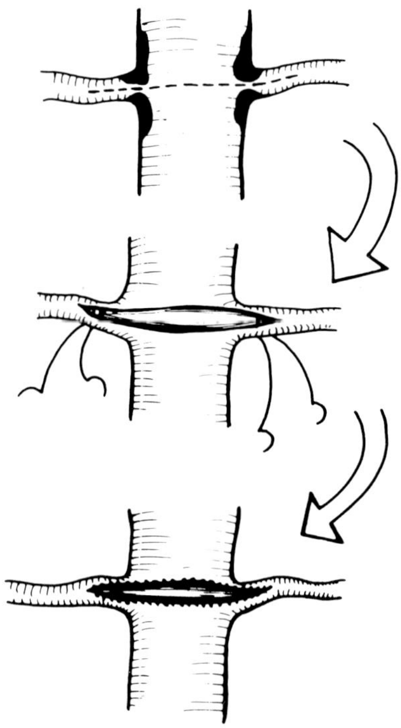

Fig. 7. Following mobilization of the juxtarenal aorta and both renal arteries bilateral renal and aortic endarterectomy is performed through a transverse incision extending beyond the lesion in each renal artery. This allows visualization of the distal end of the endarterectomy. When necessary, the distal intima can be sutured down with mattress sutures prior to closure of the arteriotomy with a vein patch.

The aorta is crossclamped below the renal arteries and a wedge of aortic wall excised to create a large orifice for the vein graft. This is especially important if the aorta is thickened or calcified by extensive atherosclerosis. Again, the anastomotic diameter should be at least three times the vein graft diameter to prevent late suture-line stenosis and subsequent thrombosis. The graft is usually brought behind the renal vein on the left and behind the vena cava on the right. However, there are instances in which the anatomy of the renal arteries is such that a course anterior to the left renal vein or anterior to the vena cava on the right seems more appropriate.

In contrast to the end-to-side bypass technique, we usually first construct the proximal (aortic) anastomosis when performing an end-to-end renal artery bypass. After the proximal anastomosis is completed the renal artery is ligated proximally and transected. The renal artery and graft are then spatulated to provide an anastomotic diameter at least three times the diameter of the renal artery (Fig. 4). Again, a continuous suture line using 6–0 or 7–0 monofilament polypropylene is employed for this anastomosis.

Thromboendarterectomy

In some cases of bilateral atherosclerotic occlusions of the renal artery origins, simultaneous bilateral endarterectomy may be the most applicable procedure. Although transaortic endarterectomy has been advocated by others,[6] we prefer the transverse incision (Fig. 7). This arteriotomy is carried across the aorta and out the renal artery to a point beyond the stenosis. With this method, the distal intima can be assessed directly and tacked down with mattress sutures under direct vision if necessary. Following completion of the endarterectomy, the arteriotomy is closed with a vein patch to ensure that the proximal renal artery is left widely patent.

Renal Artery Reimplantation

Many patients will have a somewhat redundant renal artery after it has been dissected from the surrounding retroperitoneal tissue. When the renal artery stenosis is limited to its origin and the vessel is redundant, the renal artery can simply be transected and reimplanted, following spatulation, into the aorta at a slightly lower level (Fig 8). Occasionally, this can even be done in small children and thereby abolish the necessity of using a graft (Fig. 9).

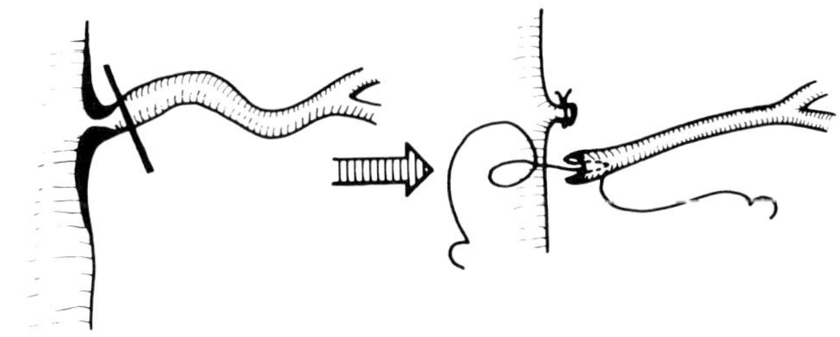

Fig. 8. Renal reimplantation is performed by suture ligation of the origin of the renal artery after transection. After excising a "button" of aorta just below the renal artery, the renal artery is spatulated and reattached to the aorta using 6–0 monofilament polypropylene sutures.

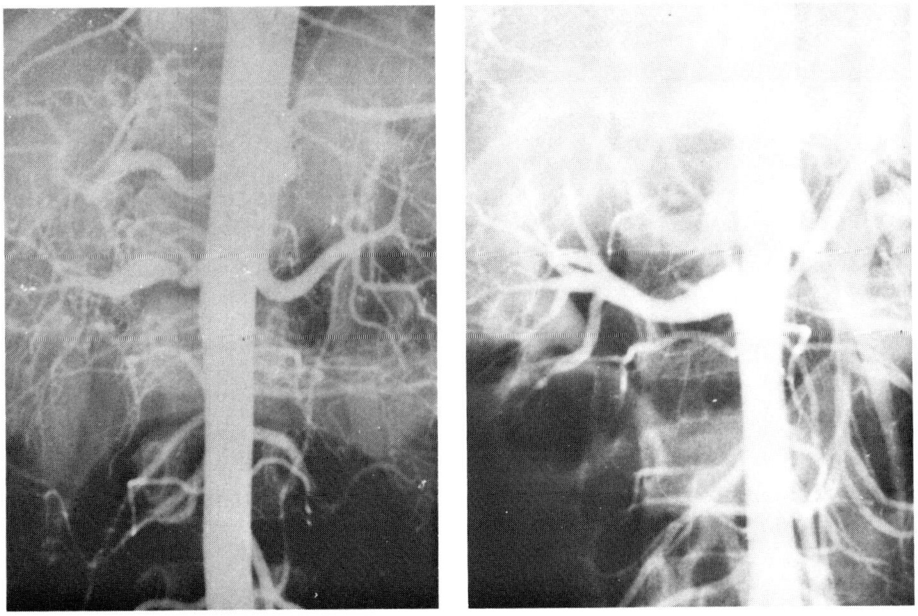

Fig. 9. Preoperative and postoperative arteriogram in a 5-year-old child with proximal renal artery stenosis. The renal artery lesion was managed by reimplantation after spatulating the renal artery to allow an anastomotic diameter larger than the size of an adult's renal artery origin.

REFERENCES

1. Dean RH: Indications for operative management of renovascular hypertension. Journal of South Carolina Medical Assn p 523, December 1977
2. Dean, RH: Operative management of renovascular hypertension, in Bergan JJ, Yao JST (Eds): Surgery of the Aorta and its Body Branches. New York, Grune and Stratton, 1979, p. 377
3. Dean RH, Foster JH: Criteria for the diagnosis of renovascular hypertension. Surgery 74:926, 1973
4. Wylie EJ, Perloff DL, Stoney RJ: Autogenous tissue revascularization techniques in surgery for renovascular hypertension. Ann Surg 170:416, 1969
5. Kauffman JJ, Maxwell M, Maloney PJ: Synthetic bypass grafts in the treatment of renal artery stenosis. Surg Gynecol Obstet 126:53, 1968
6. Stoney RJ: Transaortic renal endarterectomy. Vascular Surgery. Philadelphia, WB Saunders Co, PA, 1977, p. 1001

Renal Artery Aneurysmectomy

James C. Stanley, Walter M. Whitehouse, Jr.

Renal artery aneurysms represent unusual vascular lesions. These aneurysms are frequently associated with renal artery stenoses. Renovascular hypertension due to coexisting occlusive disease affects as many as 40 percent of cases[1] and is an exceedingly important factor in planning appropriate therapy for these aneurysms. Only three reports on renal artery aneurysms describing individual operative experiences with 25 or more patients exist in the English literature.[1–3] Brief descriptions of vascular reconstructive approaches to these aneurysms have been included in previous reviews,[1–5] yet many operations continue to be associated with an unacceptable incidence of complications leading to nephrectomy. Carefully planned and expertly executed arterial reconstructive procedures may better the results of surgical therapy.

Eighty-six patients harboring a total of 111 renal artery macroaneurysms, excluding dissections and fibrodysplastic mural dilations, have been encountered at the University of Michigan Medical Center. Clinical manifestations and the basis for surgical treatment of renal artery aneurysms have been detailed in an earlier report.[1] The operative techniques described in the following text have been derived from an experience with 62 elective surgical procedures for renal artery aneurysmal disease in 56 patients. Specific operations are dictated by the aneurysm location, size, and configuration.

OPERATIVE EXPOSURE (FIGS. 1 AND 2)

The authors' preferred approach to the renal vessels has been by way of an anterior abdominal wall supraumbilical transverse incision. This particular incision is carried across both rectus muscles from the midclavicular line on one side to the opposite midaxillary line. A rolled sheet under the flank on the side of the aneurysm enhances operative exposure. The same incision, extended into both flanks, is used when bilateral renal reconstructive procedures are contemplated. Transverse abdominal incisions facilitate handling of instruments in a direction perpendicular to the longitudinal axis of the body and are of particular benefit in renal artery reconstructive procedures. This small but definite technical advantage of the transverse incisions, rather than their healing properties, has caused us to favor them over midline vertical incisions.

The right renal artery and vein, as well as the inferior vena cava and aorta, are exposed by reflecting the colon and duodenum medially. This is accomplished by incising the lateral parietes, from the hepatic flexure to the cecum, and separating the mesocolon from retroperitoneal structures by both blunt and sharp dissection. Care is required to avoid entering Gerota's fascia anterior to the kidney. As this dissection progresses, the duodenum, which overlies the upper portion of the right kidney, and the proximal pancreas are carefully displaced to the left in an extended Kocher-like maneuver. Excellent visualization of the upper abdominal vena cava and vessels to the right kidney is thus provided.

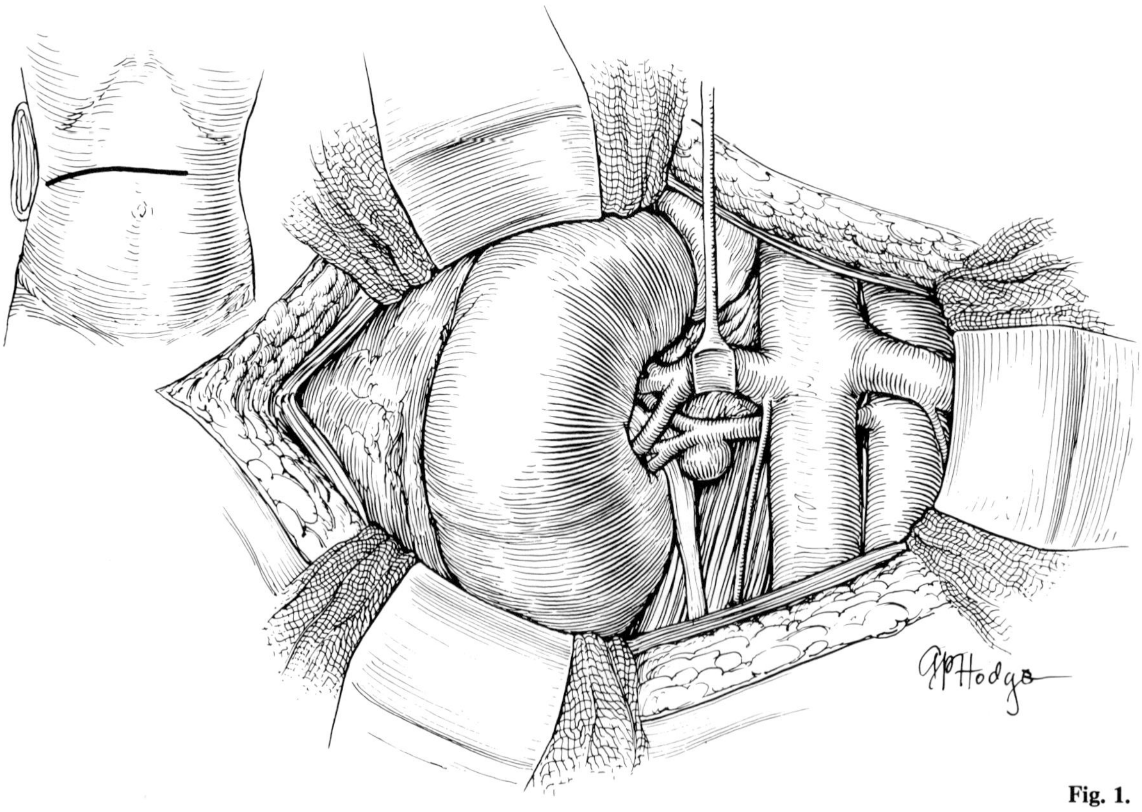

Fig. 1. Right renal artery.

The proximal renal artery, as well as vessels beyond the aneurysm, are then clamped, and the aneurysm is resected. The proximal renal artery is ligated. The between the cava and renal hilum. Dissection of the renal artery is usually facilitated by retraction of the renal vein superiorly. By blunt and sharp means, the renal artery is initially isolated in its midportion just lateral to the vena cava. Although an aneurysm may often be palpable in the hilum of the kidney, in general it is unwise to approach it directly. If one dissects the more proximal renal artery first, and then commences to expose the more distal vessels, troublesome injury to small arterial and venous branches may be more easily avoided. Although rupture of renal artery aneurysms during operative dissection is rare, dislodgment of mural debris with distal embolization may occur if these lesions are not handled with care. Renal artery branches may be encircled with fine polyethylene tubing for retraction purposes. Use of elastic bands for vessel retraction or occlusion is considered potentially harmful because of unrecognized tension that may occasionally be applied to them. Vessel occlusion is best achieved with precision microvascular clamps.

In the case of fusiform aneurysms involving the proximal right renal artery, exposure may be obtained by careful circumferential dissection of the inferior vena cava just below the renal veins. It is then possible to retract the cava to the right and expose the right renal artery at its aortic origin.

Exposure of the left kidney and renal vessel follows a retroperitoneal dissection similar to that performed on the right, with reflection of the viscera, including the left colon medially. The tail and body of the pancreas are easily elevated, without undue tension, over the superior pole of the kidney. Only rarely does a low-lying or large spleen obscure the operative field. It is the authors' contention that this retroperitoneal approach through a transverse incision offers better visualization of the renal vessels than does direct exposure of these structures through an incision in the mesocolon at the root of the mesentery. The proximal and midrenal arteries lie beneath the renal vein on the left. Exposure often requires mobilization of the latter vein with ligation and transection of the gonadal branch inferiorly and multiple small adrenal venous branches superiorly.

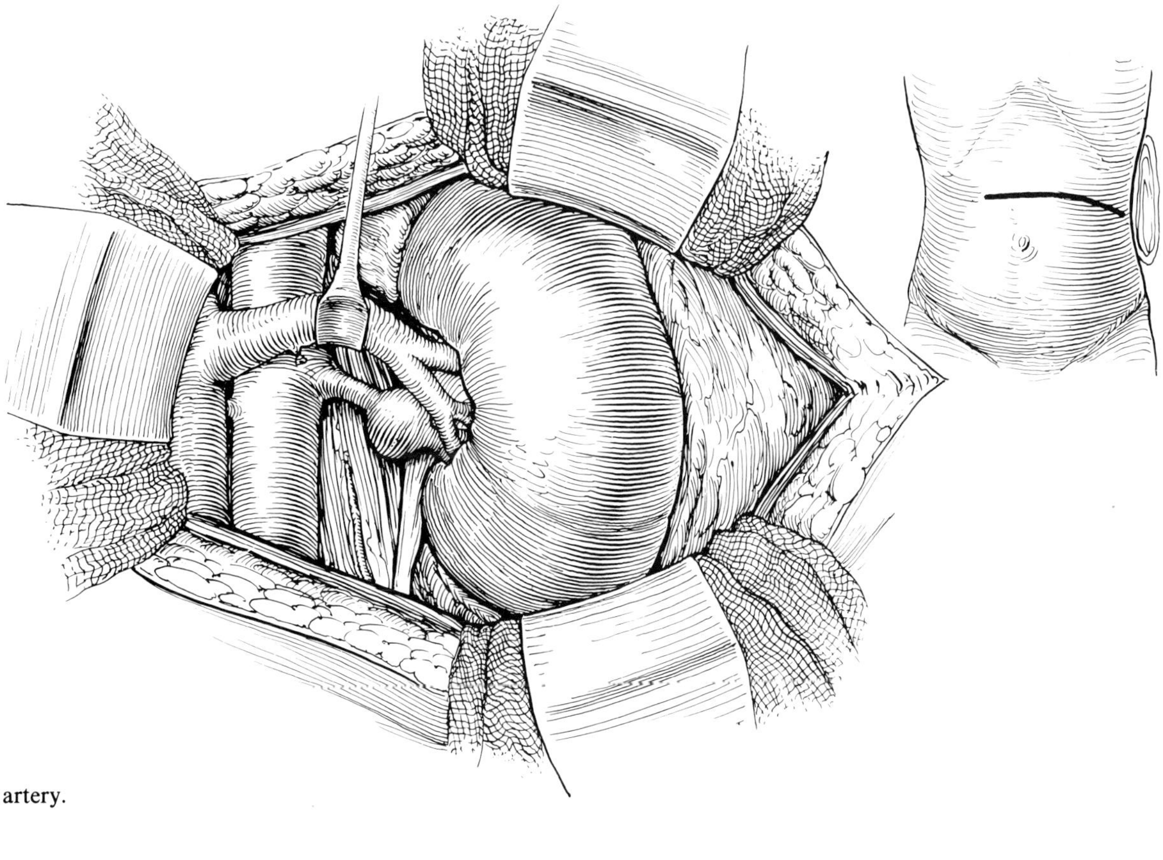

Fig. 2. Left renal artery.

PRIMARY CLOSURE (FIG. 3)

Solitary renal artery aneurysms involving the main renal artery and occasionally primary segmental branch bifurcations may be excised and closed in a simple primary fashion. Once exposure of the renal artery has been obtained, systemic anticoagulation is achieved by the intravenous administration of sodium heparin, 150 U/kg. Regional heparinization is not considered effective.

Microvascular clamps, developing tensions ranging from 30 to 70 gm, are preferred over conventional vascular clamps for occluding vessels in juxtaposition to the aneurysm. They have less potential to cause vessel wall injury, and obscuration of the operative field is less likely because of their small size. Application of these devices should be such that the blades, rather than the handles, are positioned towards the aneurysm. This reduces nuisance entanglements of suture material in the microvascular clamp handles as the reconstruction progresses.

The aneurysm is excised after systemic heparinization and clamping of all vessels. A simple continuous suture closure of the arterial defect, using a fine cardiovascular braided polyester suture or a monofilament polypropylene suture, usually suffices. The authors prefer suture ranging in size from 6–0 to 8–0 depending on the caliber of the vessel being reconstructed. The completed arteriorrhaphy should not encroach on the renal artery lumen. Although a small rim of aneurysmal tissue may be incorporated in the vessel closure, approximated tissue must include normal arterial wall.

At the completion of the aneurysmectomy and reconstructive procedure, the anticoagulated state is reversed using protamine sulfate. An empiric dose of the latter drug, 1.2 mg for every 100 units of previously administered heparin, is usually given to this end. In patients not receiving massive blood transfusions or having preoperative coagulopathies, activated clotting times are probably a more objective means of assessing the amount of protamine sulfate needed to achieve adequate reversal of the heparin effect.

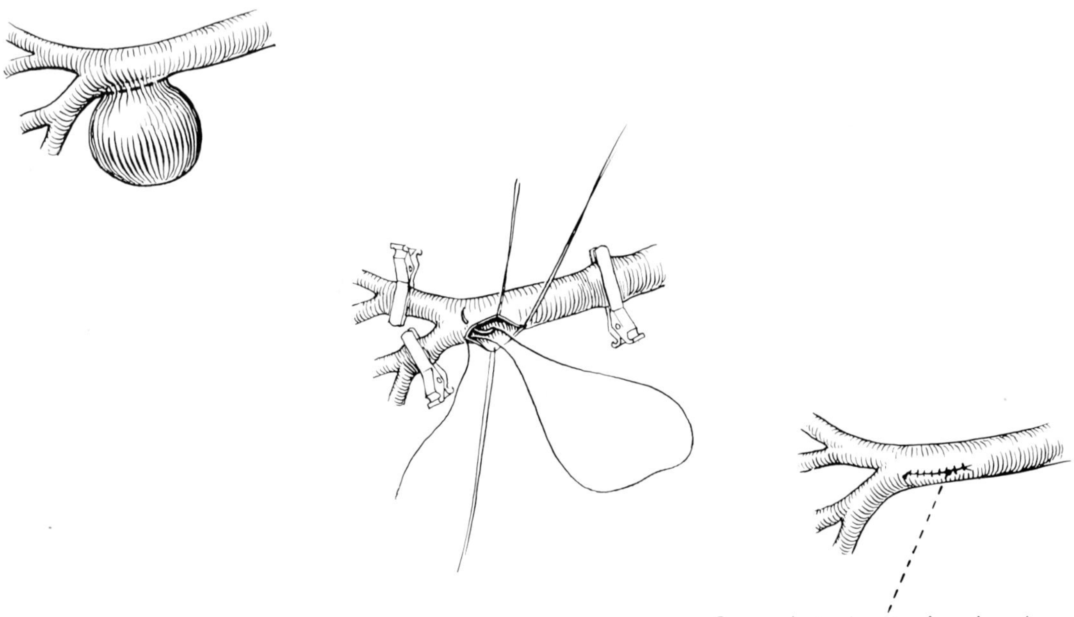

Fig. 3. Aneurysmectomy, primary closure.

PATCH GRAFT CLOSURE (FIG. 4)

Closure of defects following aneurysmectomy, particularly with broad-based saccular lesions occurring at bifurcations, will occasionally require the use of a patch graft to prevent vessel stricture. In these instances the diseased aneurysmal wall should be excised completely, even if this necessitates arteriotomies onto primary or secondary segmental branches.

Vein patches are preferred to prosthetic materials when dealing with these small vessels. Autogenous saphenous vein is the preferred source of such a patch. Segments larger than that actually needed are procured, so that they may be handled about margins which ultimately will be excised as the defect is closed. In this manner the vein material remaining will have been minimally traumatized during the arterioplasty.

The initial sutures should be placed in the apex of segmental branch arteriotomies. This facilitates visualization of the patch graft and vessel margins and lessens the likelihood of luminal compromise in the closure. Magnification may enhance the precision of suture placement. Fine, 6–0 to 8–0, cardiovascular polyester suture can be accurately placed one stitch at a time, without developing tension on previously placed stitches. This type of suture is favored over polypropylene suture, which with too much tension may cause a purse-string narrowing of circular-type anastomoses. The completed arterioplasty must neither compromise blood flow nor be so redundant as to be aneurysmal itself.

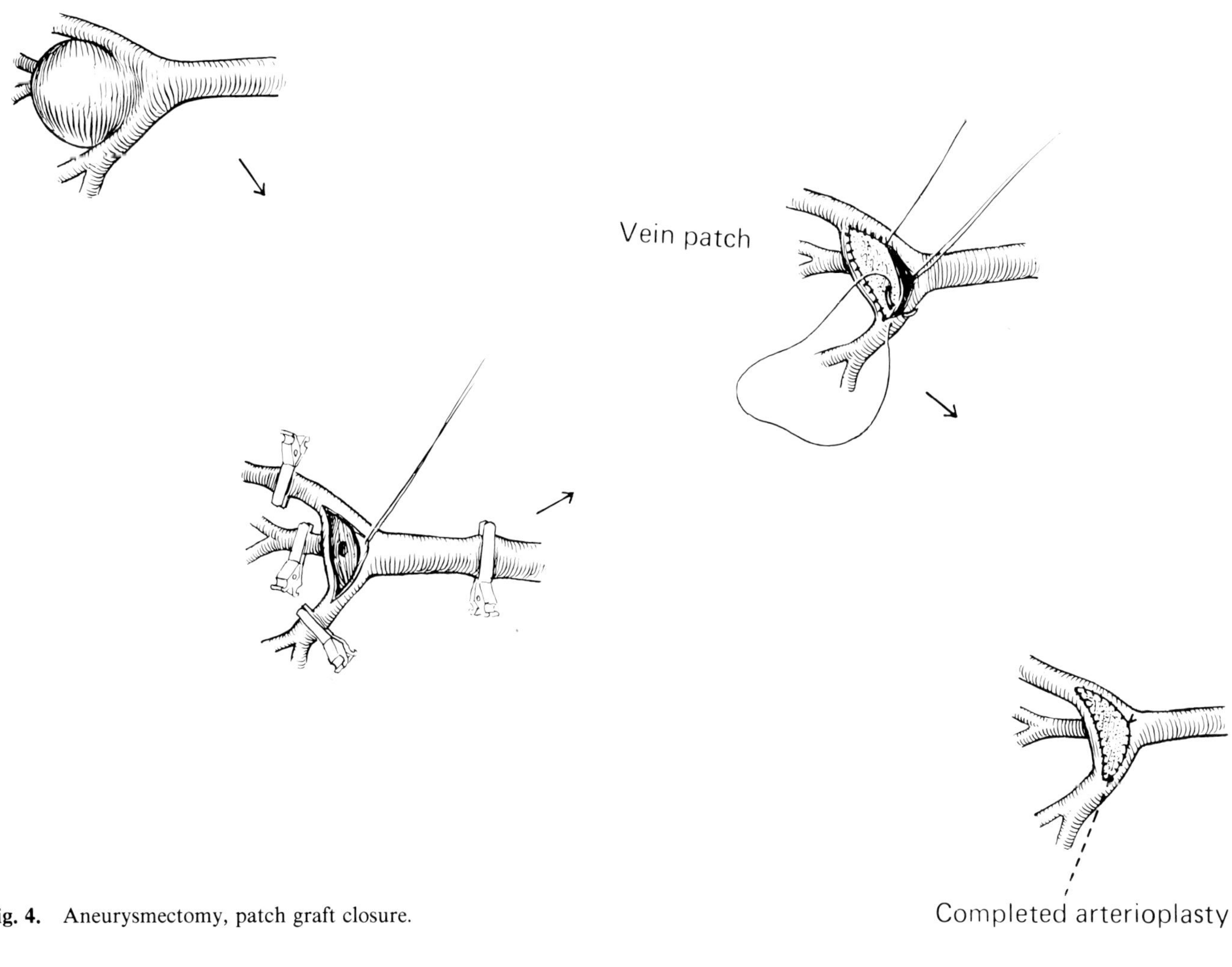

Fig. 4. Aneurysmectomy, patch graft closure.

AORTORENAL BYPASS (FIG. 5)

Main renal artery aneurysms without involvement of the segmental vessels account for less than 15 percent of these lesions. Although excision and placement of an interposition graft seems logical, fashioning a proximal renal artery-to-graft anastomosis is usually more difficult than creation of an aorta-to-graft anastomosis. Proximal main renal artery aneurysms, as well as distal aneurysms occurring with concomitant arteriosclerotic or fibrodysplastic stenoses, are best treated by conventional aortorenal bypsss graft procedures. Aortorenal bypasses have been performed on 269 reported occasions in treating patients at the authors' institution with renal artery stenoses and dissections, as well as aneurysms.[5–7] Despite occasional graft failure,[8] autogenous saphenous vein is preferred over prosthetic grafts because of the precise manner with which difficult anastomoses with small arteries may be fashioned. However, prosthetic grafts have proven durable in reconstructing larger vessels.

Vein grafts are carefully procured, gently handled, and irrigated with cold heparinized blood prior to implantation. They are not distended with irrigation solutions, and disturbance of adventitial tissue is kept to a minimum as the graft is prepared. After systemic heparinization, a side-biting vascular clamp is placed on the aorta adjacent to or just below the inferior mesenteric artery. An aortotomy is usually created such that its length is approximately three times the vein graft diameter. The vein graft should always be spatulated. The aortic-graft anastomosis is performed using a continuous suture, usually of 4–0 or 5–0 polypropylene. The initial stitch is placed through the apex of the spatulated graft and superior aspect of the aortotomy. Once this anastomosis has been completed, attention is directed to performance of the distal anastomosis. The aortic clamp is usually left in place during creation of the distal anastomosis, as to remove this clamp and place another occluding device on the vein graft may cause significant injury to the latter conduit.[8]

The proximal renal artery, as well as vessels beyond the aneurysm, are then clamped, and the aneurysm is resected. The proximal renal artery is ligated. The graft-to-renal-artery anastomosis is performed in an end-to-end fashion. This anastomosis is facilitated by spatulation of the renal artery on its anterior aspect, and of the vein graft on its posterior aspect. The renal artery spatulation allows visualization of this vessel's interior such that inclusion of intima with each stitch is easily accomplished. Initial suture placements, usually with 6–0 polyester, are through the apex of the spatulated vessel and to the margin of the opposite vessel. These are tied, and with traction, used as stay-sutures. The anastomosis is completed using continuous-suture technique. Spatulated anastomoses are somewhat ovoid, with increased suture-line circumferences. Upon healing they are less likely to produce late strictures than are nonspatulated end-to-end anastomoses. Similarly, isolated segmental renal artery aneurysms requiring revascularization are often most easily handled using reversed autogenous saphenous vein grafts carried from the aorta to the segmental vessel. Maintenance of normal blood flow to the remainder of the kidney occurs through the uninvolved renal vasculature.

The most direct route for aortorenal vein grafts to the right kidney is in the retrocaval position. In general, this lessens the likelihood of distal anastomotic kinking, sometimes seen when grafts are carried anterior to the inferior vena cava and down to the renal pelvis. However, the choice of antecaval or retrocaval positioning of the graft must be individualized.

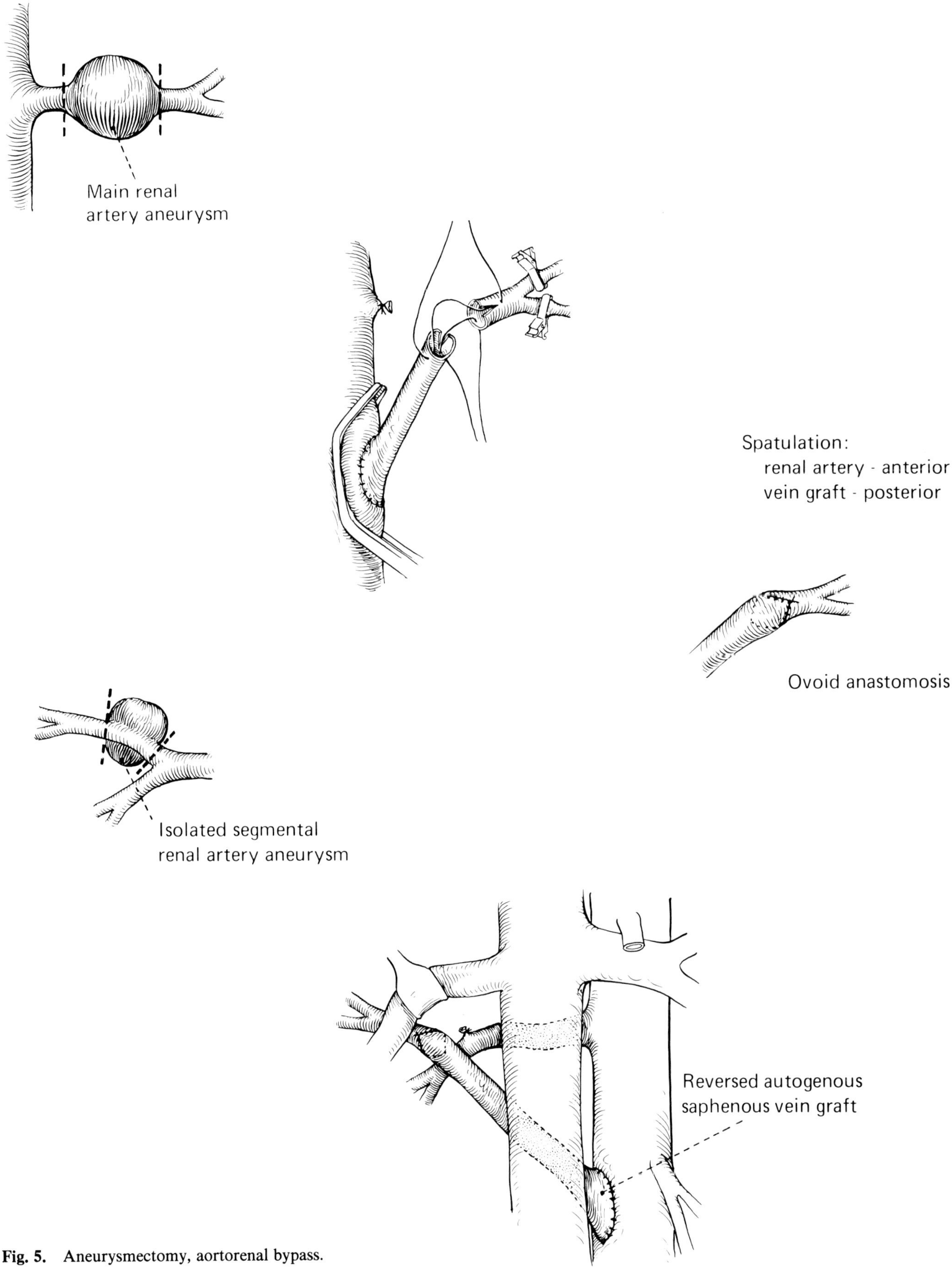

Fig. 5. Aneurysmectomy, aortorenal bypass.

REIMPLANTATION (FIG. 6)

Renal artery aneurysms, in 80 to 90 percent of cases, involve branches of the main renal vessel. Approximately 10 percent of these lesions are so intimately involved with the segmental branches that treatment of the aneurysm includes reconstruction of the vessels. In many instances reimplantation to the parent vessel is the preferred manner of managing these small branches. Solitary-vessel involvement is not uncommon, and direct reimplantation may occasionally be favored over aortorenal bypass. Limited spatulations in the longitudinal axis of the renal vessels to be anastomosed will allow creation of a more generous anastomosis.

Multiple branch involvement frequently requires initial approximation by lateral anastomosis of small branches prior to reimplantation. The technique of spatulating opposing segmental vessels and creating a common orifice prior to implantation is exceedingly important. Although such procedures may be successfully performed in situ using standard microsurgical techniques, they are in certain instances best performed as ex vivo repairs.[9] This is particularly relevant if in situ reconstruction is anticipated to cause renal ischemia exceeding 40-to-60-minutes duration. Reimplantations are more prone to subsequent anastomotic strictures than patch graft arterioplasty or aortorenal revascularizations and should be performed only by those who are experienced in small-vessel reconstructions. Magnification may be required to affect precise creation of these small anastomoses. Simple ligature obliteration or clipping of small aneurysms involving segmental vessels has not been advocated in the literature.

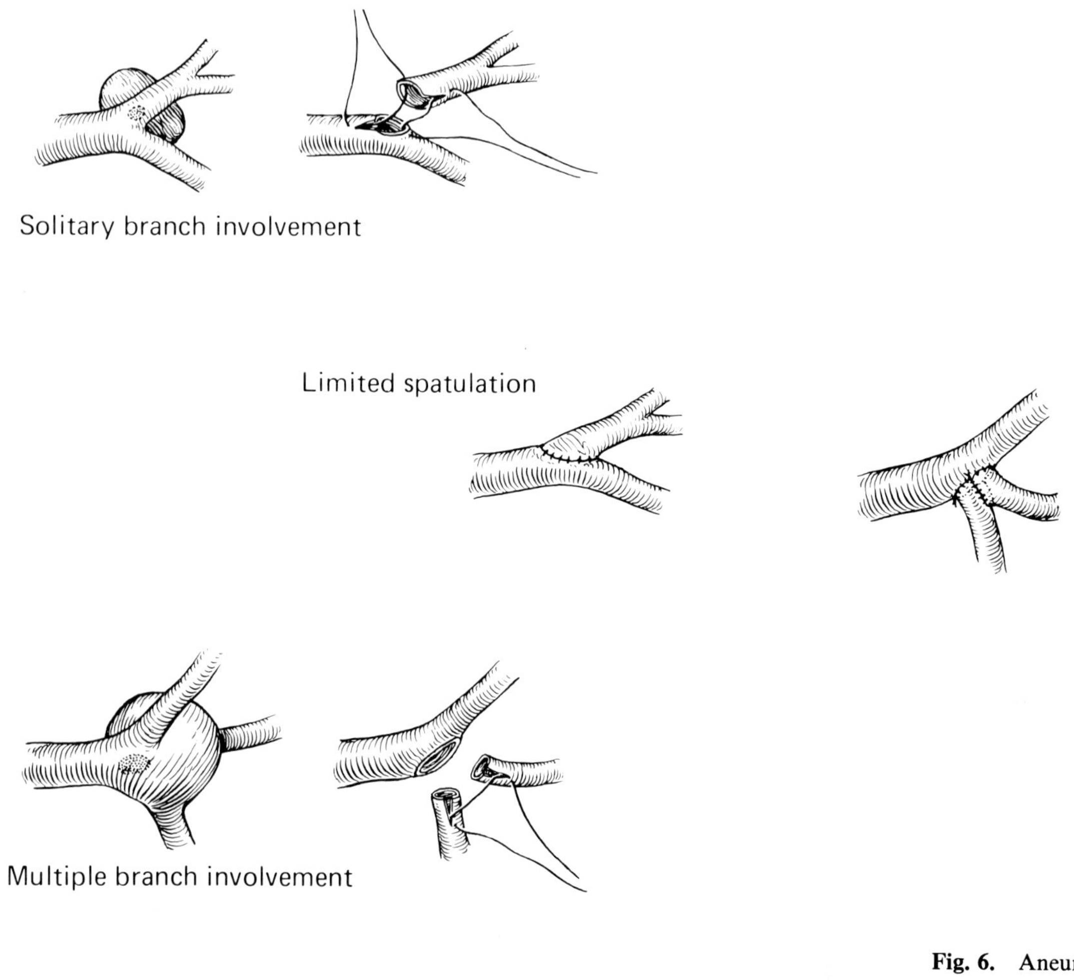

Fig. 6. Aneurysmectomy, reimplantation.

ANEURYSMECTOMY AND AORTORENAL BYPASS TO A COMMON ANASTOMOTIC ORIFICE (FIG. 7)

When multiple segmental vessels arise from an aneurysm involving the distal main renal artery, aneurysmectomy often leaves a defect requiring a rather complex reconstruction. In most instances, lateral anastomoses of branches may be performed following spatulation of their adjacent walls. Such anastomoses begin with the initial suture being placed at the apex of the spatulated vessels. This allows creation of a rather generous orifice of the compounded segmental arteries. This orifice is further enlarged with another limited spatulation, usually on its superior or anterior aspect, so as to create an ovoid graft-to-renal artery anastomosis. Completion of a distal aortorenal graft anastomosis in these cases is then undertaken in a conventional manner as previously described.

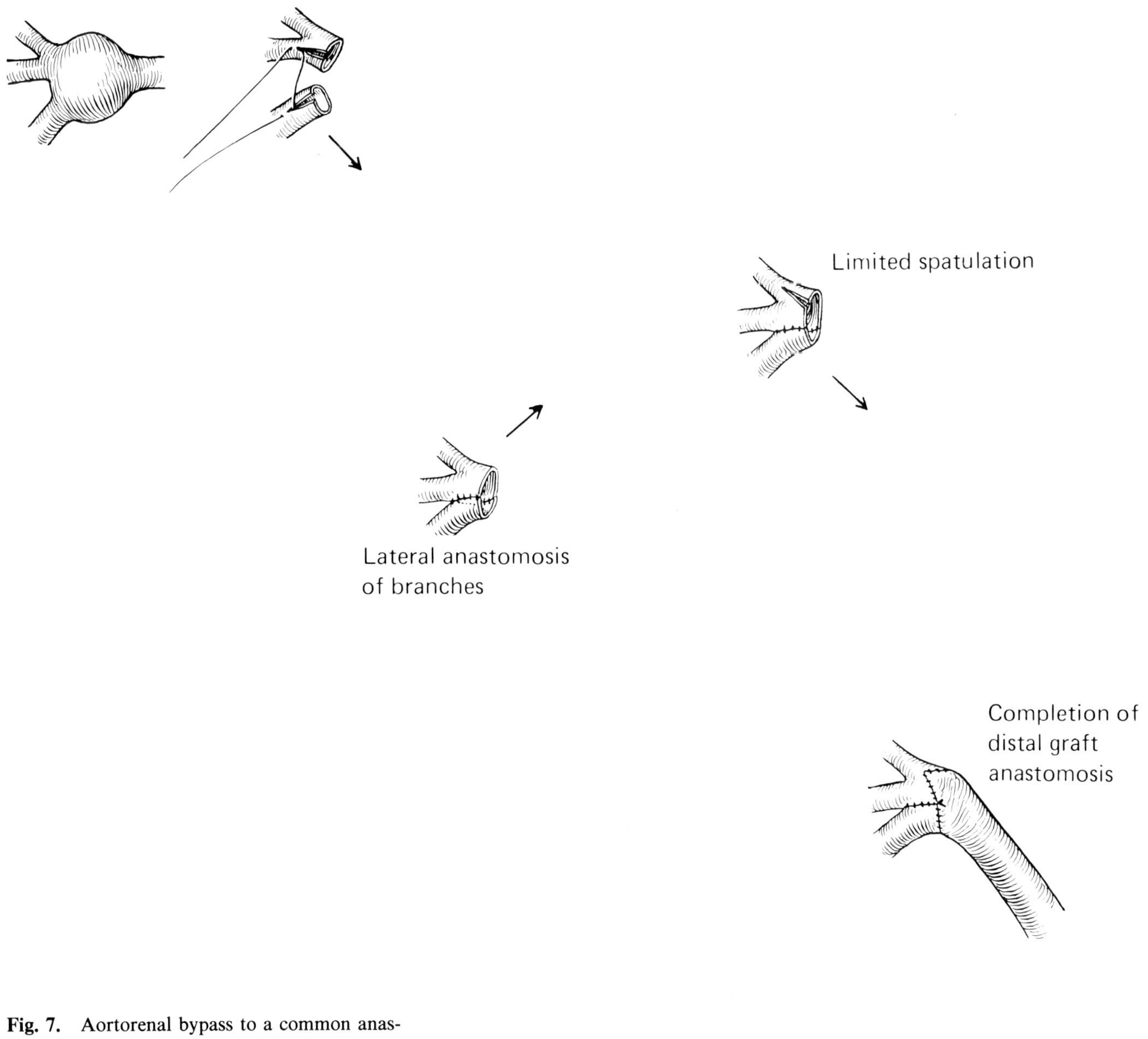

Fig. 7. Aortorenal bypass to a common anastomotic orifice.

ANEURYSMECTOMY AND COMPOUND AORTORENAL BYPASS WITH INDIVIDUAL BRANCH ANASTOMOSES (FIG. 8)

Occasionally aneurysms are best managed by implantation of multiple segmental vessels to a conduit arising in an end-to-side fashion from the aorta. Anastomosis of inferior segmental vessels, end-to-side to proximal autogenous saphenous vein aortorenal graft, followed by end-to-end anastomosis of the distal graft to a second superior segmental vessel, has been used successfully in managing select aneurysms.[10] In a similar fashion, autologous internal iliac artery with its bifurcation intact may be used in reconstructing multiple branches of the distal renal artery. This particular graft material may be most useful in treating aneurysms affecting children and adolescent patients, where dilation of vein grafts is a recognized late complication. However, when using internal iliac artery for reconstructions, one must be certain that this vessel does not harbor occult arteriosclerotic or fibrodysplastic stenotic disease. Compound reconstructions such as these to individual segmental branches may be performed in situ, although ex vivo reconstructions are often necessary in complicated cases.

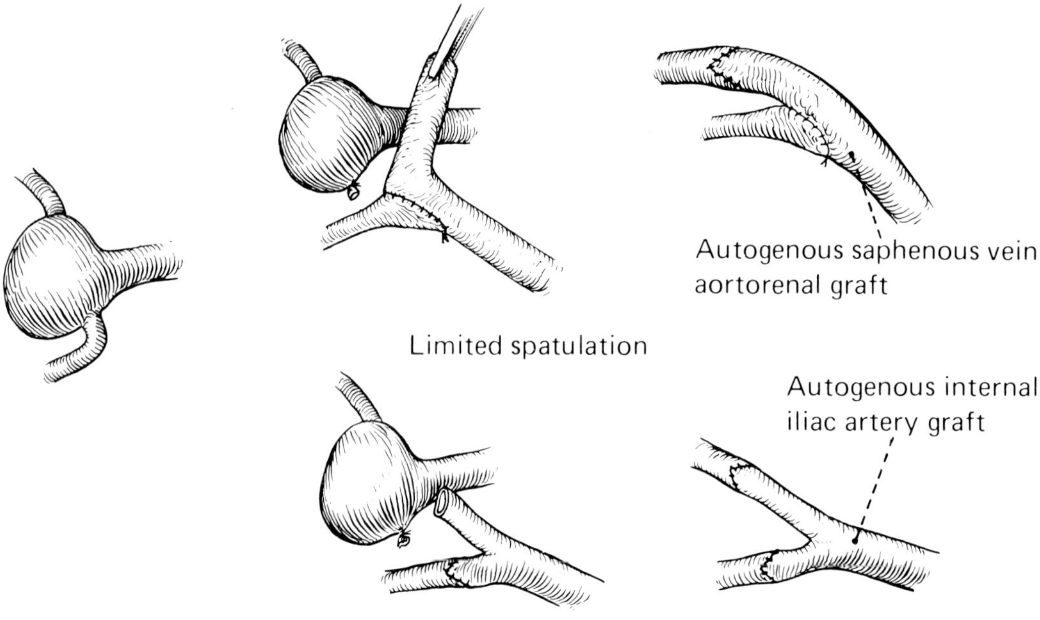

Fig. 8. Compound aortorenal bypass with individual branch anastomoses.

REFERENCES

1. Stanley JC, Rhodes EL, Gewertz BL, Chang CY, Walter JF, Fry WJ: Renal artery aneurysms: Significance of macroaneurysms exclusive of dissections and fibrodysplastic mural dilations. Arch Surg 110:1327–1333, 1975
2. Poutasse EG: Renal artery aneurysms. J Urol 113:443–449, 1974
3. Soussou ID, Starr DS, Lawrie GM, Morris GC Jr: Renal artery aneurysm: Long-term relief of renovascular hypertension by in situ operative correction. Arch Surg 114:1410–1415, 1979
4. DeBakey ME, Lefrak EA, Garcia-Rinaldi R, Noon GP: Aneurysm of the renal artery: A vascular reconstructive approach. Arch Surg 106:438–443, 1973
5. Hageman JH, Smith RF, Szilagyi DE, Elliott JP: Aneurysms of the renal artery: Problems of prognosis and surgical management. Surgery 84:563–572, 1978
6. Gewertz BL, Stanley JC, Fry WJ: Renal artery dissections. Arch Surg 112:409–414, 1977
7. Stanley JC, Fry WJ: Surgical treatment of renovascular hypertension. Arch Surg 112:1291–1297, 1977
8. Stanley JC, Ernst CB, Fry WJ: Fate of 100 aortorenal vein grafts: Characteristics of late graft expansion, aneurysmal dilation, and stenosis. Surgery 74:931–944, 1973
9. Stoney RJ, Silane M, Salvatierra O Jr: Ex vivo renal artery reconstruction. Arch Surg 113:1272–1278, 1978
10. Ernst CB, Stanley JC, Fry WJ: Multiple primary and segmental renal artery revascularization utilizing autogenous saphenous vein. Surg Gynecol Obstet 137:1023–1026, 1973

Ex-Vivo Repair of the Renal Artery for Renovascular Hypertension

William K. Ehrenfeld, Oscar Salvatierra, Jr., Ronald J. Stoney

The patient is hydrated preoperatively with one-half normal saline instituted 12 hours before operation in order to achieve a urinary output of at least 1 cc/min prior to induction of anesthesia. A full-length midline abdominal incision is used to expose the aorta, renal vessels, and kidney. The ipsilateral colon is mobilized and retracted medially to allow retroperitoneal exposure of the kidney and ureter. Gerota's fascia is incised and the kidney is freed of perinephric fat. The main portions of the renal artery and vein are mobilized from the aorta and vena cava, respectively. The polar-branch renal arteries are dissected after the kidney is placed on the perfusion apparatus. The ureter is mobilized circumferentially together with its vascular supply to the point where it crosses the iliac artery.

The renal artery and vein are divided and the kidney is exteriorized onto the patient's abdomen. The kidney is flushed through the renal artery with cold Ringer's lactate with additives until the venous effluent is clear. The renal artery or arteries are cannulated with appropriate perfusion cannulae after the kidney is placed on the perfusion platform resting on the lower abdomen (Fig. 1). A probe is in contact with the surface of the kidney for continuous temperature monitoring. Additional dissection of the renal vasculature is extended into the hilar area more easily since the vessels are distended by the continuous perfusion at a pressure of 60/40 mm Hg and flow rate of 90–150 cc/min.

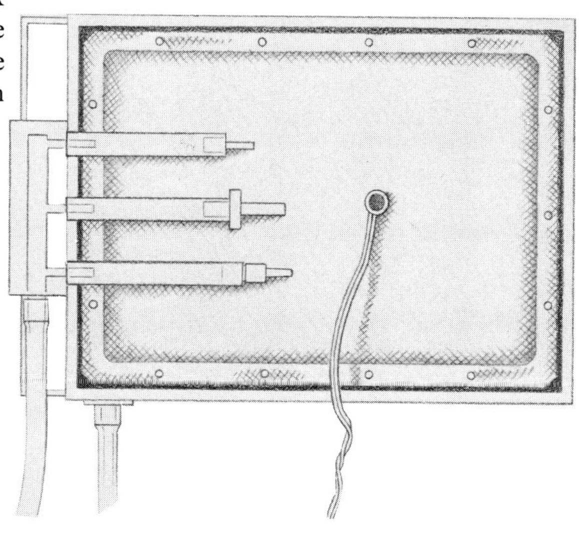

Fig. 1. A perfusion platform is placed on the patient's lower abdomen.

The ipsilateral internal iliac artery is then harvested as the renal autograft replacement artery. A tongue of atherosclerosis is occasionally present in this artery and its branches, but this can easily be removed. There is no need to restore vascular continuity at the donor site.

The diseased renal artery and its branches are replaced with the autograft by serially dividing the renal artery branches and anastomosing them branch-to-branch to the internal iliac artery autograft, using interrupted 6–0 or 7–0 vascular suture technique (Fig. 2A–C). Perfusion preservation is maintained to the entire kidney except for that segment dependent on the isolated branch artery then undergoing anastomosis to the autograft. The reconstructed renal artery branch and its parenchymal segment are sequentially perfused through the cannulated autograft while the next branch artery is temporarily excluded from perfusion to allow a secure anastomosis to the appropriate autograft branch (Fig. 2D, E). If a renal artery branch cannot be matched to the autograft configuration for an end-to-end anastomosis, the end of this branch can be beveled and attached to the side of the autograft at an appropriate site. A special bore is useful in creating an ostium that matches the diameter of the branch artery.

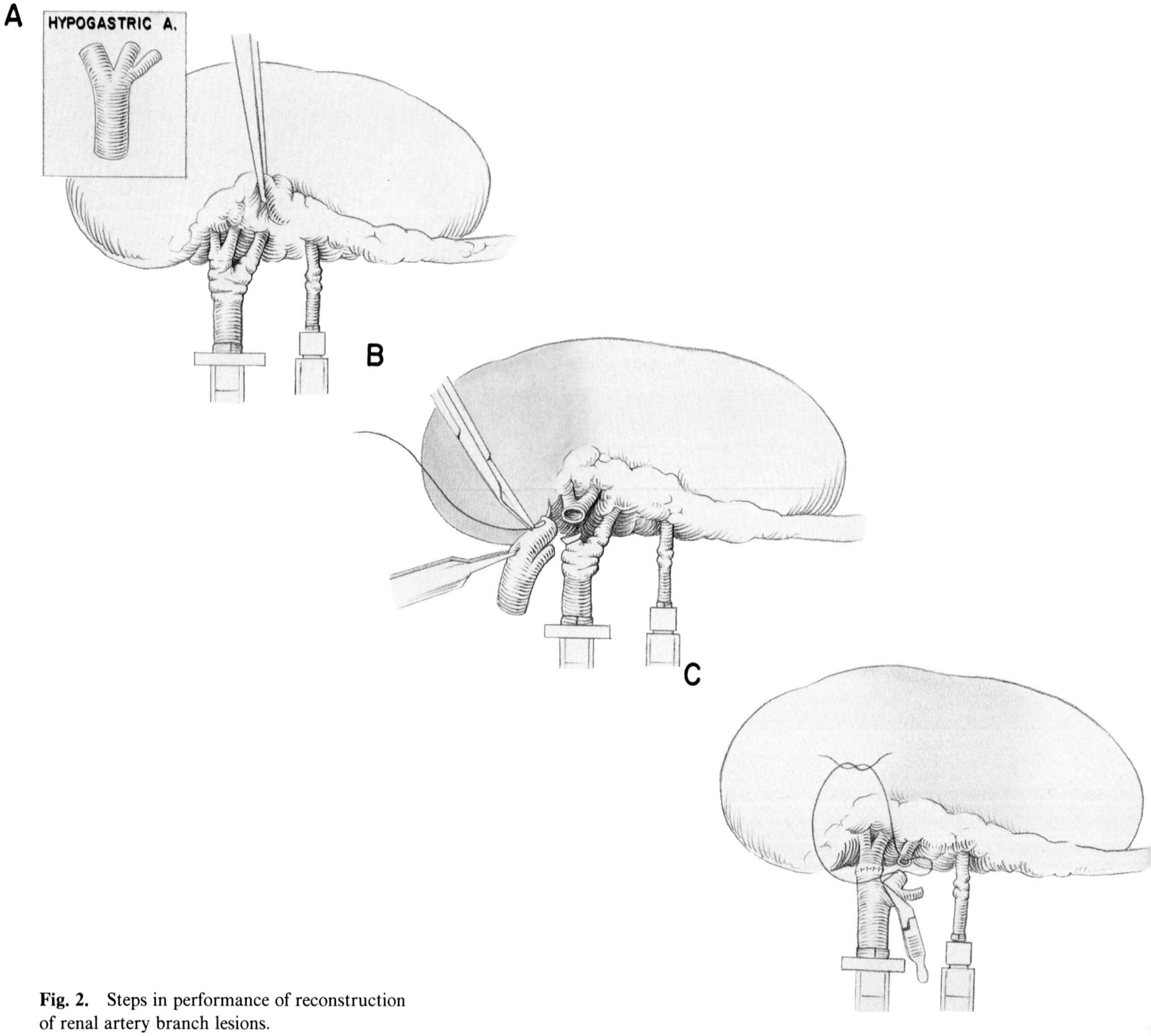

Fig. 2. Steps in performance of reconstruction of renal artery branch lesions.

D

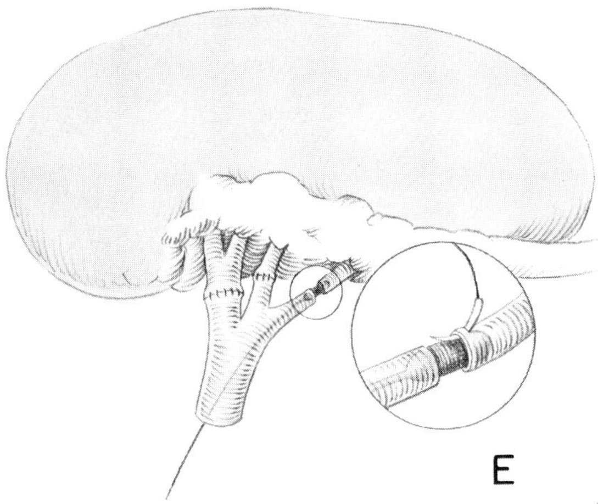

E

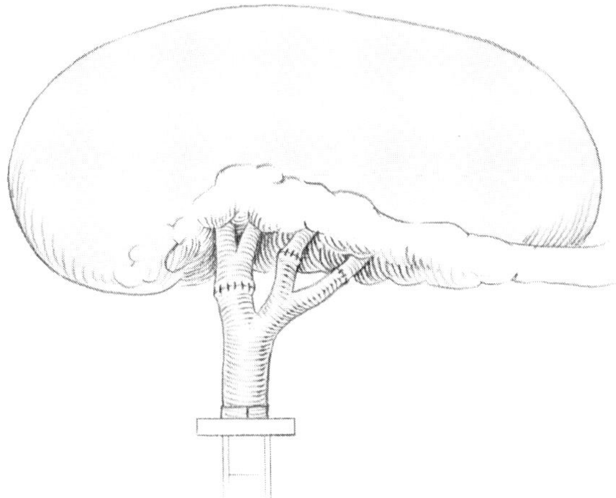

After all of the renal artery branches have been transposed to the autograft, the kidney is maintained on perfusion while the appropriate sites on the vena cava and aorta are prepared for reimplantation into the original renal fossa. The renal vein is reanastomosed on the left, and on the right it is attached to the side of the vena cava slightly below the oversewn stump of the right renal vein. The renal artery autograft is usually anastomosed to the side of the aorta, 2 to 4 cm caudad to the original renal artery orifice that has been oversewn. To facilitate the arterial anastomosis, the aorta is doubly clamped to isolate a 2 to 3–cm segment. A circular defect is created in the posterolateral wall of the aorta that approximates the diameter of the autograft. The end of the autograft is then anastomosed to the circular defect with interrupted 5–0 vascular sutures.

There are several distinct advantages of continuous hypothermic perfusion preservation in ex vivo renal artery reconstruction:[1–5]

1. Dissection of the renal arterial vascular tree as it ramifies into primary and secondary branches is greatly simplified, since they are distended with the continuous perfusion. This distension greatly facilitates the dissection and skeletonization of the vascular tree when considerable hilar and perivascular cicatricial reaction exists from previous arterial reconstructive procedures.

2. Perfusion preservation permits immediate and exact identification of an injury occurring to the small vessels during dissection and allows precise repair.

3. Continuous cold perfusion of most of the kidney throughout the procedure maintains a constant core temperature and only that portion of the kidney parenchyma supplied by the branch artery being anastomosed to the arterial autograft is temporarily excluded from perfusion. This method permits precise reconstruction and eliminates concern regarding the limits of ischemia.

4. At the end of the reconstruction, perfusion pressure is set at the patient's systolic pressure so that any branch-vessel anastomotic leaks can be identified and controlled before the repaired kidney is removed from the perfusion circuit. If hemostasis were left to the end of reimplantation, the small branch arteries could be injured during repair because their location deep in the renal hilus could prevent adequate exposure.

The precision of ex vivo anatomic repair has been demonstrated in our series by the patency of 56 out of 58 renal artery branch repairs shown on postoperative renal arteriograms. Postoperative tubular necrosis in the operated kidney has been avoided in almost 90 percent of our 26 patients, as verified by normal isotopic renograms on the first postoperative day. In the remaining instances, only mild transient impairment of function in the operated kidney was observed.

REFERENCES

1. Levinson SA, Ehrenfeld WK: Replacement of renal artery aneurysm with branched hypogastric artery autograft. Am J Surg 124:685–686, 1972.
2. Belzer FO, Salvatierra O Jr, Perloff D, Grausz H: Surgical correction of advanced fibromuscular dysplasia of the renal arteries. Surgery 75:31–37, 1974
3. Belzer FO, Salvatierra O Jr, Palubinskas A, Stoney RJ: Ex-vivo renal artery reconstruction. Ann Surg 182:456–463, 1975
4. Salvatierra O Jr, Olcott IV C, Stoney RJ: Ex-vivo renal artery reconstruction using perfusion preservation. J Urol 119:16–19, 1978
5. Stoney RJ, Silane M, Salvatierra O Jr: Ex-vivo renal artery reconstruction. Arch Surg 113:1272–1278, 1978

Operative Procedures in Acute Mesenteric Infarction

John J. Bergan

The syndromes of acute mesenteric artery occlusion are becoming increasingly well known. For mesenteric artery embolism, catastrophic abdominal pain in a patient with cardiac arrhythmia or other cardiac source of an embolus accompanied by bowel emptying is well established.[1] When, in addition, findings of leukocytosis and history of prior embolism[2] are present, a clinical diagnosis seems secure but can be supplemented by urgent mesenteric arteriography.[3] An arteriogram will show occlusion of the superior mesenteric artery in the region of the midcolic. Unfortunately, the syndrome of mesenteric artery thrombosis is more obscure: It mimics bowel obstruction, causing abdominal distension, and is treated much as bowel obstruction.[4] Only the hallmarks of profound leukocytosis and appearance in the patient of an acute devastating illness lead to a working diagnosis of mesenteric thrombosis. This can be confirmed by urgent arteriography, during which occlusion of the superior mesenteric artery adjacent to the aorta is found. Such occlusion of a mesenteric artery may be accompanied by celiac axis occlusion,[5] as is common in arteriosclerotic thrombotic obliteration of the mesenteric vessels, or it may occur alone, as is common in acute mesenteric artery embolism. Obviously, a history of postprandial abdominal pain and weight loss will not occur in patients with an embolus to the mesenteric artery, but these symptoms may be a precursor of mesenteric infarcation due to thrombosis.

SURGERY

Surgery for acute mesenteric infarction is now characterized by reconstruction of major blood vessels.[6–8] No longer is bowel resection alone acceptable therapy.

Exposure of the abdominal contents is best attained by a long midline incision extending from near the xiphoid to the pubis. Bowel ischemia may be the first and most obvious finding. The pattern of such ischemia becomes important in establishing a firm diagnosis. Total infarction of the entire jejunum, ileum, and portions of the colon will be the hallmark of thrombotic occlusion at the origin of the superior mesenteric artery. In contrast, sparing of the first portions of jejunum is an indication that embolic occlusion of the superior mesenteric artery is present. Patchy, segmental necrosis of the small bowel may be due to showers of emboli or to severe spasm occurring in conjunction with nonorganic mesenteric occlusion.

Once the pattern of intestinal ischemia has been noted, the mesenteric artery can be palpated by placing four fingers of the hand behind the root of the mesentery, with the thumb opposite and anterior to the mesenteric root. Pulsations will be present in the most proximal portion if mesenteric embolism has occurred. In contrast, the root of the mesentery will be pulseless if thrombotic obliteration of the mesenteric artery is the cause of the severe ischemia. Nonorganic occlusion will be characterized by pulses throughout the mesenteric root with no pulses in the arcade vessels.

Surgical therapy is dictated by the underlying cause of occlusion. Thrombotic occlusion of the mesenteric artery calls for an aortomesenteric graft. The aorta is approached by dividing the ligament of Treitz and the superior attachments of the duodenum in the fourth and third portions. The aorta is skeletonized and encircled in its infrarenal portion and occluded by crossclamping. Distal occlusion is obtained by anterioposterior clamping in the region of the inferior mesenteric artery without complete aortic mobilization. The aorta is incised in its anterior portion. If the aortic wall is quite stiff, a button is removed. An anastomosis from the end of the saphenous vein to the side of the aorta is completed using running 6–0 prolene.

The mesenteric artery is approached in the medial portion of the intestinal mesentery. It is skeletonized and freed of autonomic nerve fibers, and the first jejunal branches are carefully preserved. A linear arteriotomy allows passage of a No. 3 Fogarty catheter and extraction of thrombi from the distal arborizations of the mesenteric artery. Irrigation with heparinized saline solution facilitates thrombus removal. An end-to-side anastomosis is carried out with continuous 6–0 prolene.

Following revascularization and after waiting a suitable period of time (usually no more than 20 minutes), the intestine itself is inspected. Pulsation in arcade vessels is suggestive of intestinal revascularization. The use of a Doppler probe on the antimesenteric border of the bowel will allow objective evaluation of pulsations reaching the intestine itself. Such an examination is extremely reliable.

At the time of the first operation in surgery of acute mesenteric infarction, a decision must be made for or against a second-look procedure, which is a general surgical operation designed to remove necrotic bowel. There are no physical findings or laboratory determinations in the postoperative period that will aid in making this decision. If a second look is decided upon, the abdomen is closed in a single layer to facilitate re-exploration. If a second look is decided against, the abdomen is closed in the usual fashion, in layers.

The second-look procedure should be preceded by adequate hydration and fluid replacement as well as correction of blood loss. The patient coming to the operating room for a second-look procedure is frequently in better physical condition than at the first operation. If revascularization is necessary at this stage, the patient's outlook is most probably hopeless.

Fig. 1. (A) A long midline incision gives access to the visceral vessels while arterial reconstruction is contemplated in acute mesenteric infarction.
(B) The aorta is best exposed by an incision into the retroperitoneum and across the ligament of Treitz to detach the superior attachments of the fourth and third portions of the duodenum.
(C) The site chosen for the aortic anastomosis is usually superior to the inferior mesenteric artery. The superior mesenteric artery is approached in the medial aspect of the intestinal mesentery. Its first, second, and third jejunal branches are carefully preserved.
(D) Aortomesenteric grafting is best done with a short segment of saphenous vein that is not encroached upon by the duodenum. As indicated, the aorta can be crossclamped while other vessels are controlled with atraumatic slings.

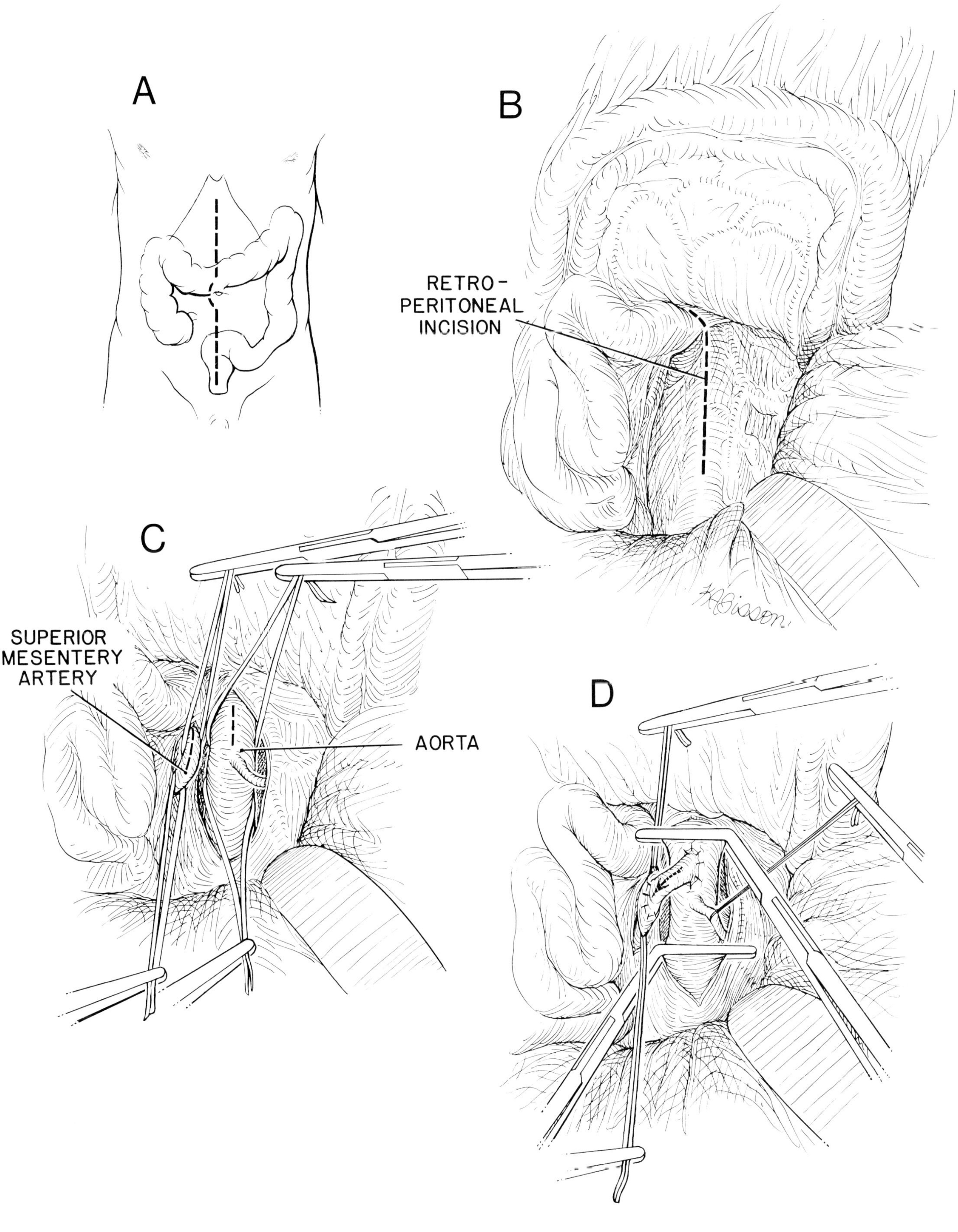
A
B
RETRO-
PERITONEAL
INCISION
C
SUPERIOR
MESENTERY
ARTERY
AORTA
D

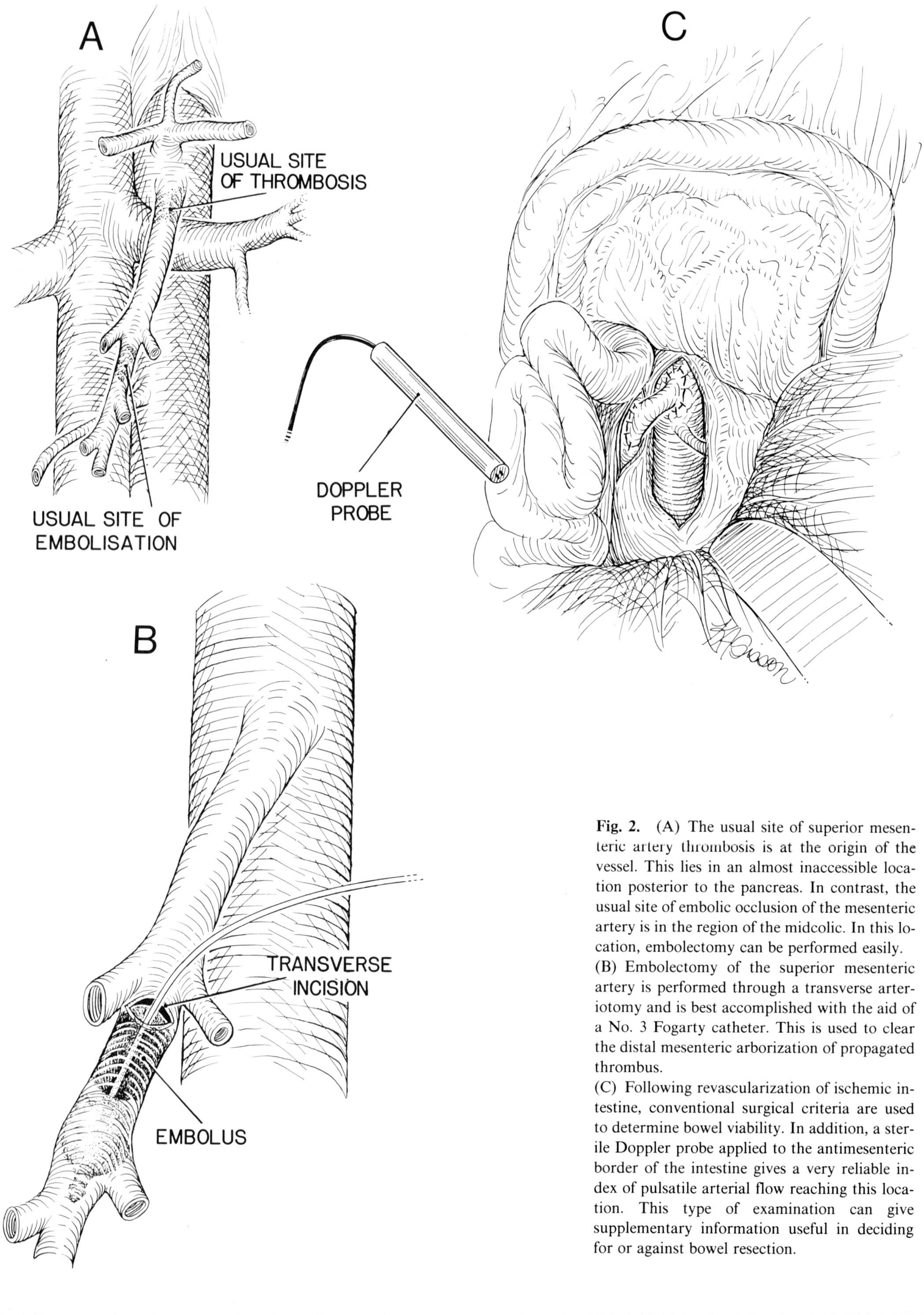

Fig. 2. (A) The usual site of superior mesenteric artery thrombosis is at the origin of the vessel. This lies in an almost inaccessible location posterior to the pancreas. In contrast, the usual site of embolic occlusion of the mesenteric artery is in the region of the midcolic. In this location, embolectomy can be performed easily.
(B) Embolectomy of the superior mesenteric artery is performed through a transverse arteriotomy and is best accomplished with the aid of a No. 3 Fogarty catheter. This is used to clear the distal mesenteric arborization of propagated thrombus.
(C) Following revascularization of ischemic intestine, conventional surgical criteria are used to determine bowel viability. In addition, a sterile Doppler probe applied to the antimesenteric border of the intestine gives a very reliable index of pulsatile arterial flow reaching this location. This type of examination can give supplementary information useful in deciding for or against bowel resection.

REFERENCES

1. Klass AA: Embolectomy in acute mesenteric occlusion. Ann Surg 134:913, 1951
2. Bergan JJ: Acute mesenteric ischemia, in Bergan JJ, Yao JST (eds): Surgery of the Aorta and its Body Branches. New York, Grune & Stratton Inc, 1979, p 477
3. Boley SJ, Sprayregan S, Siegelman SS, et al: Initial results from an aggressive roentgenological and surgical approach to acute mesenteric ischemia. Surgery 82:848, 1977
4. Bergan JJ, Dean RH, Conn J Jr, et al: Revascularization in treatment of mesenteric infarction. Ann Surg 182:430, 1975
5. Cheine J: Complete obliteration of the celiac and mesenteric arteries: Viscera receiving their blood supply through extraperitoneal system of vessels. J Anatomic Physiol 3:65, 1868
6. Krausz MM, Manny J: Acute superior mesenteric arterial occlusion: A plea for early diagnosis. Surgery 83:482, 1979
7. Ottinger LW: The surgical management of acute occlusion of the superior mesenteric artery. Ann Surg 188:721, 1978
8. Bergan JJ: Recognition and treatment of superior mesenteric artery embolization. Geriatrics 24:118, 1969

Surgical Treatment of Chronic Visceral Arterial Insufficiency

John J. Bergan

A firm diagnosis of chronic visceral ischemia is based upon the correlation of patient symptomatology with angiographic demonstration of pathologic lesions of the celiac axis and superior mesenteric artery.

In chronic visceral ischemia, weight loss is virtually always present. Careful questioning will reveal abdominal discomfort, in the form of nauseating cramp associated with food intake. Studies of malabsorption have been disappointing in establishing a firm diagnosis in such patients. Muscular peristaltic activity in an intestinal vascular bed perfused at low pressure because of proximal arterial stenosis produces extraluminal pressure in excess of intraluminal arterial perfusion pressure. The resultant intestinal ischemia creates a stimulus toward muscular spasm, which aggravates the situation further. This vicious cycle is perceived by the patient as severe but vaguely located abdominal pain, the end product of which is food fear, the small meal syndrome, and weight loss.[1,2,3]

SURGICAL TREATMENT

Exposure of the visceral vessels is best obtained via the standard transabdominal midline incision, which extends from the xiphoid to the pubis. While a number of procedures are available to the surgeon,[4,5] in fact the most reliable procedure is the simplest: This consists of bypass grafting from the infrarenal abdominal aorta to the superior mesenteric artery or celiac axis branches, as dictated by the pathologic lesions present.[6]

Exposure of the infrarenal abdominal aorta is achieved by dividing the ligament of Treitz and all of the superior and posterior attachments of the third and fourth portions of the duodenum.[7,8] The abdominal aorta is most normal in its immediate infrarenal location, and can be encircled immediately below the renal arteries. Each of the lumbar arterial branches can be controlled by soft clamps or traction sutures or slings, and the aorta immediately superior to the inferior mesenteric artery is crossclamped in an anteroposterior direction to avoid aortic encirclement.

Approach to the celiac axis is best gained by retraction of the liver in a superior direction and placement of the gastrocolic omentum on a stretch by retraction of the stomach in an inferior direction. The lesser sac is entered by incising the peritoneum. The posterior surface of the lesser sac is similarly opened to expose the celiac axis. Dense sympathetic fibers from the solar plexus are cut sharply to expose the celiac axis in its entirety from the anterior surface of the abdominal aorta through its branchings.

Many variations of the celiac axis occur that defy classification. However, the celiac trunk can be visualized as the common origin of three vessels: the left gastric, the splenic, and the common hepatic arteries. Of these, the splenic and common hepatic are the largest and may be used alternatively for the revascularization of this arborization. Therefore, skeletonization of the three vessels is done to select the most appropriate site for anastomosis of the graft. Each of the vessels is controlled by soft rubber slings, which are then used for distal arterial occlusion. Proximal occlusion is usually not necessary with total occlusion of the celiac trunk.

Construction of the tunnel from the infrarenal aorta to the lesser omental sac is accomplished by lifting the pancreas forward and passing a finger anterior to the left renal vein through the retropancreatic fusion fascia to the lesser omental bursa and the celiac axis. A clamp can then follow and pass the graft from the inferior to superior locations in readiness for the anastomosis.

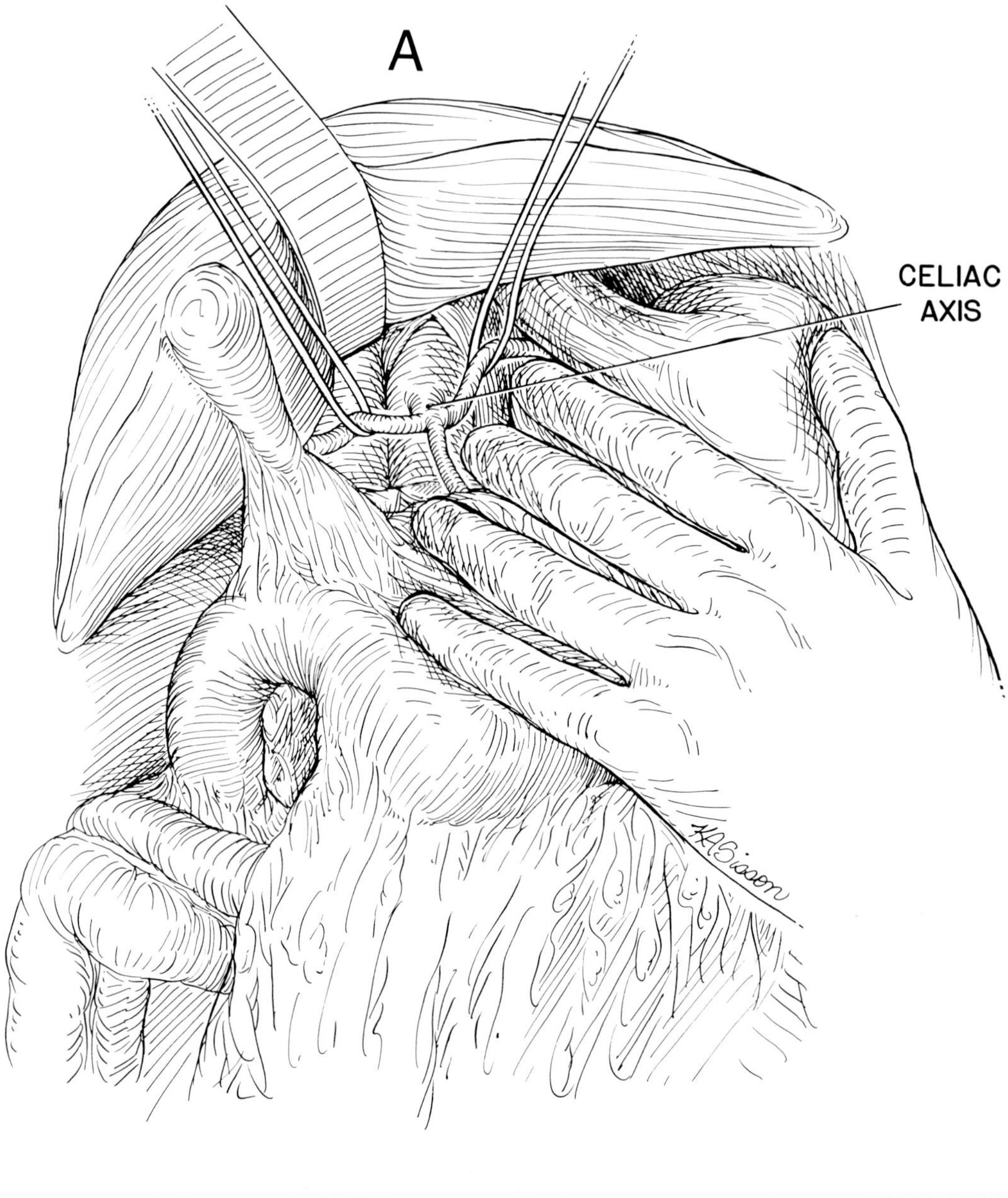

Fig. 1. (A) With the liver retracted in a superior direction and the stomach in an inferior direction, the lesser sac is opened by incising the peritoneum, and the celiac axis is exposed. This arborization varies greatly, but the celiac trunk can be thought of as a common origin of three vessels: the left gastric, the splenic, and the common hepatic artery.
(B) Construction of the tunnel from the infrarenal aorta to the lesser omental sac is accomplished by lifting the pancreas forward and passing a finger anterior to the left renal vein, through the retropancreatic fusion fascia to the lesser omental bursa and the celiac axis.

B

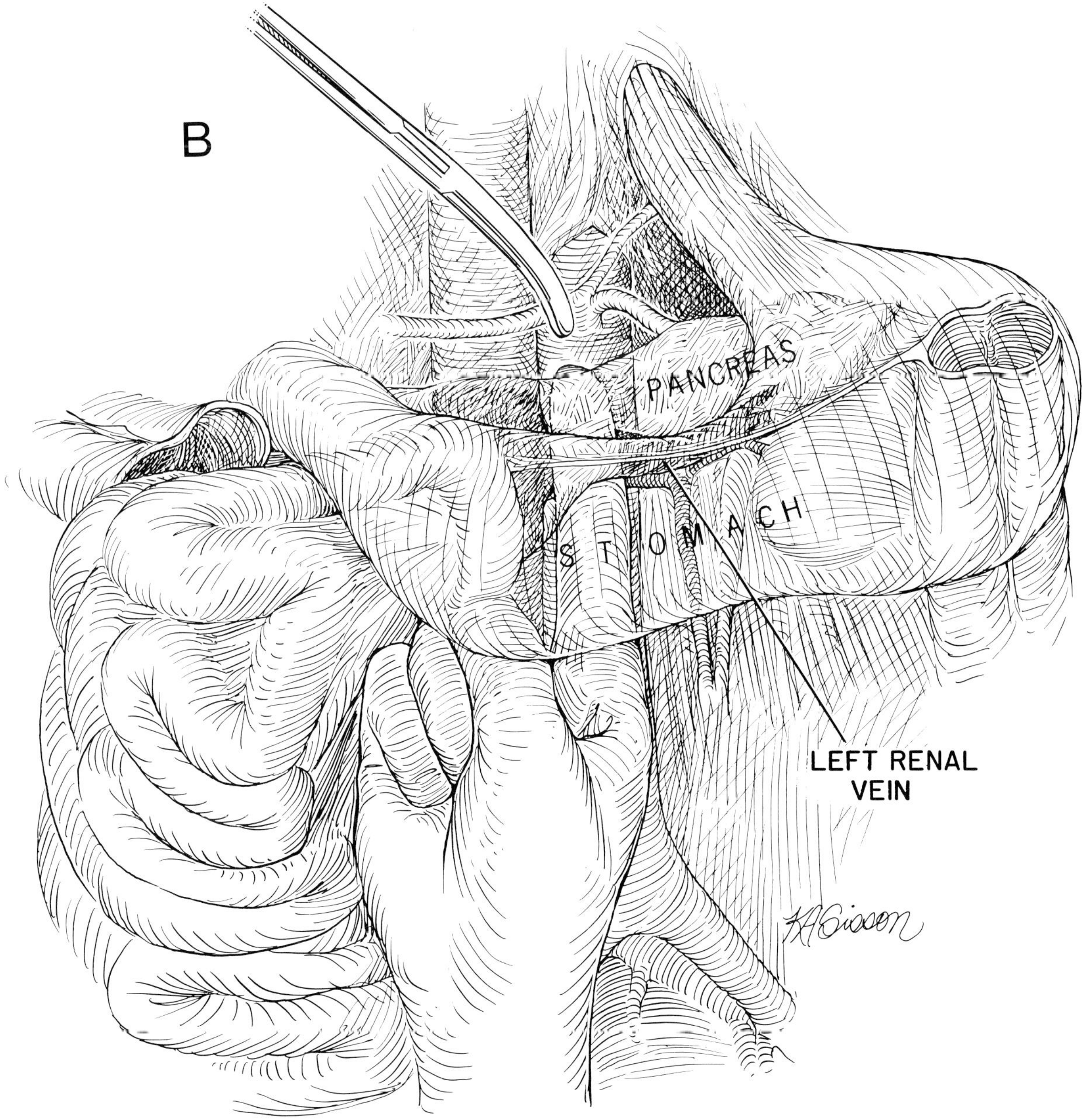

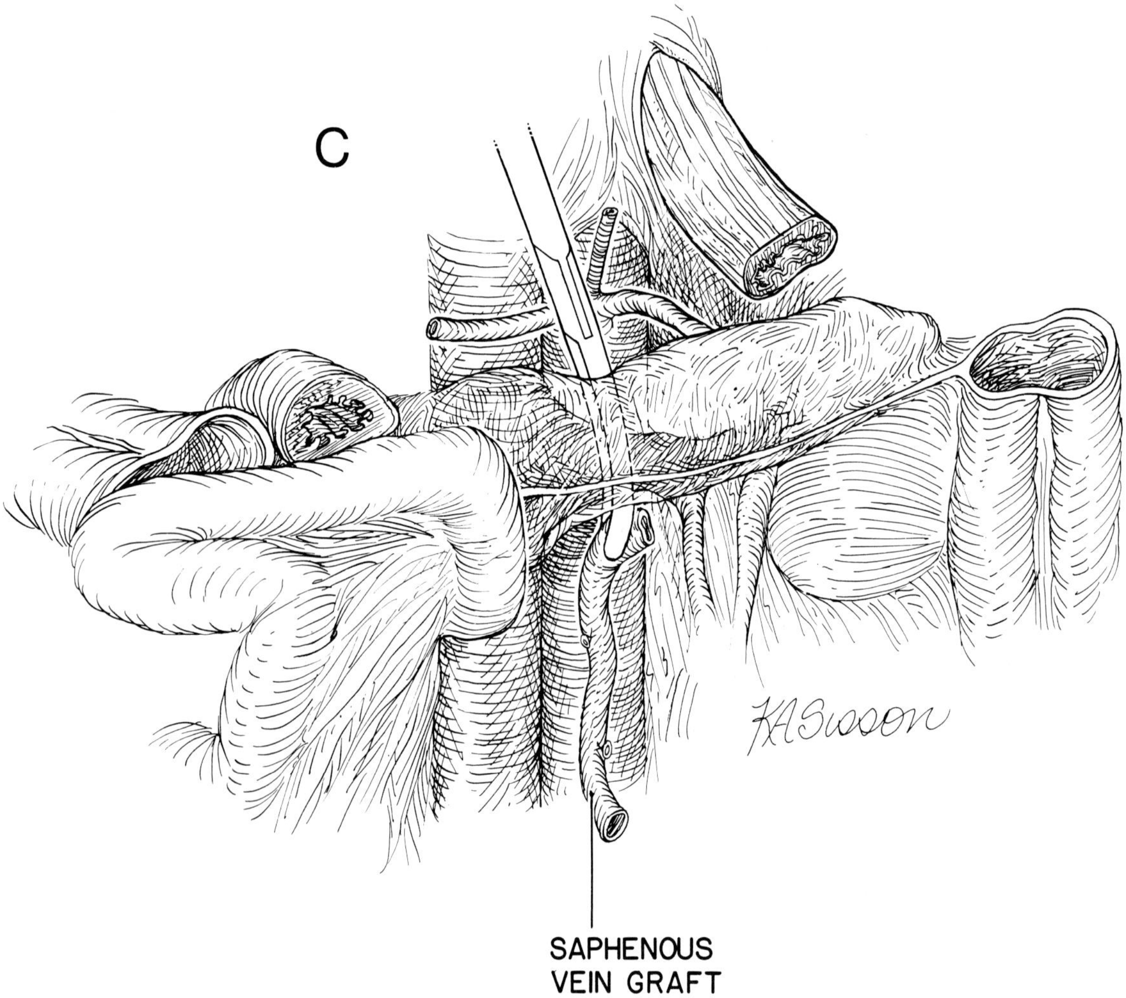

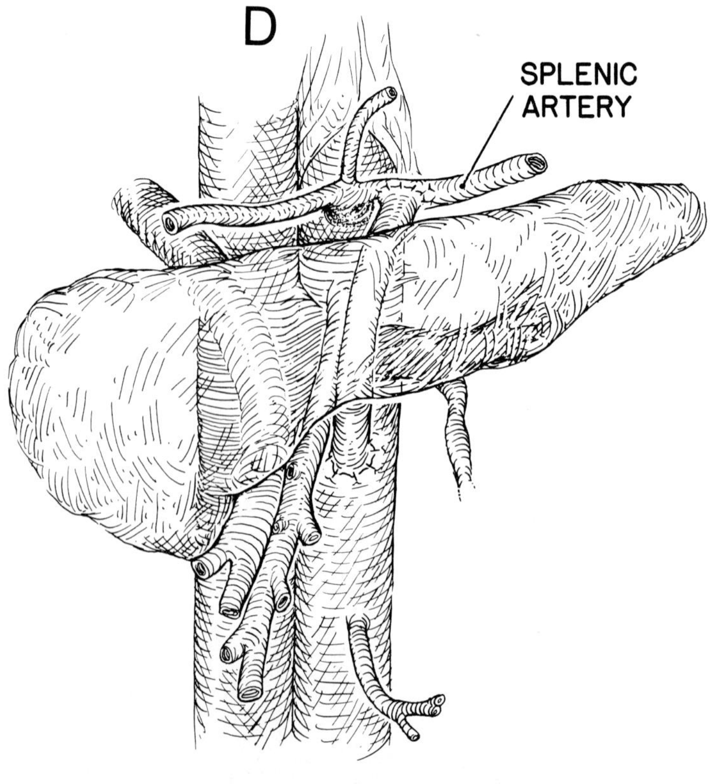

(C) Saphenous vein is the graft material of choice in reconstructions of visceral vessels. The saphenous vein graft can be passed through the retropancreatic tunnel with the aid of a vascular clamp.
(D) Revascularization of the celiac axis territory can be accomplished by anastomosis to the splenic artery or the common hepatic artery. In either instance, assurance must be made that blood will flow across the celiac axis into the entire arterial bed.

Anastomosis to the aorta is carried out when total aortic occlusion exists above and below the selected area. Anastomosis to the splenic artery or common hepatic artery is done with 6–0 prolene, with proximal and distal control and an end-of-graft to side-of-recipient vessel approximation.

Exposure of the superior mesenteric artery is achieved by freeing this vessel from the root of the mesentery and the extensive surrounding network of sympathetic nerve fibers. The proximal portion of the artery is avoided, even though this is the site of the occlusion. Primary branches supplying the jejunum are controlled and preserved. An area of the superior mesenteric artery proximal to major branchings is selected because at this point the artery is of maximum size. Once control is obtained, the artery may be opened in linear fashion and a vein graft anastomosed to the vessel in an end-to-side fashion using 6–0 prolene suture.

The aortic anastomosis is made in a manner similar to that described in anastomosis of the celiac artery graft; that is, the anterior surface of the aorta is incised after proximal and distal clamping, a button of aorta is excised if the aortic wall is stiff, and the anastomosis effected with a continuous suture of 6–0 prolene. The graft is laid in place so that there will be no kinking once the mesentery is returned to its proper location. This precaution is of major importance.

Although successful mesenteric revascularization can be done by correcting one of the two lesions present, it is best to place two grafts to correct celiac artery occlusion and superior mesenteric artery insufficiency if both of these vessels are involved. The reason for this is that mesenteric artery reconstructive surgery is difficult, and one of the grafts may occlude in the remote postoperative period. The second graft can serve as the supplier of the entire visceral circulation, so that the operation can be a physiologic success even if hemodynamic failure occurs in one of the grafts.

Postoperative angiography is essential for assessment of the reconstruction. It is only through such angiography that the surgeon can ascertain the results of the surgical technique.

REFERENCES

1. Bergan JJ, Yao JST: Acute intestinal ischemia, in Rutherford RB (ed): Vascular Surgery. Philadelphia, WB Saunders Co, 1977, p 825
2. Bergan JJ: Chronic intestinal ischemia, in Rutherford RB (ed): Vascular Surgery. Philadelphia, WB Saunders Co, 1977, p 843
3. Bergan JJ, Yao JST: Visceral ischemic syndromes: Obstruction of the superior mesenteric artery, celiac axis, and inferior mesenteric artery, in Sabiston DC Jr (ed): Davis-Christopher Textbook of Surgery. Philadelphia, WB Saunders Co, 1977, p 1987
4. Stoney RJ, Ehrenfeld WK, Wylie EJ: Revascularization methods in chronic visceral ischemia caused by atherosclerosis. Ann Surg 186:468, 1977
5. Stoney RJ, Olcott C IV: Visceral artery syndromes and reconstructions. Surg Clin North Am 59:637, 1979
6. van Dongen RJAM: Photographic Atlas of Reconstructive Arterial Surgery. New York, Springer-Verlag, 1979, p 292
7. Cooley DA, Wukasch DC: Techniques in Vascular Surgery. Philadelphia, WB Saunders Co, 1979, p 113
8. Hershey FB, Calman CH: Atlas of Vascular Surgery, ed 3. St. Louis, CV Mosby Co, 1973, p 273

SURGERY OF THE UPPER EXTREMITY

Transaxillary Extrapleural Thoracic Sympathectomy

David B. Roos

The transaxillary *extrapleural* thoracic sympathectomy offers advantages over the older sympathectomy techniques by avoiding "keyhole" exposure of the sympathetic chain, open thoracotomy requiring chest-tube drainage, and a painful postoperative incision. Exposure of the thoracic sympathetic chain is achieved by performing the standard first-rib resection described in the previous chapter. After completing that operation, the surgeon then peels the parietal pleura off the mediastinum, using a slow, sweeping motion of the fingertips while applying pressure with the palm to collapse the apex of the lung. After the pleura has been stripped off the mediastinum to the level of the fourth rib and veterbra, the sympathetic chain is easily felt as it passes vertically along the vertebral bodies and over the head or neck of each rib. The stellate ganglion is readily located by palpation between the subclavian artery and the T-1 root of the brachial plexus on the neck of the first rib that has just been resected. Using long thoracic scissors, the stellate ganglion and lower rami communicantes are carefully dissected from investing areolar tissue, and the chain is exposed down to the level of the third rib and vertebra. A careful search is made for the nerve of Kuntz, the intrathoracic nerve of variable size and location that passes from the second intercostal nerve to the first vertebral nerve (T-1 root) above, but about two centimeters *lateral* to the sympathetic chain. For complete sympathetic denervation of the upper extremity, Kuntz recommended that his somatic nerve be divided or resected in addition to the sympathetic chain because it contains sympathetic nerve fibers passing from the spinal cord through the second intercostal nerve, then up to the first vertebral nerve which forms the lower trunk of the brachial plexus, thus bypassing the sympathetic chain. Because all the ascending axones of the sympathetic nerves eventually supplying the upper extremity pass through the second thoracic ganglion, it is important to resect that ganglion but unnecessary to resect the first or third thoracic ganglion if the postganglionic gray fibers from the stellate ganglion to the brachial plexus are divided. The preganglionic white rami, which pass from the spinal cord to the sympathetic chain medial to the chain, will be resected at the level of T-2 when the second ganglion is removed, but the white rami medial to the stellate ganglion should be undisturbed to prevent Horner's syndrome. To prevent development of Horner's syndrome, the large stellate ganglion itself should not be held with forceps, elevated, or disturbed in any way.

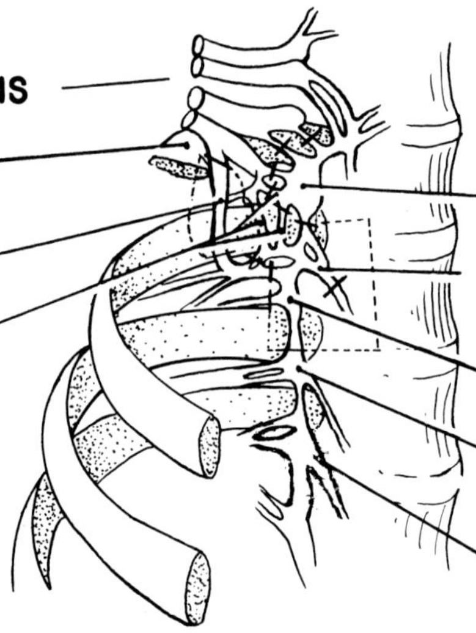

Therefore, I believe the optimal surgical sympathectomy for the upper extremity may be achieved by dividing the sympathetic chain immediately below the stellate ganglion and just above the T-3 ganglion, removing this small part of the chain containing the T-2 ganglion, and then dividing or resecting Kuntz's nerve lateral to the chain as well as the gray rami that pass from the stellate ganglion to the brachial plexus. This "selective sympathectomy" for the upper extremity is outlined in dotted lines in the accompanying sketch.

Occasionally, a small aberrant branch of the subclavian artery may pass posteriorly directly across the stellate ganglion and impair exposure. If present, this vessel should be clipped and divided to achieve maximal exposure of the sympathetic chain. I believe, however, clips should *never* be applied to the sympathetic chain, ganglia, or rami themselves, as they never bleed or "regrow." Clips should be applied to vessels only, and not to live nerve tissue. By avoiding crushing clips on the remaining sympathetic tissue, postsympathectomy pain may be short-lived or avoided altogether. Since I stopped using crushing clips on live sympathetic nerve tissue 18 years ago, I have had no cases of postsympathectomy neuralgia and no complications caused by avoiding the clips.

After completing the resection of the second thoracic ganglion, Kuntz's nerve, and appropriate gray rami, hemostasis is obtained by sponge pressure or clips applied to small vessels. The wound is irrigated with sterile saline during lung inflation to check the pleura. The indications for chest tube and the overall closure after the sympathectomy are identical to that described for the standard first rib resection. Because the transaxillary extrapleural technique for thoracic sympathectomy avoids entering any body cavity, surgical trauma is relatively slight and postoperative pain is usually mild. Therefore, this procedure may be performed bilaterally during the same anesthesia, if indicated.

BIBLIOGRAPHY

1. Atkins HJB: Sympathectomy by the axillary approach. Lancet 1:538, 1954
2. Goetz RH, Marr JAS: The importance of the second thoracic ganglion for the sympathetic supply of the upper extremity with a description of two new approaches for its removal. Clin Proc 3:102, 1944
3. Goetz RH: Sympathectomy for the upper extremities, in Dale WA (ed): Management of arterial occlusive disease. Chicago, Year Book Publishers, 1971
4. Kuntz A: Distribution of the sympathetic rami to the brachial plexus: Its relation to sympathectomy affecting the upper extremity. Arch Surg 15:871, 1927
5. Palumbo LT: Upper dorsal sympathectomy without Horner's syndrome. Arch Surg 71:743, 1955
6. Pick J: The autonomic nervous system. Philadelphia-Toronto, JB Lippincott Co, 1970
7. Roos DB: Transaxillary extrapleural thoracic sympathectomy. Surg Techniques Illus 2:3, 1971
8. Roos DB: Sympathectomy for the upper extremities: Anatomy, indications, and techniques, in Rutherford R (ed): Vascular Surgery. Philadelphia, WB Saunders Co, 1977

Bypass Grafting for Upper Extremity Ischemia

James S.T. Yao, William R. Flinn,
Charles S. O'Mara, John J. Bergan

Unlike arterial occlusive disease of the lower extremity, ischemia due to atherosclerotic disease of the upper extremity is seen infrequently.[1,2] Causes for chronic upper-extremity ischemia also differ from those of lower-extremity ischemia. Trauma, iatrogenic catheter injury,[3,4] and penetrating[5] or blunt force[6,7] are important causes of upper-extremity ischemia. Aneurysms with thrombus formation, distal embolization,[8] arteritis,[9] radiation injury, fibromuscular dysplasia,[3] or drug abuse[10] can also cause this problem. Brachial artery occlusion due to unrecognized emboli or late manifestation of embolic events also may be a cause of upper-extremity ischemia. Clinical presentation of upper-limb ischemia includes exercise pain in forearm muscles and tissue loss or gangrene of the digits.

Revascularization of the upper extremity may be achieved by vein patch with thrombectomy and/or endarterectomy, especially when iatrogenic injury is present. In treating chronic severe ischemia, a bypass graft is often necessary. This is especially true when extensive occlusive process or multiple occlusions exist. Garrett et al[1] were the first to report use of an autogenous vein bypass graft for upper-extremity ischemia. Subsequently, others have reported good results with bypass grafting.[3,11]

Arteriography is necessary to allow the extent of the bypass procedure to be planned. Depending on the extent of the angiographic evidence of thrombosis, bypass grafting usually consists of axillary-to-distal-brachial or brachial-to-ulnar, radial or interosseus artery reconstructions, at either the elbow or wrist level. Exposure of the distal subclavian artery to ensure adequate inflow is sometimes necessary if an extended thrombotic process is seen in the entire segment of the axillary artery. In this circumstance, the distal subclavian artery can be exposed as described in the chapter "Carotid-Subclavian Bypass" by Flanigan and Yao.

SURGICAL PROCEDURE

The patient is placed in a supine position with the hand and upper arm positioned at 90 degrees abduction and resting on an arm board. The arm must be draped free in sterile fashion using a stockinette, so that an incision on the inner aspect of the upper arm can be made easily if necessary. This position allows palpation of distal pulses (radial, ulnar, brachial) to ascertain the success of the operation.

Exposure of the Axillary Artery

An horizontal incision is made approximately 6 to 8 cm in length about 2 fingerbreadths below the clavicle (Fig. 1A). This is similar to exposure of the axillary artery for axillary-femoral bypass (see chapter "Axillary-Bifemoral Bypass Graft" by Rutherford). The pectoralis major muscle fibers between the clavicular and sternocostal heads are split horizontally parallel to the skin incision. After division of the pectoralis minor close to its insertion, the axillary artery is easily exposed. Great care must be taken to avoid injury to the surrounding structures, such as the axillary vein, which lies inferiorly, and the lateral cord of the brachial plexus, which is located above the artery. Exposure of the axillary artery may be facilitated by dividing the pectoralis nerve (Fig. 1B); this procedure causes no motor loss. The lateral thoracic artery (Fig. 1B) must be identified and looped with a silastic tape for control of bleeding during the arteriotomy. After exposure of the axillary artery proximally and distally for about 4 cm, the artery is ready for the bypass procedure.

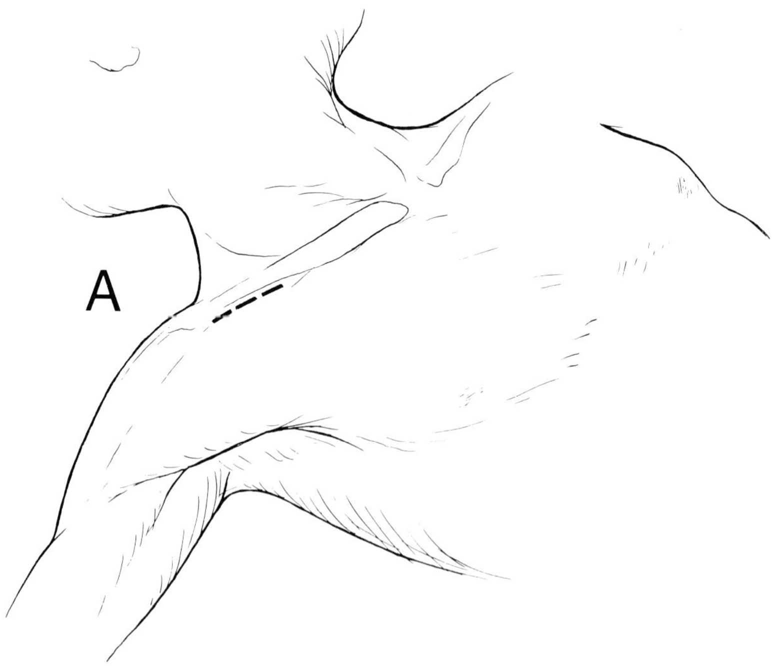

Fig. 1. (A) Skin incision for axillary-to-brachial, ulnar, radial artery bypass.
(B) Exposure of the axillary artery is greatly facilitated by dividing the pectoris minor muscle at the insertion.

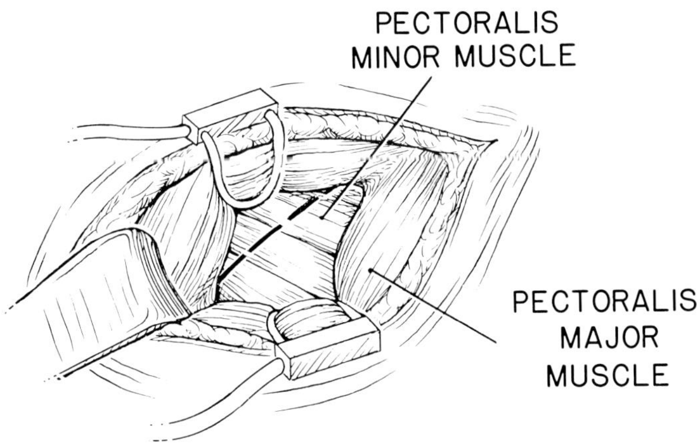
PECTORALIS
MINOR MUSCLE
PECTORALIS
MAJOR
MUSCLE

B

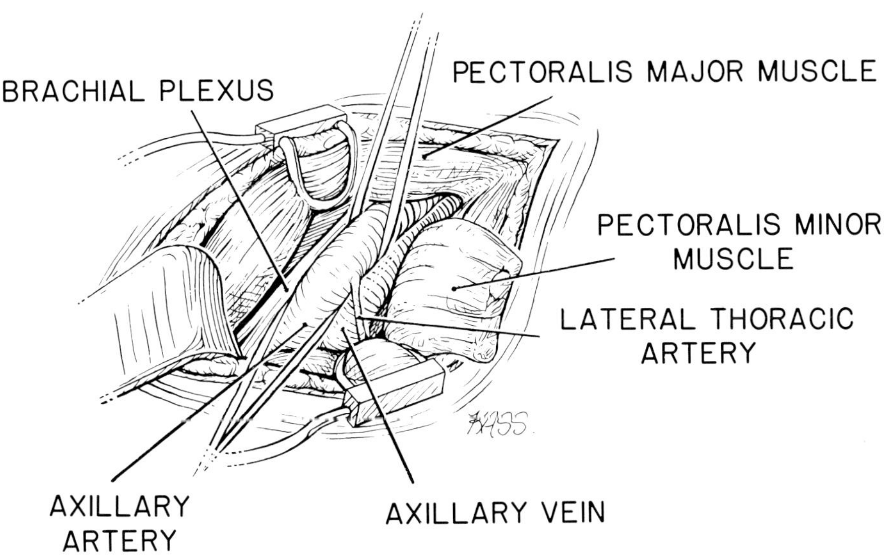
BRACHIAL PLEXUS
PECTORALIS MAJOR MUSCLE
PECTORALIS MINOR
MUSCLE
LATERAL THORACIC
ARTERY
AXILLARY
ARTERY
AXILLARY VEIN

Exposure of the Brachial Artery

The arm is placed in abduction with the forearm and hand in supination. An incision of 6 to 8 cm is made medially along the posterior border of the biceps muscle (Fig. 2A). After medial and lateral retraction of muscle, the brachial artery is identifiable. The sheath of the neurovascular bundle is then entered through an avascular area. The artery is normally surrounded by the median nerve and medial cutaneous nerve of the forearm (Fig. 2B). A 4-cm segment of brachial artery is exposed, which can be used either to accept a vein graft from the axillary artery or as the proximal supply of a brachial-to-radial or brachial-to-ulnar bypass.

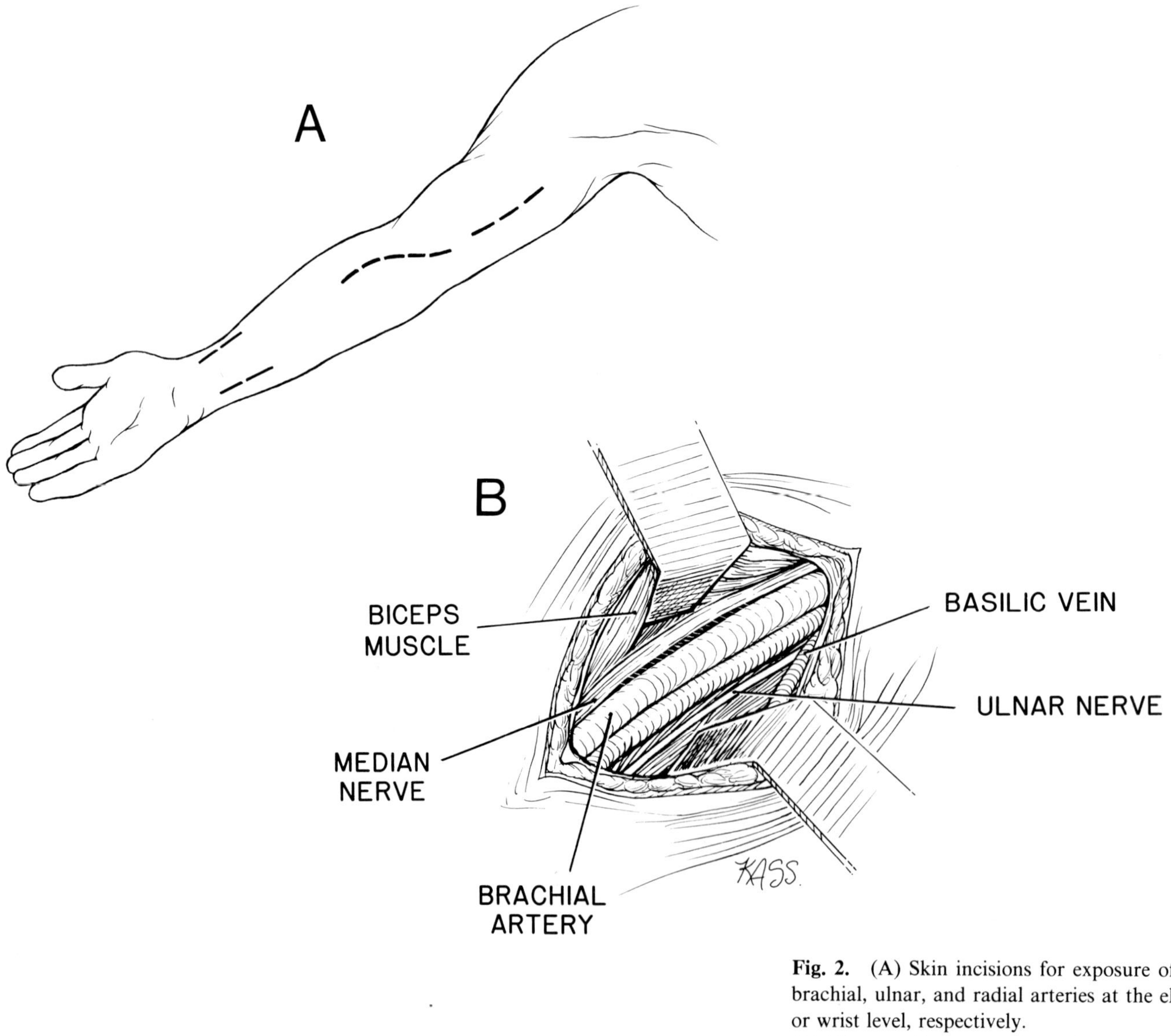

Fig. 2. (A) Skin incisions for exposure of the brachial, ulnar, and radial arteries at the elbow or wrist level, respectively.
(B) The brachial artery is readily identifiable after the sheath of the neurovascular bundle is entered.

Exposure of the Radial, Ulnar, or Interosseous Artery

Depending on the nature of the occlusion, the radial or ulnar artery can be exposed and used for bypass at either the elbow or the wrist. At the elbow, the radial or ulnar artery is exposed simply by extending the incision across the elbow joint as depicted in Figure 2B. The lacertus fibrosus (bicipital aponeurosis) of the biceps muscle can be retracted laterally to facilitate the exposure of these two major branches. If necessary, the bicipital aponeurosis may be divided. The brachial vein is seen between the artery and the medial nerve. The recurrent radial artery, a small branch, may be seen (Fig. 3) and must be identified for control of back-bleeding. Either the ulnar or radial artery may be used as the recipient for the bypass. If both ulnar and radial arteries are occluded, the interosseous artery may be used. The interosseous artery can be identified as a branch arising from the ulnar artery under the interosseous membrane. If distal bypass is necessary at the wrist level, either the ulnar (Fig. 4) or the radial artery may be exposed by a short (4-cm) longitudinal incision over the wrist (Fig. 5).

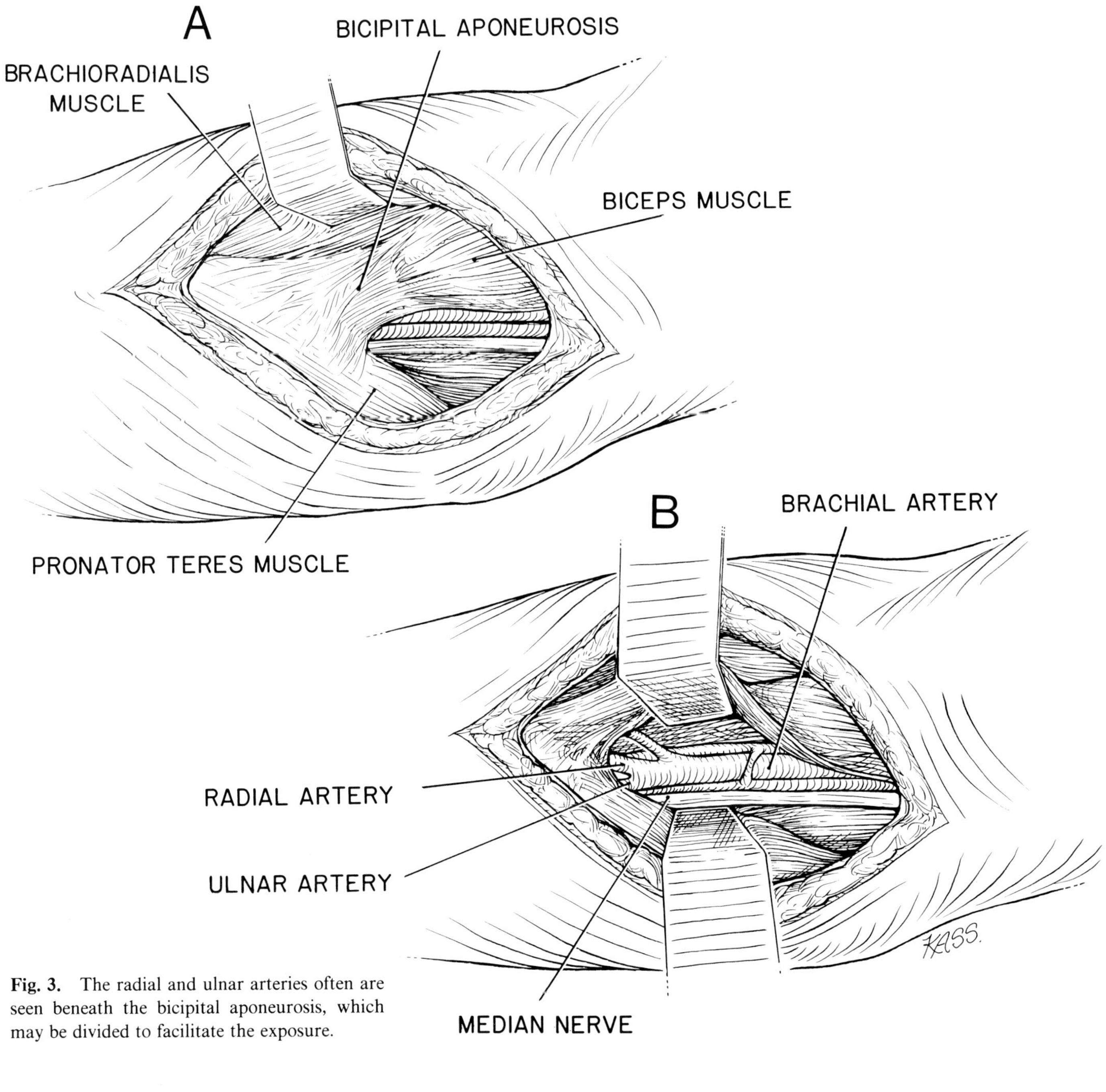

Fig. 3. The radial and ulnar arteries often are seen beneath the bicipital aponeurosis, which may be divided to facilitate the exposure.

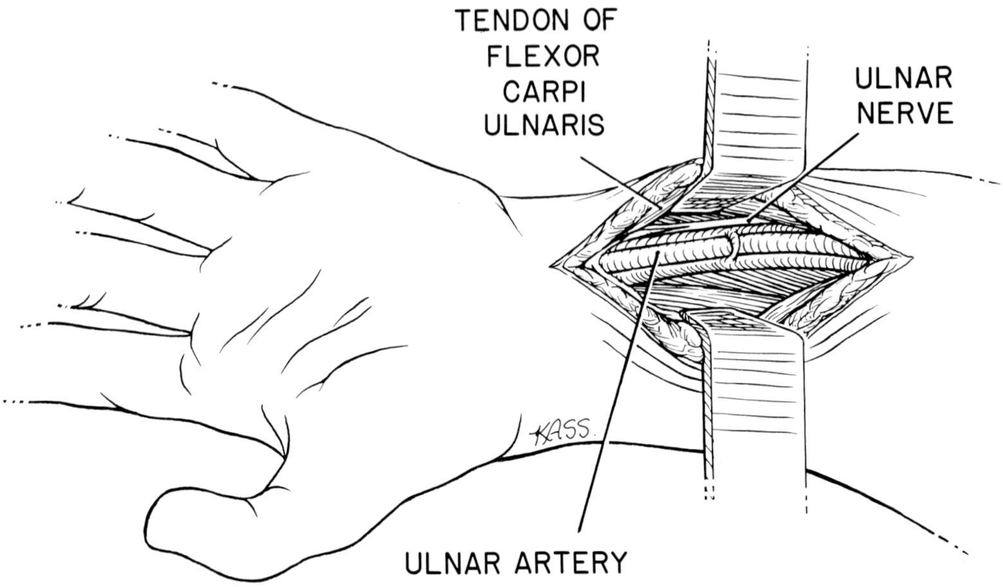

Fig. 4. Exposure of the ulnar artery.

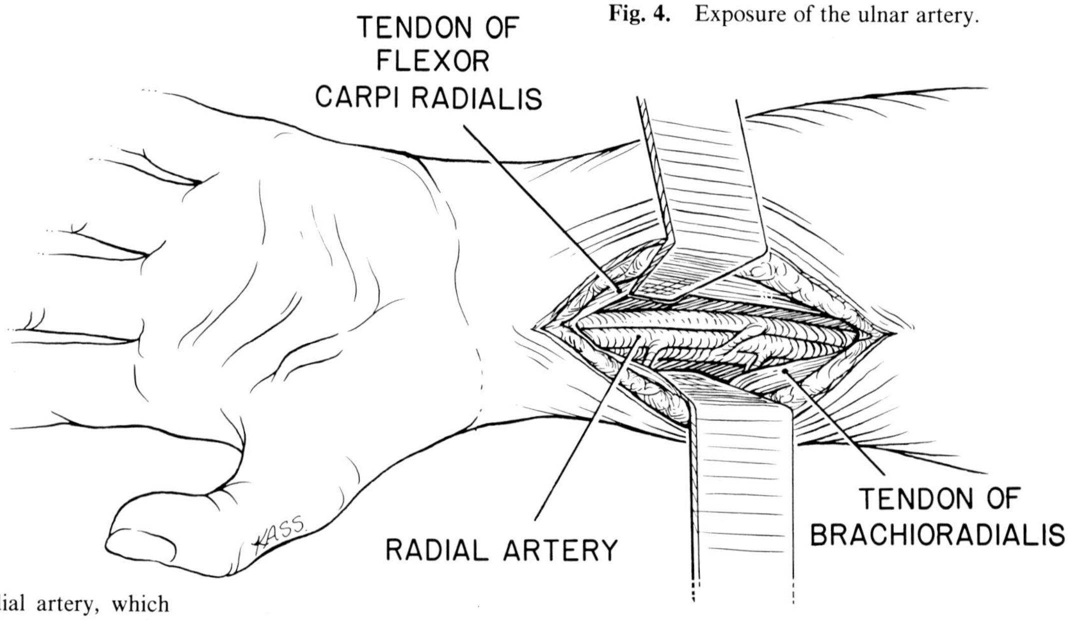

Fig. 5. Exposure of the radial artery, which lies between the brachioradialis tendon and the flexor carpi radialis tendon.

Bypass procedures in the upper extremity are normally done with autogenous vein harvested from the lower limb. If saphenous vein is not available, the cephalic vein from the contralateral arm may be used as a substitute. Expanded polytetrafluoroethylene (PTFE) is used only when the autogenous veins are not available. Tunneling of the bypass graft is made to follow the normal pathway of the artery. The bypass graft is seldom placed subcutaneously. The graft is sutured end-to-side using 6–0 prolene sutures.

REFERENCES

1. Garrett HE, Morris GC, Howell JF, et al: Revascularization of upper extremity with autogenous vein bypass graft. Arch Surg 91:751, 1965
2. Laroche GP, Bernatz PE, Joyce JW, et al: Chronic arterial insufficiency of the upper extremity. Mayo Clin Proc 51:180, 1976
3. Wood PB: Vein graft bypass in axillary and brachial artery occlusion causing claudication. Br J Surg 60:29, 1973
4. Machleder HI, Sweeney JP, Barker WF: Pulseless arm after brachial artery catheterization. Lancet 1:407, 1972
5. Sachatello CR, Ernst CB, Griffen WO: The acutely ischemic upper extremity: Selective management. Surgery 76:1002, 1974
6. Abbott WM, Darling RC: Axillary aneurysm secondary to crutch trauma. Am J Surg 125:515, 1973

7. Tullos HS, Erwin WD, Woods GW, Wukasch DC, Cooley DA, King JW: Unusual lesions of the pitching arm. Clin Orthop 88:169, 1972
8. Perry SP, Massey CW: Bilateral aneurysms of the subclavian and axillary arteries. Radiology 61:53, 1953
9. DePalma RG, Moskowitz RW, Holden WD: Peripheral ischemia and collagen disease. Arch Surg 105:313, 1972
10. Maxwell TM, Olcott C IV, Blaisdell FW: Vascular complications of drug abuse. Arch Surg 105:875, 1972
11. Gross WS, Flanigan DP, Kraft RO, Stanley JC: Chronic upper extremity arterial insufficiency: Etiology, manifestations and operative management. Arch Surg 113:419, 1978

Transaxillary First Rib Resection for Thoracic Outlet Syndrome

David B. Roos

The anatomic relationships of the important structures in the thoracic outlet are shown schematically (Fig. 1) from the right axillary view. The anterior scalene muscle separates the outlet into an anterior compartment, containing the subclavian vein, and a posterior compartment, containing the subclavian artery and brachial plexus. The subclavius muscle crosses over the vein and inserts into the costal cartilage, forming the anterior boundary of the thoracic outlet. The middle scalene muscle attaches on top of the posterior third of the first rib, just behind the brachial plexus, and forms the posterior wall of the outlet. The posterior scalene muscle does not participate anatomically or physiologically in the thoracic outlet, as it inserts entirely on the second rib.

The patient is turned and supported in the straight lateral position, and the second assistant elevates the brachium from the thorax, holding the forearm in a double wrist-lock grip. This affords the most comfortable and efficient leverage for elevating the shoulder girdle intermittently to provide deep exposure in the outlet for the surgeon (Fig. 2). The assistant should avoid grasping the brachium with both hands to elevate the shoulder. This will tire him quickly, and cause postoperative arm pain for the patient. Because the arm and shoulder need to be moved at times during the operation to alter the exposure, and in order to relax periodically the tension on the neurovascular structures, I prefer manual elevation and control of the limb rather than sustained elevation by a fixed device.

The transverse incision is made over the third rib below the hairline of the axilla, between the anterior edge of the latissimus dorsi muscle and the posterior edge of the pectoralis major muscle. The incision should be placed in the axillomammary crease in women, demonstrated by depressing the shoulder and elevating the breast towards the axilla. In men, this same natural skin line is located by forcefully elevating the shoulder towards the ceiling and making the incision at the level where the skin abruptly turns upward from the lateral rib cage to cover the axilla. In women, the incision is 8 to 10 cm in length, depending on the size of the patient. In men, it is 2 to 3 cm longer than in women, because the distance from the axilla to the posterior aspect of the first rib is considerably greater in the larger male shoulder girdle.

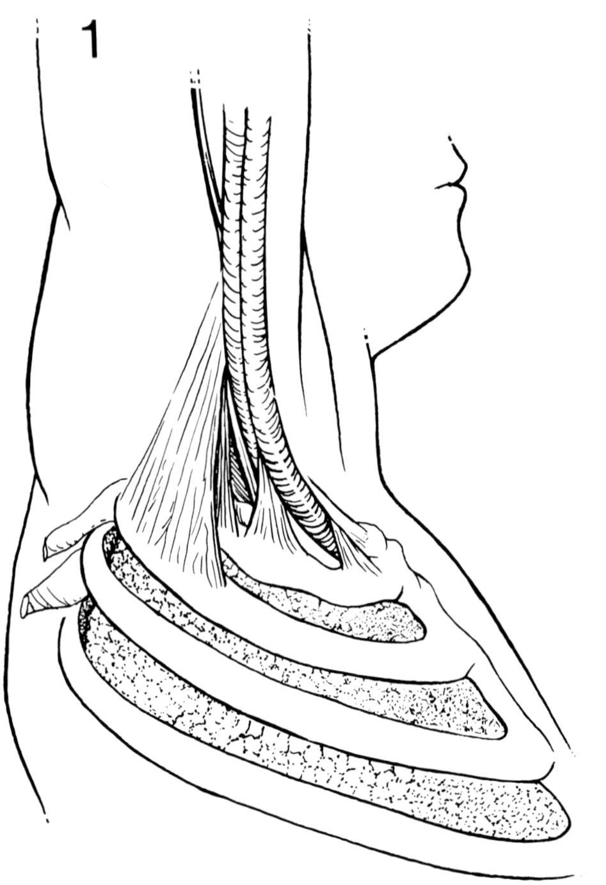

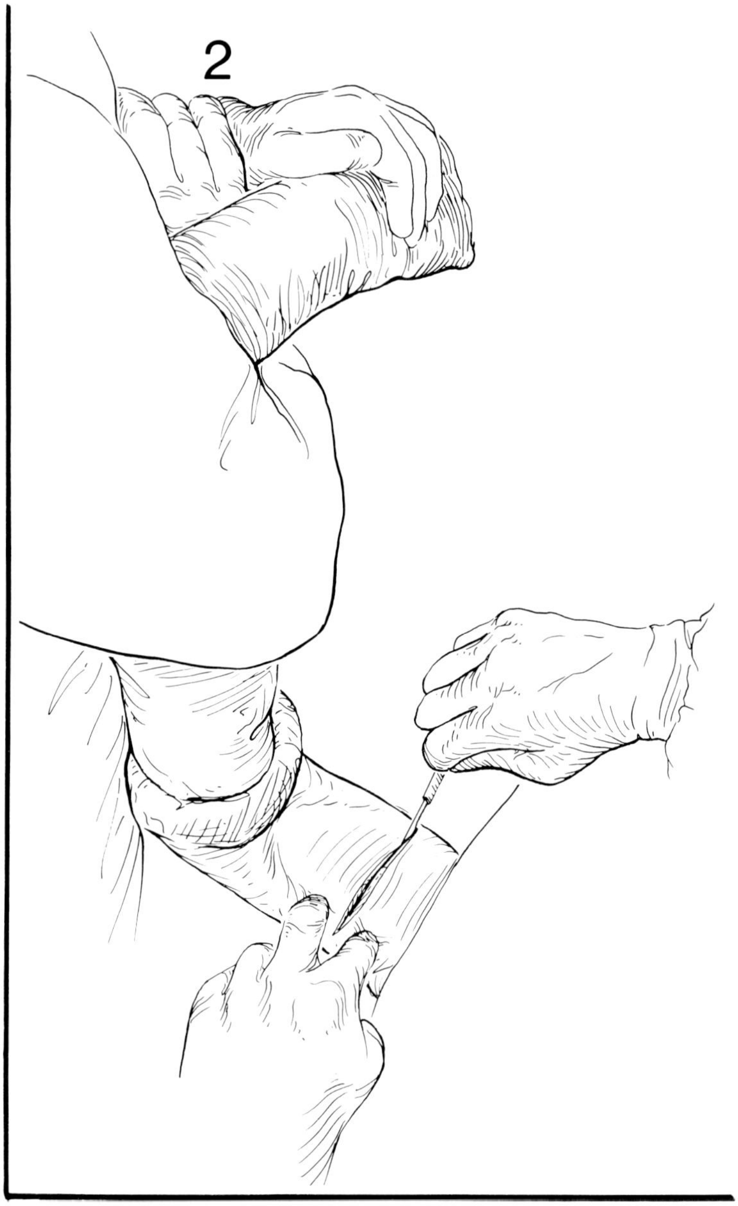

Fig. 1. Schematic representation of the anatomic relationships of the important structures in the thoracic outlet from the right axillary view.

Fig. 2. The patient is turned and supported in the straight lateral position, and the second assistant elevates the brachium from the thorax, holding the forearm in a double wrist-lock grip.

After developing the incision down to the third rib, the wound is held open by Gelpi retractors. The first structure encountered in forming the axillary tunnel is the thoracoepigastric vein in the midaxillary line below the subcutaneous fascia. It is often accompanied by the smaller lateral thoracic artery. These vessels should be clamped, divided, and tied to permit deeper development of the tunnel. The second structure encountered is the intercostobrachiocutaneous nerve, a pure sensory nerve that supplies the skin surfaces of the axilla and inner brachium. It usually leaves the chest wall as a single nerve from under the second rib in the midaxillary line and crosses the axillary tunnel vertically, but it may have multiple origins from other intercostal nerves as well. This nerve should be preserved, preferably with accompanying vein and fat, to avoid stripping it as that may cause postoperative burning pain in the axilla and inner brachium for several weeks. Even normal surgical trauma to this nerve usually causes some hypoesthesia in these areas for several months, but this gradually fades as the nerve recovers, if it is left intact.

3

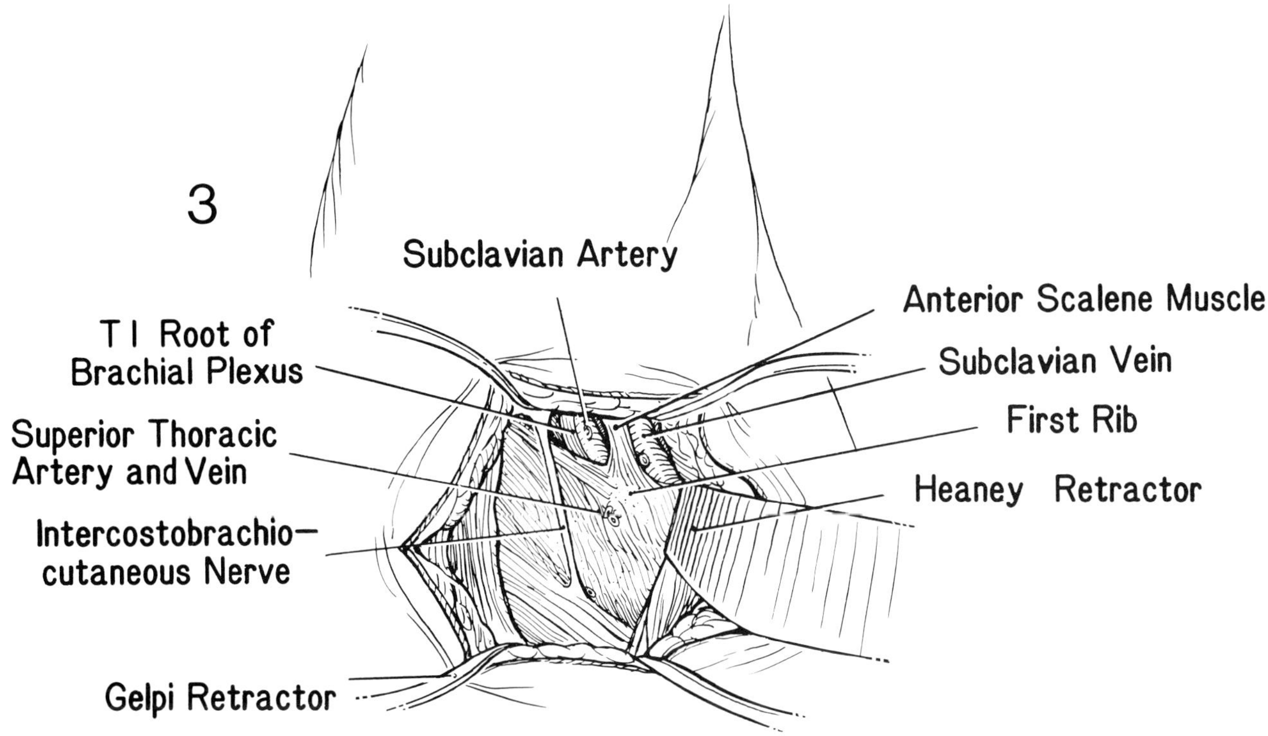

Fig. 3. The subclavian artery and vein and the brachial plexus are reflected upward from the first rib as dissection continues to expose all the major structures of the outlet.

The third set of structures encountered in developing the axillary tunnel are the superior thoracic artery and vein, which also cross the tunnel vertically as they pass from the parent axillary vessels above to the first intercostal space below. These small vessels should be anticipated, dissected free, and then clamped, divided, and tied to avoid troublesome bleeding in the tunnel before complete exposure is achieved. A right-angled Heaney retractor is used gently to draw the pectoralis major and minor muscles anteriorly to increase deep exposure.

After dividing and tying the superior thoracic artery and vein if they are present, the surgeon will encounter a cul-de-sac of fascia separating the axilla from the neck and thoracic outlet. This fascia is carefully opened by finger dissection or by spreading with long scissors, but cutting at this stage must be strictly avoided because the major neurovascular structures are on the opposite side of this fascial plane. The opening into the outlet is extended by blunt dissection anteriorly to the subclavius tendon and posteriorly to the middle scalene muscle. This maneuver will then reveal the contents of the thoracic outlet. The primary landmark is the anterior scalene muscle, which can be easily felt and freed circumferentially from other tissue by finger dissection. The subclavian artery and vein, and the brachial plexus are then carefully reflected upward from the first rib as finger dissection continues to expose all the major structures of the outlet (Fig. 3).

4

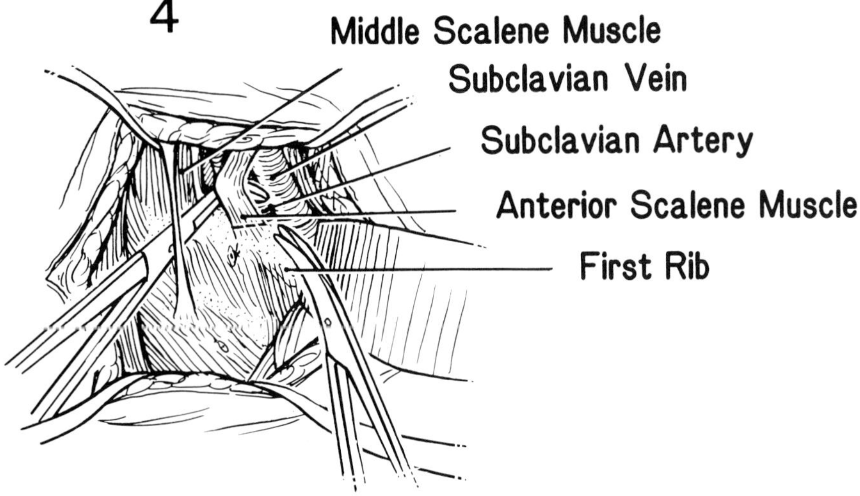

Fig. 4. The anterior scalene muscle should be separated from the artery with a right angled hemostat and pulled laterally, then divided at its attachment onto the first rib.

As the subclavian artery passes medial to the anterior scalene muscle in its course from the mediastinum to the aperture between the scalene muscles, the anterior scalene muscle should be separated from the artery with a right-angled hemostat and pulled laterally, then divided at its attachment onto the first rib (Fig. 4). This maneuver protects the artery from being cut with the anterior scalene muscle. The subclavius tendon is then carefully dissected from the investing fat just under the head of the clavicle by spreading with scissors in the direction of the tendon but not cutting until the subclavian vein is safely separated from the exposed tendon. This is one of the most hazardous parts of the operation, and if these two structures cannot be clearly separated, division of the tendon should be abandoned to avoid the risk of opening the subclavian vein in an area that affords poor proximal control.

The middle scalene muscle is then pushed off the first rib with a periosteal elevator or raspatory (Fig. 5), but the bone should not be scraped with the instrument. The periosteum of the rib should remain on the bone and be resected to avoid leaving periosteal cells behind, which may form dense scar tissue that could bind the neurovascular structures crossing the bed of the first rib into a fibrotic entrapment. I prefer the Matson raspatory for this maneuver because it has a safe, rounded end that will not injure the brachail plexus or tear the pleura as easily as other raspatories. The surgeon should guide the tip of the instrument with the fingers of the left hand for maximum control and safety. After the middle scalene muscle is completely separated from its attachment to the posterior third of the first rib, the intercostal muscle between first and second ribs is separated along with the pleura from the lateral surface and under surface of the rib, but again the surgeon should try to leave the periosteum on the bone to be resected. An extraperiosteal rib resection may increase the incidence of pneumothorax, but that minor complication is so easily treated with a chest tube at the time of closure that it is far more preferable than the potential later complications of scar tissue entrapment that may result if a subperiosteal resection is performed.

After freeing the pleura and dropping it to the level of the second rib, a hooked raspatory (Overholt No. 1) is passed under the first rib and used as a blunt knife to slice off Sibson's fascia and remnants of the scalene muscles from the inner edge of the first rib. The congenital bands usually found in patients requiring this operation can be divided with the same instrument during this maneuver.

A specially designed brachial plexus root retractor or a tonsil suction tip is then placed gently against the C-8 and T-1 roots of the plexus, as the right-angled rib shear is set as far posteriorly as possible (Fig. 6). The retractor keeps the roots from slipping into the jaws of the rib shear on the deep or "blind side" at the moment the surgeon resects the rib. A right-angled rib shear fits the desired level and angle of resection near the transverse process of the vertebra better than a straight Bethune shear. The rib must be resected as far back of the plexus as possible, about 1 to 2 cm from the transverse process, in order to avoid leaving a hooked stump of rib that may rub against the plexus or catch the roots in scar tissue from the periosteum at the line of resection. The rib is then resected anteriorly with a straight or 45-degree angled rib shear as close to the costal cartilage as possible. The bone is then removed, preferably with some muscle fragments still attached on each surface to indicate resection of the periosteum with the rib. The anterior and posterior stumps remaining are palpated, then shortened to the appropriate length, and smoothed with rongeurs (Sauerbruch) so that no sharp corners or spicules remain to stab the plexus, vein, or pleura. Great care must be used when shortening the posterior stump 1 cm from the transverse process supporting it to avoid nipping or severing the T-1 root of the plexus. Again, the root retractor or a tonsil suction tip should be used on the deep "blind side" to protect the nerves from the jaws of the rongeur.

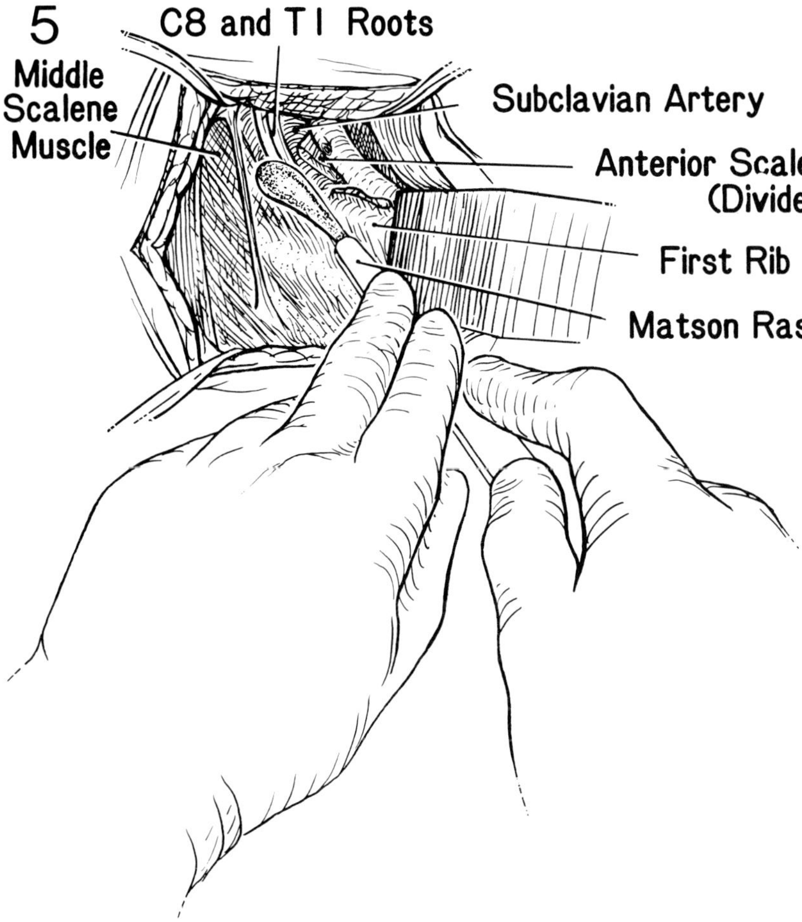

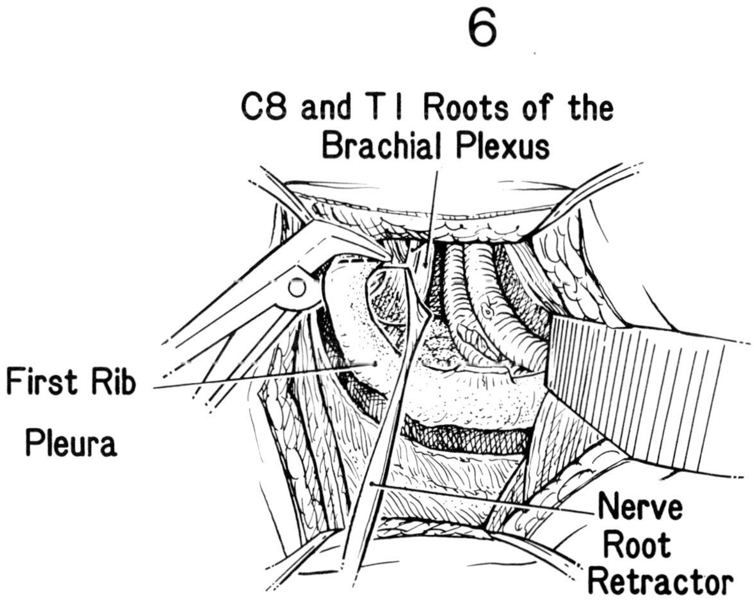

Fig. 5. The middle scalene muscle is then pushed off the first rib with a periosteal elevator or raspatory.

Fig. 6. A specially designed brachial plexus root retractor or a tonsil suction tip is then placed gently against the C-8 and T-1 roots of the plexus, as the right-angled rib shear is set as far posteriorly as possible.

After the remaining rib stumps are shortened and smoothed, a careful search is made for the various types of anomalous fibromuscular bands that are usually present in patients requiring this operation. Using long packing forceps, these bands and redundant middle scalene muscle are put on the stretch and completely resected to prevent them from reattaching to Sibson's fascia over the pleura and causing recurrent symptoms. Before closure, I shorten the anterior scalene muscle by grasping the divided end with a right-angled hemostat and forcefully stretching the muscle back down from its retracted position in the neck (Fig. 7). It is then divided as high as the surgeon can safely work between the subclavian artery and vein, being on the lookout for the phrenic nerve, which is rarely seen during this maneuver. Frequently, a prominent, taut slip of anterior scalene muscle is found to pass anteriorly under the vein and to be attached to the back of the sternum even after the rib is removed. This slip should be carefully separated from the vein with the right-angled hemostat, divided over the hemostat, and then fully resected to decompress the vein and prevent reattachment of the scalene muscle. After completion of these maneuvers, which must be performed with meticulous technique to avoid disastrous bleeding, the wound is ready for closure.

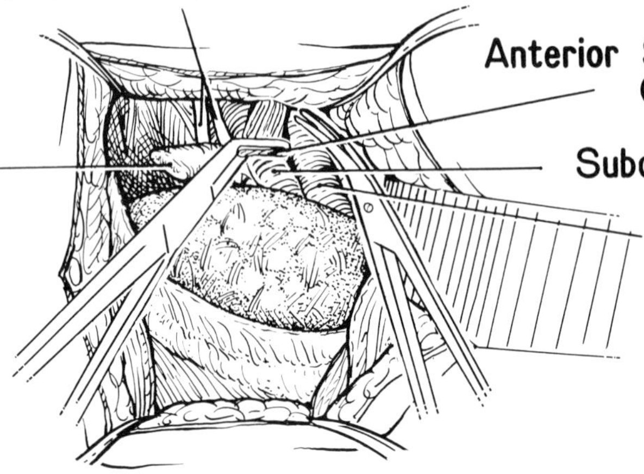

Fig. 7. The divided end of the anterior scalene muscle is grasped with a right-angled hemostat and forcefully stretched down from its retracted position in the neck, then divided as high as the surgeon can safely work.

The large cavity in the shoulder and neck region created by the operation is filled with sterile saline twice to rinse out fat, bacteria, clots, and any foreign material (ie, glove powder), as well as to check for holes in the pleura. If a stream of bubbles with expiration or a disappearing fluid level with inspiration is seen, a hole exists in the pleura and a chest tube should be inserted. I prefer placing the tube directly in the hole and bringing the tube over the second rib and out the middle of the incision rather than tunneling the tube under the second rib inside the thoracic cavity. If the hole in the pleura is obvious when the operation is completed, saline should be avoided as it will run into the thorax and cause chemical pleuritis with postoperative fever and chest pain. If there is no rent in the pleura, the wound is filled with saline to the skin level to displace the large air pocket of the shoulder girdle and to minimize postoperative subcutaneous emphysema. The shoulder is lowered, and the subcutaneous fascia of the axilla is closed with continuous absorbable suture (snugly around the chest tube if one is present). The skin is closed with continuous absorbable subcuticular suture, also snugly around the chest tube. If no chest tube is present, I prefer a plastic spray dressing, but a gauze and tape dressing is used when a chest tube has been inserted. Because there has been no injury or leak of the lung itself in these cases, the chest tube may be removed in the recovery room when the patient has good breath sounds, no longer expells bubbles in the drainage bottle, and has a fully expanded lung on portable chest film. The patient should avoid exercising, straining, and physical therapy of the arm for 6 weeks postoperatively to minimize pain, muscle spasm, and scar tissue formation.

Drawings by Sandy Marvin, some of which are after Frank Robinson in Surgical Techniques Illustrated, Vol 3, No 3, pg 4–11, summer, 1979.

BIBLIOGRAPHY

1. Rainer WG, Vigor W, Newby JP: The surgical treatment of thoracic outlet compression. Am J Surg 116:704, 1968
2. Roos DB: Experience with first rib resection for thoracic outlet syndrome. Ann Surg 173:429, 1971
3. Roos DB: Congenital anomalies associated with thoracic outlet syndrome. Am J Surg 132:771, 1976
4. Urschel HC Jr, Razuk MA: Management of thoracic outlet syndrome: Current concepts. N Engl J Med 286:1140, 1972

FEMORAL AND INFRANGENICULATE ARTERIAL BYPASS

Femoropopliteal Bypass

Henner Muller-Wiefel

Femoropopliteal arterial reconstruction has become a widely accepted procedure for revascularization of the ischemic lower extremity. However, it has retained certain specific problems and has remained a test of skill and the quality of technique of the surgeon.

The preferred material for arterial replacement in the femoropopliteal system is reversed saphenous vein. The bypass may be carried out above the knee or as an infragenicular procedure, but in the majority of cases it is necessary to place the distal anastomosis in the lower third of the popliteal artery, as this is ordinarily the last to be involved by arteriosclerosis (Fig. 1A).

The patient is placed in supine position with the thigh rotated externally and the knee flexed between 30 and 60 degrees, supported by a rolled sterile sheet. This allows the procurement of the vein graft and exposure of the femoral and popliteal arteries. In cases where it is not evident preoperatively that there will be a good vein in the diseased leg, it is advisable to prepare the contralateral extremity in case an additional saphenous vein segment is needed.

The operation starts with the dissection of the distal part of the popliteal artery in order to check local operability and runoff conditions. A skin incision about 10 to 15 cm in length is placed just below the knee joint on the medial aspect of the leg, parallel to and behind the posteromedial surface of the tibia. Care must be taken not to damage the saphenous vein in its immediate proximity to the skin in this sector.

The crural fascia is incised longitudinally and the medial head of the gastrocnemius muscle is retracted posteriorly away from the tibia. The tendon of the semitendinosus, gracilis, and semimembranosus muscles may be divided for better exposure. If necessary, attachments of the soleus muscle to the tibia are divided for a few centimeters. The popliteal artery lies lateral to the vein. It is mobilized by incision of the vascular sheath and separation of the neighboring structures. It is encircled with soft rubber tapes.

The second step is the harvesting and preparation of the vein graft. It may be procured through one or two long skin incisions from the groin down to the lower leg or by multiple short incisions. The latter is our preferred technique, since wound healing is more secure with a series of small incisions than with a single, long one (Fig. 1D). It is important to place the skin incisions directly over the course of the vein to avoid extensive undermining of the skin. The removal of the vein graft starts in the groin, where the upper end of the saphenous vein is detached from the femoral vein at their junction. For this purpose, it is advisable to choose a separate incision running medially from that one which exposes the femoral artery in the groin. The preservation of lymphatic tissue achieved by this technique reduces wound healing problems significantly. (Fig. 1B, 1C).

The saphenous vein is then mobilized by sharp and blunt digital dissection. All tributaries are carefully identified and divided between fine nonabsorbable 5–0 sutures. Ligatures on the graft side are carefully tied away from the vein wall to avoid narrowing of the lumen, which may happen when adventitia of the main trunk is caught (Fig. 1E). The optimal length of the tributary stump is 1 mm. Branches remaining too long will cause local dilatation with possible thrombus formation in the cul-de-sac (Fig. 1E). If one dissects off the majority of excess adventitia from the vein wall while it is still in situ, this will save time.

Near the knee, bifid vein trunks are usually present. Occasionally, it may be difficult to decide which of the large tributaries is the main channel. It may be necessary to trace both. When the vein is dissected through the incision that was performed in order to reach the distal part of the popliteal artery, it is mandatory to approach the vein from the deep side of the wound in order to avoid undermining of the skin. Cutaneous vascularity here is very tenuous.

The total length of the harvested grafts should always be a little longer than the actual distance between the planned anastomoses. In order to be suitable for use, the vein must be of satisfactory size and quality. It should be free of phlebosclerosis and not contain areas of fibrous thickening from old phlebitis. If such areas are present, it is better to procure a longer graft and to excise and discard the altered segments. When needed, the contralateral saphenous vein may be used as well.

Fig. 1. (A) The three incisions for exploration of the arteries when a femoropopliteal bypass has to be constructed. The distal anastomosis generally is located below the knee (1), the central one in the groin (3). The distal thigh incision (2) is used for short femoropopliteal bypasses, and is also an adjunct for creating the tissue tunnel in which the vein graft will run. The tunnel between points 1 and 2 is performed bidigitally from both sites between the two heads of the gastrocnemius muscle.
(B) I prefer two different incisions in the groin for exploration of the femoral artery and dissection of the saphenous vein to protect lymphatic tissue.
(C) The inguinal incision runs a bit laterally from the arterial pulse, so that the block of lymph nodes can be removed medially without opening lymphatic vessels.
(D) The harvesting of the greater saphenous vein can be done from multiple short or two long skin incisions over the course of the vein.
(E) Tributaries of the saphenous vein graft must be ligated with a nonabsorbable suture leaving a stump 1 mm in length. Technical mistakes include too-long stumps forming a cul-de-sac, ligations too near the main stem catching adventitial tissue and narrowing the trunk, and finally, too much traction resulting in tearing of the vein graft.

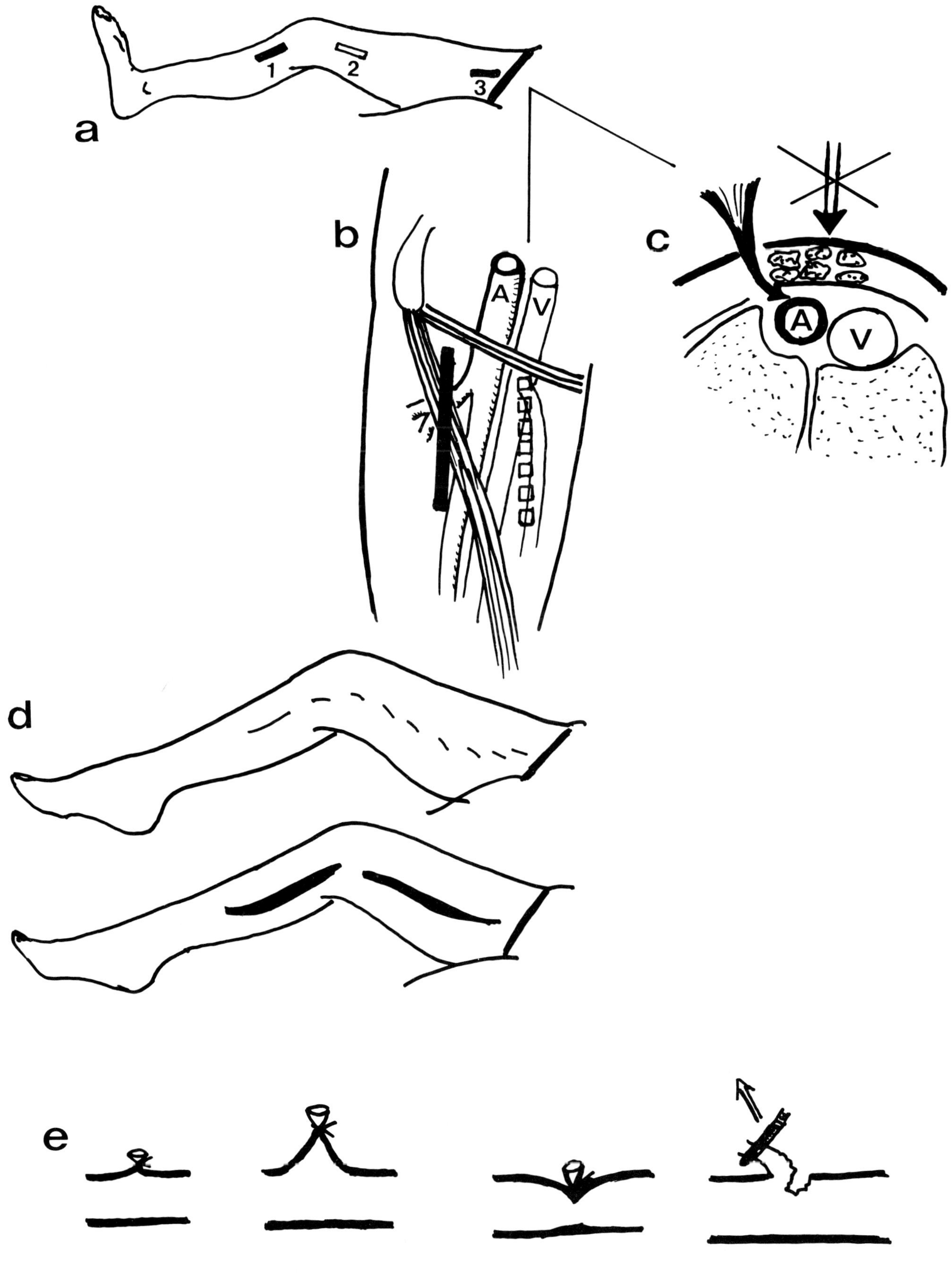
a
1
2
3
b
A
V
c
A
V
d
e

The vein should have an external diameter of at least 4 mm when gently dilated, in order to tolerate the inevitable wall hypertrophy, which will happen when the vein is subjected to arterial pressure. The ideal caliber is between 5 and 6 mm. Grafts with a diameter larger than 7 mm relatively often dilate and show a greater incidence of thrombosis.

When the vein is removed from its bed in adequate length, the final preparation of the graft will follow. A ballpoint cannula is inserted at the distal end of the vein and fixed by a ligature. With the help of a syringe filled with cool, heparinized saline solution, the transplant is irrigated, and residual liquid blood and clots are expelled. After that, a bulldog clamp is placed at the upper end of the transplant, and the vein is then gently distended by filling it with iced, heparinized saline solution (5,000 U/200ml). During the process of harvesting, the venous graft always goes into a state of vasoconstriction, so that it frequently looks too narrow for a good bypass. Gentle hydraulic pressure, however, will reestablish the normal size. Overdistension must be avoided (Fig. 2A).

During this procedure, it is usual to find additional tributaries that have been divided but not yet ligated. It is advantageous to perform this dilatation in segments, using a second soft clamp or the assistant's thumb. Each tributary is ligated as it is discovered. If a tributary has been divided so close to the main trunk that it cannot be ligated, it must be secured with a fine mattress suture of 6–0 or 7–0 prolene.

Major adventitial tissue left on the vein is pulled off with a fine thumb forceps. Constricting bands, usually at the site of improperly placed ligatures, should be eliminated. A fine pair of scissors may be helpful (Fig. 2B). Underwater distension of the vein allows passage of the tip of one blade of the scissors under the narrowing adventitia. Care must be taken not to damage the thin wall of the graft.

Occasionally, an aneurysm or localized weakness of the vein wall is encountered. Such an area should be closed with a running, everting, mattress suture (Fig. 2C). Magnifying lenses may be helpful at this stage.

The vein graft should be handled with extreme care during all procedures. Strong arterial clamps are to be avoided because of potential intimal damage. The ends of the graft may be clamped if they are cut away later. When the preparation is finished, the vein should be placed in a basin containing cool heparinized saline solution so that it will not dry out. The cannula can be left in place to indicate the former distal end of the graft.

The third step of the bypass procedure is the implantation of the reversed graft. We recommend construction of the distal anastomosis first, which will usually be to the distal third of the popliteal artery. Prior to performing any anastomoses, systemic heparin is administered in a dose of approximately 100 U/kg. We also use local heparinized saline solution in the distal arterial bed every 20 to 30 minutes during the operation.

The calf incision is kept open by a self-retaining retractor, and the gastrocnemius head is retracted by the assistant. A longitudinal arteriotomy is made medially in the popliteal artery, the length of which is at least twice, better three times, the diameter of the artery. The artery is opened initially over a length of 3 mm by a stab incision with a small-bladed sharp knife (Fig. 2D). Enlargement of the arteriotomy is done with a fine pair of angled scissors. Bleeding can be controlled with very soft, atraumatic vascular clamps or, better, stretched rubber tapes. It is very important not to injure the intima of the popliteal artery or to mobilize plaque.

The arteriotomy is spread open with a vascular forceps, and the arterial lumen is controlled. A small arteriosclerotic plaque on the posterior wall is left undisturbed. The surgeon must ensure that the runoff is adequate. If there is a relevant stenotic area some centimeters distally, the arteriotomy must be enlarged to this level and a circumscribed endarterectomy considered. One must pay careful attention so that there will not be a major intimal step which might be dissected by the bloodstream.

Fig. 2. (A) The harvested vein is filled up with heparinized saline solution and distended moderately to detect leaks as well as to control caliber adequacy.
(B) Constricting adventitial tissue bands may be divided with a pair of scissors.
(C) Circumscribed dilatations can be corrected by a continued mattress suture.
(D) The longitudinal arteriotomy is best performed with a small stab knife.
(E) Preparation of the end of the vein graft to be anastomosed with the artery. The graft is split longitudinally and trimmed by cutting off the edges.
(F) The anastomosis starts with a double-armed prolene suture at the inner corner. Both suture lines run over the circumference and meet at the middle.

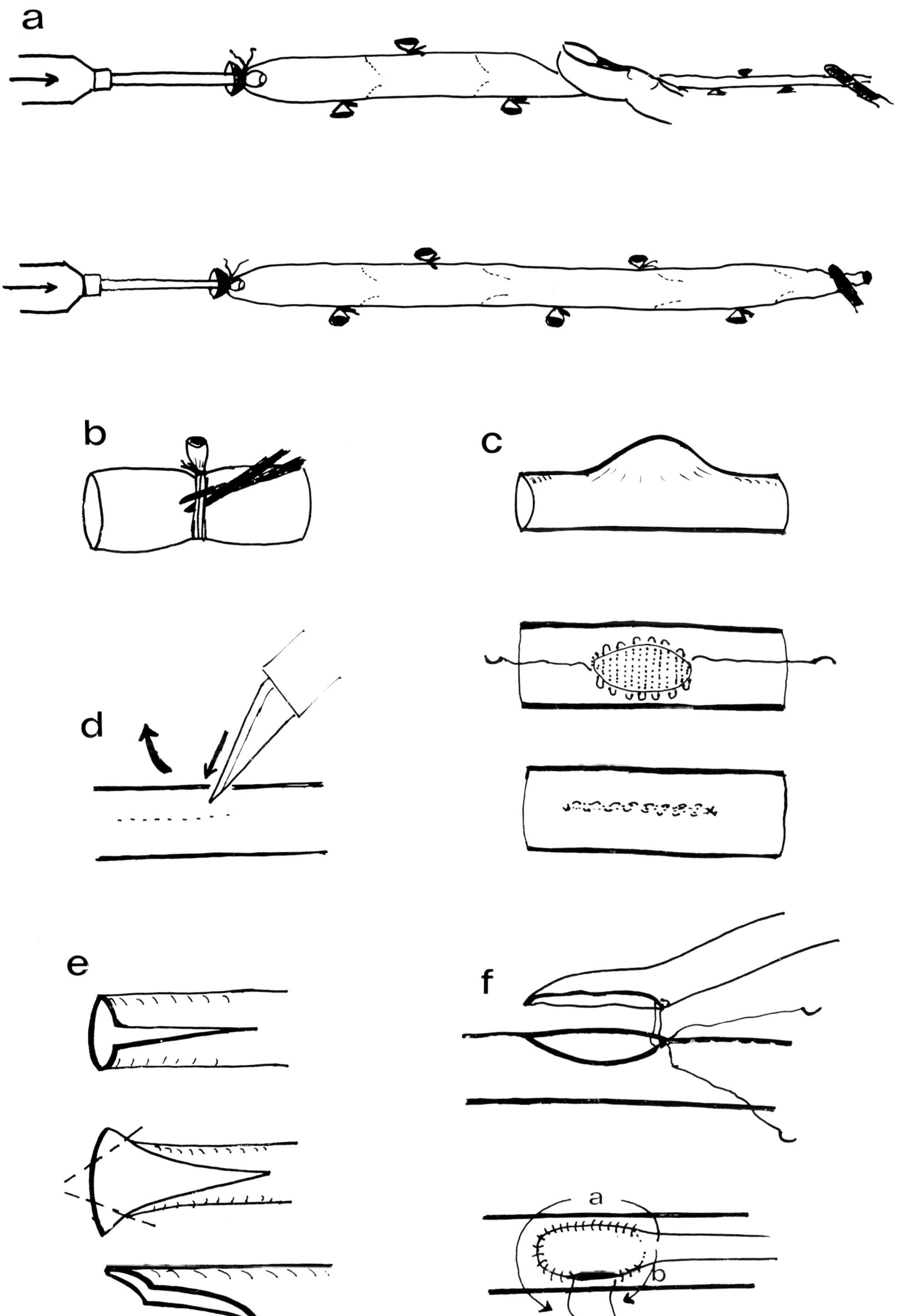
a
b
c
d
e
f
a
b
A
B

The venous graft now is removed from the heparinized saline bath, and its former proximal end is trimmed by resecting 1 cm. The vein wall is split longitudinally for a distance corresponding to the length of the popliteal arteriotomy. Small sections of the corners of the graft cuff are removed. It is important to leave a small transverse section at the tip of the graft tongue and not make the cut very pointed, to facilitate a more perfect anastomosis (Fig. 2E).

Additionally, it is advantageous to keep the graft tongue a bit longer than needed. This will allow the assistant to pick it with the forceps during the suturing, and before completion of the anastomosis this altered tip can be cut away (Fig. 3A).

The suture line is then carried out with double-armed 6–0 or 7–0 prolene suture. Magnifying lenses may be helpful for complete control of the distal anastomosis and assurance that there is no significant narrowing. The suture starts at the proximal corner of the anastomosis, and the needles go from the outside of the vein graft to the inside of the vessel, while a small forceps is placed in the lumen of the vein. As these sutures are pulled through, it is important to prevent adventitial tissue from being caught in the suture, as this would kink or narrow the proximal part of the anastomosis (Fig. 3B). After the central mattress suture is completed by stitching the needles from the inside of the artery to the outside, an intima-to-intima approximation of venous graft and artery is present. The needles should pass 1 mm from the edge of the anastomosis.

The procedure is continued by everting stitches from vein to artery, running from the central edge over three quarters of the anastomotic circumference. Passing the needles from vein to artery greatly reduces the danger of separating the media or intimal plaque from the arterial wall (Fig. 2F). Before the final one-fourth of the anastomosis is completed, it is my practice to calibrate the outflow of the anastomosis with coronary artery dilators, to check the backflow from the crural vasculature, and to pass a Fogarty catheter gently distally to ensure patency of the distal arterial tree and remove any clot that might have formed. Heparinized saline solution is instilled again. Under repeated control of the artery, the remaining one-fourth of the anastomotic circumference is completed with the second free suture from the central edge so that both sutures will meet at the midpoint, where the first one stopped. Both ends are here ligated together (Fig. 2F).

After completion of the distal anastomosis, the graft is filled again with heparinized saline solution from the other end to ensure free flow and to identify major leaks that can be sutured. Clamps or controlling rubber tapes are now removed from the popliteal artery, and the anastomosis is gently packed with oxidized cellulose sponge to stop bleeding from small leaks.

The central anastomosis is normally performed to the femoral bifurcation in the groin, either as an end-to-side connection with the common femoral or as an end-to-end anastomosis with the superficial femoral artery. Exposure of the inguinal arteries is done by a longitudinal incision placed a bit lateral to the palpable pulse to preserve lymphatic tissue and prevent wound healing complications (Fig. 1B, C).

The tissue tunnel for the graft is run from the calf incision to Hunter's canal behind the knee joint and the popliteus muscle in order to let the bypass cross the popliteal space in an orthotopic manner. An additional incision at the medial part of the lower third of the thigh that opens Hunter's canal allows the bidigital nontraumatic construction. The mobile end of the vein that is still filled with heparin solution is closed with a small bulldog clamp, and a large, curved clamp is passed from Hunter's canal between both heads of the gastrocnemius muscle to the infrapopliteal incision. The graft then is extended and pulled through to the thigh incision by seizing the bulldog clamp. Meticulous control to avoid twisting or kinking is mandatory.

Fig. 3. (A) It is advantageous to cut the "tongue" of the graft a bit longer than the anastomosis itself. This allows fixation with a small forceps and facilitates the suturing. The redundant part of the vein is cut away afterwards.

(B) A typical mistake is to catch too much of the graft wall during the first suture bite. This will result in serious narrowing of the entrance into the transplant (see arrow).

(C) The origin of a tributary can be incorporated in the anastomotic line, resulting in a wider "cobra-hood" anastomosis.

(D) The vein graft runs from the distal section of the popliteal artery below the knee through a 2-finger breadth tissue tunnel between the two heads of the gastrocnemius muscle to the additional incision that opens Hunter's canal. From here the transplant runs through a subsartorial tunnel. The surgeon must be sure that this tunnel is not placed through any fibers of the belly of the muscle, since a compression syndrome may cause graft occlusion in the early postoperative period.

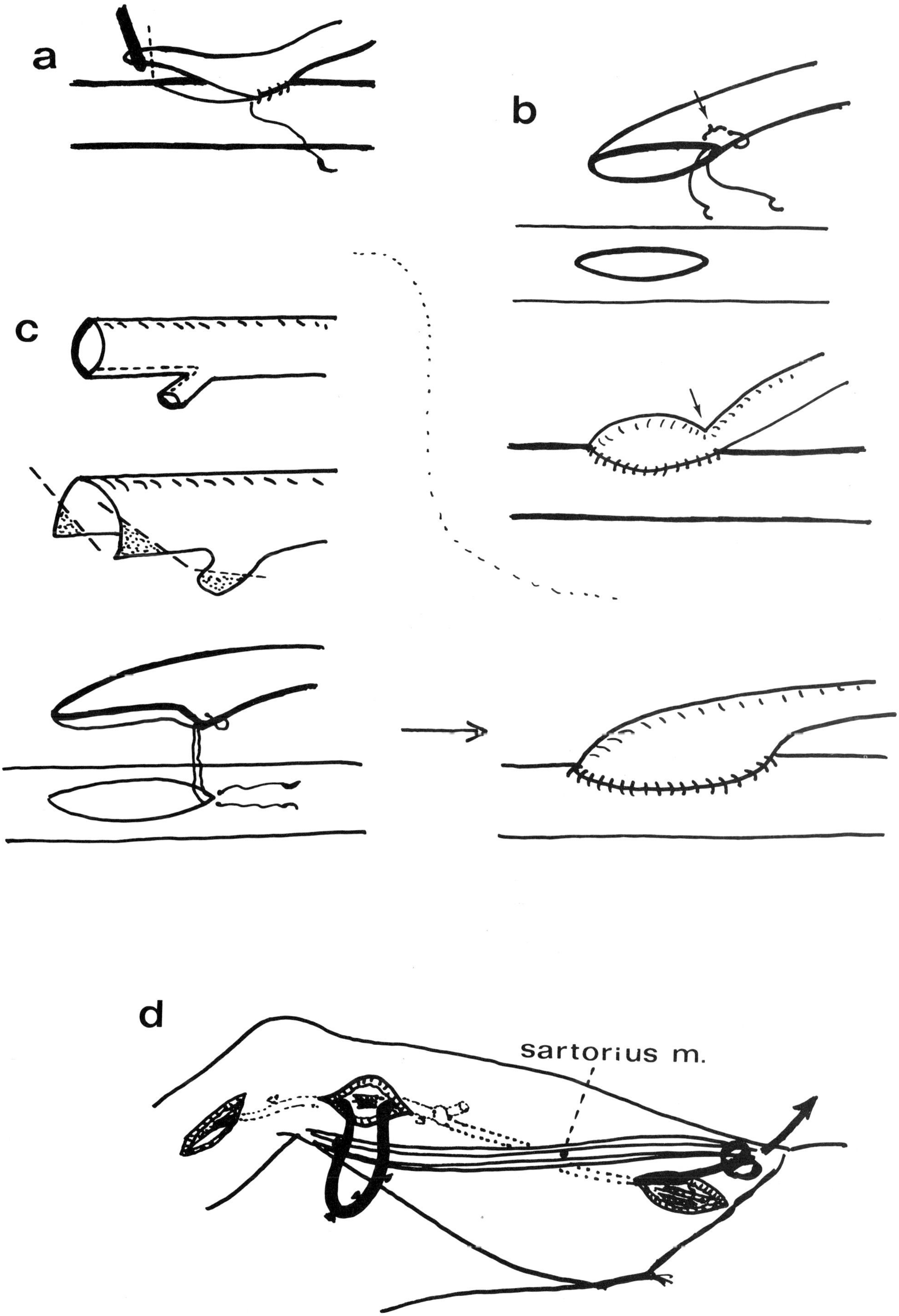
a
b
c
d
sartorius m.

From the midthigh to groin, we use a subsartorial tunnel created with a large, curved clamp. Special tunneling instruments are not necessary (Fig. 3D). When the proximal end of the venous graft has reached the groin incision, the leg is stretched and the knee brought to an 180-degree position. A correct length of the transplant without excessive tension but also without redundancy is mandatory. When the central anastomosis is constructed, the graft should be a little taut, since it will stretch a bit after releasing the clamps. Before starting the inguinal anastomosis, heparinized-saline solution is again injected into the free end. Palpation of the popliteal anastomosis assures arrival of flow.

The proximal anastomosis is performed using the same principles as described for the distal one. A 5–0 or 6–0 prolene suture will be used. From the technical point of view, this is the weakest part of the whole procedure, since the smallest diameter of the saphenous vein has to be anastomosed to the thick wall of the common femoral artery. It is very important to take delicate bites of vein and avoid incorporating too much of the vein wall into the anastomosis so as not to narrow the inflow into the graft (Fig. 3B). When there is a venous tributary near the central end of the venous graft, it can sometimes be incorporated into the anastomosis (Fig. 3C). The widened venous cuff results in a larger anastomotic caliber. For cases with a rather thick atherosclerotic arterial wall and a very thin venous wall, the surgeon may consider insertion of a venous patch graft into the arteriotomy to create better wall conditions for anastomosing the venous trunk (Fig. 4B).

Hemodynamically, an end-to-end anastomosis in the groin is preferred. The occluded superficial femoral artery is transected about 2 cm distal to the origin of the deep femoral artery, sliced longitudinally on the anterior wall, and locally endarterectomized. This incision may run proximally beyond the orifice of the profunda femoris. The venous graft, on the other hand, is sliced on the posterior wall and sutured to the artery so that an oblique anastomotic plane will result. When there is an obvious caliber difference between the femoral artery and the venous graft, we enlarge the anastomosis with an additional vein patch inserted in the anterior wall as demonstrated in Fig. 4D.

Sometimes a saphenous vein transplant that is correct in length but very tapering in its caliber is found. Here, one alternative is to transect the graft in the middle and to reunite the segments after having used the proximal one for the central anastomosis and vice versa (Fig. 4F). Another alternative is a nonreversed venous bypass, which will require destruction of the valves by passing a large polyethylene catheter down the vein. Before constructing the anastomoses, irrigation with heparinized-saline solution must prove unlimited patency of the vein. The nonreversed saphenous vein bypass can also be performed in the so-called in situ technique, a procedure that is quite uncommon in Germany. Only the proximal and distal ends of the saphenous vein are dissected free and anastomosed with the arteries after the valves have been made incompetent. Arteriovenous fistulas caused by the nonligated venous tributaries must be detected with a sterile stethoscope, a Doppler probe, or an angiogram, and must be closed by ligation of the venous branches.

When only a short vein transplant is available, the surgeon has the choice of putting the central anastomosis more distally, in the middle of the superficial femoral artery. Because of poor late results, I have decided to use a composite graft consisting of a venous and a synthetic segment, running from the groin distally. When there is no available vein at all, synthetic tubes must be used for femoropopliteal bridging. The polytetrafluoroethylene (Gore-Tex) graft is favored. The operative technique follows the same principles given above for the vein bypass, except that it is started with the proximal anastomosis.

Fig. 4. (A) The central anastomosis between vein graft and artery normally is performed end-to-side at the common femoral artery and opposite the origin of the deep femoral artery.
(B) The insertion of an autogenous vein patch to a thick-walled common femoral artery and the following anastomosis between a small-caliber graft and the patch helps create a technically more perfect anastomosis.
(C) Hemodynamically, the best type is an end-to-end anastomosis in the groin. The anastomotic plane is oblique, and both ends of graft and artery must be bevelled. Depending on local findings, one will use only the proximal stump of the superficial femoral artery (as demonstrated here) or will extend the arteriotomy to the common femoral artery, controlling as well the orifice of the profunda.
(D) To adjust a difference in caliber between graft and central stump of the artery, it is helpful to insert an autogenous vein patch into the anastomosis, as demonstrated here.
(E) Angioplasty of the proximal end of a venous graft, using two tributary branches to obtain a wider caliber of the anastomosis.
(F) When a long distance has to be bridged by a reversed saphenous vein transplant, there is sometimes a too-large difference between the calibers of vein and artery at the proximal and distal connections. Here it is advantageous to transect the graft in the middle and to use the distal portion for the proximal segment of the bypass.

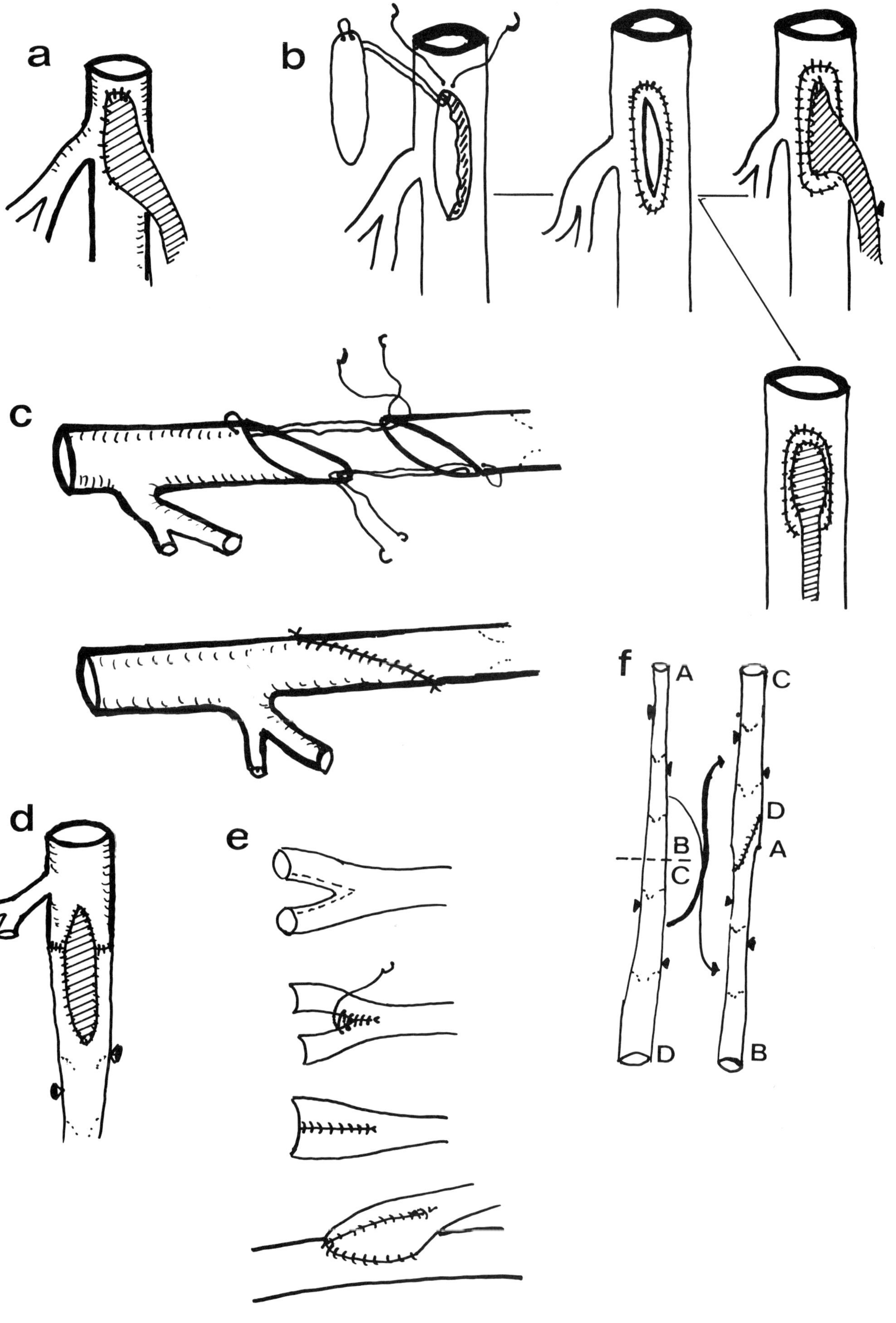
a
b
c
d
e
f
A
C
D
A
B
C
D
B

Finally, it must be emphasized that no bypass procedure should be finished without an intraoperative angiographic control. To obtain the best information on anatomy and function, the angiography should be done after releasing all clamps, with injection of the dye proximal to the central anastomosis. Twenty to 40 ml of Angiografin R will be sufficient, and normally only one film will have to be exposed. A ceiling-mounted x-ray machine, constructed by the Siemens Company especially for our operating rooms, is in use.

BIBLIOGRAPHY

1. Darling RC: Autogenous saphenous vein bypass grafts for femoropopliteal occlusive disease, in Sawyer PN, Kaplitt MJ (eds):Vascular Grafts. New York, Appleton-Century-Crofts, 1978
2. Haimovici H: Femoropopliteal arteriosclerotic occlusive disease, in: Haimovici H (ed): Vascular Surgery. New York, McGraw-Hill, 1976
3. Hershey FB, Calman CH: Atlas of Vascular Surgery. St. Louis, CV Mosby Co, 1973
4. Linton RR: Atlas of vascular surgery. Philadelphia-London-Toronto, W B Saunders Co, 1973
5. Mannick JA: Femoro-popliteal and femoro-tibial reconstructions. Surg Clin North Am 59:581–596, 1979
6. Müller-Wiefel H: Eingriffe an den Arterien, in: Breitner B (ed): Chirurgische Operationslehre, München-Wien–Baltimore, Urban & Schwarzenberg, 1978
7. Rob C (Ed): Operative Surgery, vol 3. Philadelphia, JB Lippincott, 1968
8. Vollmar J: Rekonstruktive Chirurgie der Arterien, Stuttgart, G Thieme, 1975
9. Yao JST: Femoropopliteal artery bypass, in Rutherford RB (ed): Vascular Surgery. Philadelphia-London-Toronto, WB Saunders Co, 1977

Femoral-distal Artery Bypasses

Frank J. Veith, Sushil K. Gupta

Reconstructions to arteries distal to the popliteal can be performed in the upper, middle, or lower third of the leg as well as in the ankle region or foot. The technical approaches to each of these levels will be described separately in this chapter. However, there are several generalizations applicable to any bypass that is inserted into the posterior tibial, anterior tibial, dorsalis pedis, or peroneal arteries.

These are technically demanding, time-consuming procedures that should only be performed by vascular surgeons with skill, patience, and a commitment to conduct the operation with great care and attention to detail. Even if these small vessel bypasses are performed with technical perfection, 10 to 25 percent of them will fail within several days. If this occurs, the circulatory status of the involved limb may be worsened. Therefore, these operations should never be performed for intermittent claudication alone but only to salvage limbs that have gangrene, a nonhealing ulcer, or *severe* true-rest pain.

Complete preoperative angiography to identify patent arterial segments and distal obstructions is an absolute prerequisite to these operations. Occasionally this will have to be supplemented by intraoperative angiography. This may be required after an acute occlusion in which no contrast media reaches the distal vasculature. Rarely, it may be required to visualize adequately patent arteries in the distal leg and foot with occlusive disease.

These operations are usually required in elderly patients with advanced generalized arteriosclerosis and multisystem disease. Complete preoperative medical evaluation is essential, with particular attention being given to cardiac and diabetic status. Careful anesthetic management by an anesthesiologist experienced in the care of these difficult patients is important if operative (30-day) mortality is to be kept in the 3 to 5 percent range, which can be achieved.[1,2,3] Continuous epidural or light general anesthesia can be used. An arterial line should be placed for pressure and blood-gas monitoring, and hypotension should be avoided. In patients with borderline congestive failure, a Swan-Ganz catheter should be placed in the pulmonary artery and pulmonary wedge pressure monitored. All patients should have an indwelling Foley catheter, and the opposite extremity must be cushioned to prevent heel necrosis. Prophylactic cefazolin is given preoperatively and immediately after operation.

The patient's ipsilateral greater saphenous vein, if available, is presently the vascular graft of choice for small vessel bypasses. It may be difficult to obtain sufficient length of this graft, particularly if the bypass is to an artery in the distal third of the leg or beyond. For this reason, we perform the proximal anastomosis to the superficial femoral artery if it is of good quality and has a normal or only minimally narrowed lumen on preoperative angiography. Similarly, to minimize the length of saphenous vein required, we perform the distal anastomosis to the most proximal portion of any leg artery that has a direct course into the foot. Small vessel bypasses to leg arteries that are obstructed distally can occasionally remain patent, but they usually do not and should be avoided if possible. On the other hand, we would perform a bypass to an isolated popliteal segment in preference to a more distal small vessel bypass in patients without extensive gangrene or infection in the foot. We have achieved good results with such operations.[4]

If an ipsilateral segment of greater saphenous vein is not available or if it is smaller than 3.0 to 3.5 mm in its smallest diameter with gentle dilatation, a tapered (6.5 to 4.5 mm) expanded polytetrafluoroethylene (PTFE) graft may be employed. Many of these grafts have functioned from 2 to 3 years.[5] However, late patency rates with this graft are not known, and its value in comparison to saphenous vein will not be known until prospective, randomized, controlled studies are completed. Therefore, this graft should not be widely used if a saphenous vein graft is available. On the other hand, we presently use it in preference to taking a saphenous vein from the opposite leg or constructing a composite graft from several veins or from a segment of vein and a prosthetic graft.

If the ipsilateral saphenous vein is to be used, the incisions to be detailed in the sections below should be modified wherever possible so that they are placed over the course of the greater saphenous vein (Fig. 1A). In that way the undermining of the skin is minimized and flaps are of maximal thickness so that the best healing of incisions can occur. We prefer a single long vein harvesting incision, although multiple small ones can be used effectively. Most of this incision is sutured closed temporarily during performance of the bypass to avoid drying and necrosis of the subcutaneous fat. After the bypass is completed and the heparin neutralized, the vein harvest incision is reopened, all blood is removed, meticulous hemostasis is obtained, and the wound is carefully reclosed with sutures or clips.

The greater saphenous vein is mobilized by ligating all branches close to the main vessel without catching any adventitia in the ligatures. If the adventitia of the main vein is so caught, stenosis can result after it is distended. For speed, the peripheral end of branches may be clipped, but clips on the main vein should be avoided since they may be caught during tunneling and produce distortion or injury to the graft.

After the vein graft is removed, it is immersed in and distended gently with chilled (4° C) Hank's solution. This is best accomplished using a long (5-inch) plastic cannula attached to a 20-cc plastic syringe (Fig. 1F). In this way the vein can be distended and tested for leaks in segments (Fig. 1F). If unligated branches are present, they are discovered during distension and ligated. Avulsed branches leave holes in the main vein, and these must be carefully sutured with 6–0 silk so as to avoid any constriction of the main vein. After preparation and measurement, the vein is placed in the chilled Hank's solution until it is used. Drying and warming are avoided as much as possible even while the vein is being sutured into place.

Fig. 1. Small Vessel Bypass in the Upper and Middle Third of the Leg. This may be performed to the tibioperoneal trunk, the posterior tibial artery, or the peroneal artery, using a medial approach below the knee joint to gain access to these vessels (Part 1). The anterior tibial artery requires an additional anterior incision (Part 2).

(A) In heavy lines, the position of the incisions required to perform bypasses from the femoral artery to the tibioperoneal trunk or the posterior tibial and peroneal arteries in the upper third of the leg. The upper incision provides access to the common or superficial femoral artery. The above-knee incision allows tunneling under the sartorius muscle and along the course of the popliteal vessels behind the knee. The dashed extension to the lower incision provides access to the posterior tibial and peroneal arteries in the middle third of the leg. If the saphenous vein is to be used, all incisions should be placed over the vein as shown by the double line, and access to deeper structures obtained when needed by raising thick flaps.

(B) The below-knee incision opened through the skin, subcutaneous fat, and deep fascia of the popliteal space. The gastrocnemius muscle is retracted posteriorly. The more superficial popliteal vein is encircled with a silastic loop to facilitate dissection of the underlying popliteal artery (arrow) which can be seen disappearing deep to the fibers of the soleus muscle.

(C) A finger or right-angle clamp being placed deep to this muscle prior to cutting it at its origin from the fibrous band that attaches to the back of the tibia and fibula. This exposes the origin of the anterior tibial artery and its accompanying vein or veins.

(D) Division of these veins allows further retraction of overlying veins and exposure of the tibioperoneal trunk and its terminal branches.

(E) Tunnels are fashioned by finger dissection.

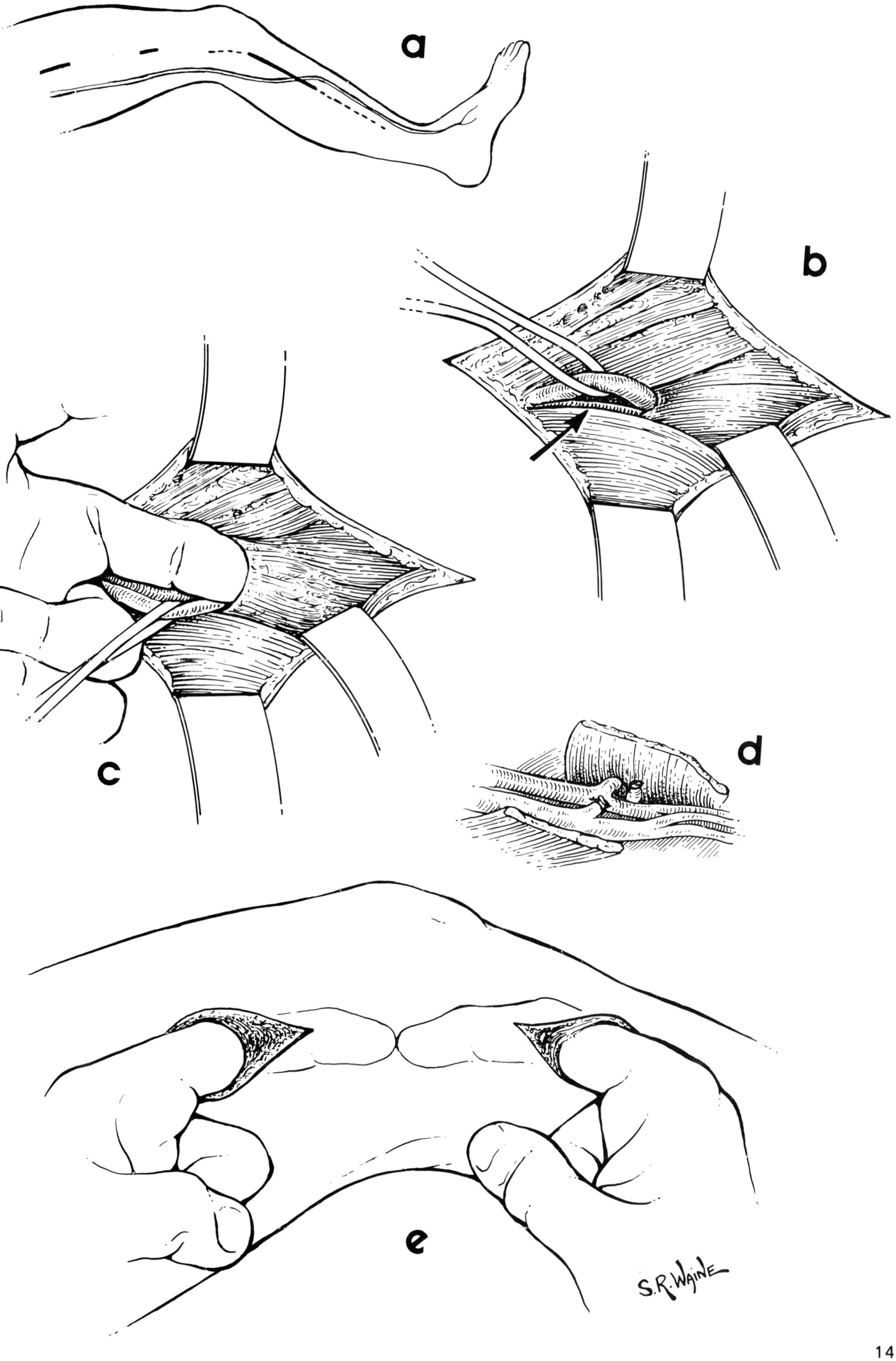
a
b
c
d
e
S.R.WAINE

After arterial mobilization and vein harvesting are completed, tunnel construction is performed. This may be carried out with blunt finger dissection (Fig. 1E and 2D), use of a plastic tube,* passage of a large gently curved clamp (Fig. 3D), or by a combination of two or more methods. When this is completed, the patient is given systemic heparin (1.5 mg/kg). The artery for distal anastomosis is elevated by gentle traction on silastic vessel loops which may be held taut by clamping them to the appropriate drapes or self-retaining retractors (Fig. 1G). Frequently such gentle traction is adequate to provide hemostasis during arteriotomy and anastomosis. If not, microvascular clips (Fig. 1G), small atraumatic vascular clamps, double looping of the vessel loops (Fig. 1G), or passage and inflation of a No. 3 balloon catheter may be used. Although it is essential to have a bloodless field so that perfect visualization can be obtained, it is important to note that any of the above hemostatic methods may damage the delicate small vessel, which may also be calcified or thick-walled. We, therefore, prefer to use whatever method requires the least force and produces the least vessel distortion, and we take as much time as necessary to perform this phase of the operation with the least trauma to the artery. Side branches, although always dissected free, are only encircled with ligatures or silastic loops when necessary, and this is not usually the case.

All arteriotomies and anastomoses must be performed with extreme care. Optical magnification with loupes (2 to $2\frac{1}{2}$ power) and headlight illumination (Design for Vision) may be helpful in providing adequate visualization, which is essential for these technically demanding procedures. Arteriotomies are usually performed with a new-bladed (No. 15 blade) scalpel (Fig. 1G), so that all layers of the arterial wall are cut evenly. This is particularly important if the artery is diseased. After the initial incision in the artery, placement of a fine mosquito clamp within the vessel can facilitate the rest of the arteriotomy (Fig. 1H) and prevent injury to the opposite wall. Fine scissors are only used if the artery is small and thin-walled (Fig. 1H). In general, the length of the arteriotomy and the anastomosis is 2 to 3 times the diameter of the graft, which in turn is $1\frac{1}{2}$ to 3 times the diameter of the recipient distal artery, although this relationship may vary if a saphenous vein graft is employed.

All anastomoses are constructed with fine monofilament polypropylene continuous sutures (6–0). Every stitch must be perfectly placed under direct vision using Castroviejo needle holders and fine atraumatic forceps, so that small even bites of intima and other layers of the arterial wall (Fig. 1I,2) are included in every stitch. We prefer to start the distal anastomosis with a double-armed toe suture and then run each side of the suture halfway down the anastomosis (Fig. 1I). Thereafter, the double-armed heel stitch is placed and tied. Each half is run to the mid-portion of the anastomosis and tied to the appropriate end of the toe stitch. Interrupted stitches at the toe of the anastomosis, which have been advocated by some, are almost never necessary if the described method is employed.

*Argyle Thoracic Catheter Container, Catalog No. Mar-5705–32.

(F) Details of vein preparation using a long cannula to permit the vein to be distended in segments so that leaks can be controlled.
(G) Elevation of the arteries by silastic vessel loops and the beginning of the scalpel incision in the artery. In this view only the taut silastic loops are required to control bleeding, except for the posterior tibial artery which also has a microvascular clip applied to it.
(H) Placement of a mosquito clamp to facilitate extension of the initial opening in the artery. Alternatively, a microvascular scissors may be used to extend the arteriotomy if the vessel is thin-walled and normal.
(I) Details of the anastomotic suturing, which is begun at the distal end and continued to the midportion of each side of the anastomosis of the artery and the saphenous vein graft.
(J) Completed distal anastomosis with the graft in place. If more distal exposure of the posterior tibial or peroneal arteries is required, further separation of the soleus muscle from the posterior surface of the tibia and its overlying muscles provides access to the neurovascular bundles. Careful dissection of the veins with ligation of crossing branches provides access to the more deeply placed arteries. These can be dissected free, taking great care to preserve all branches, so that the appropriate segment of artery can be elevated and controlled to perform the distal anastomosis.

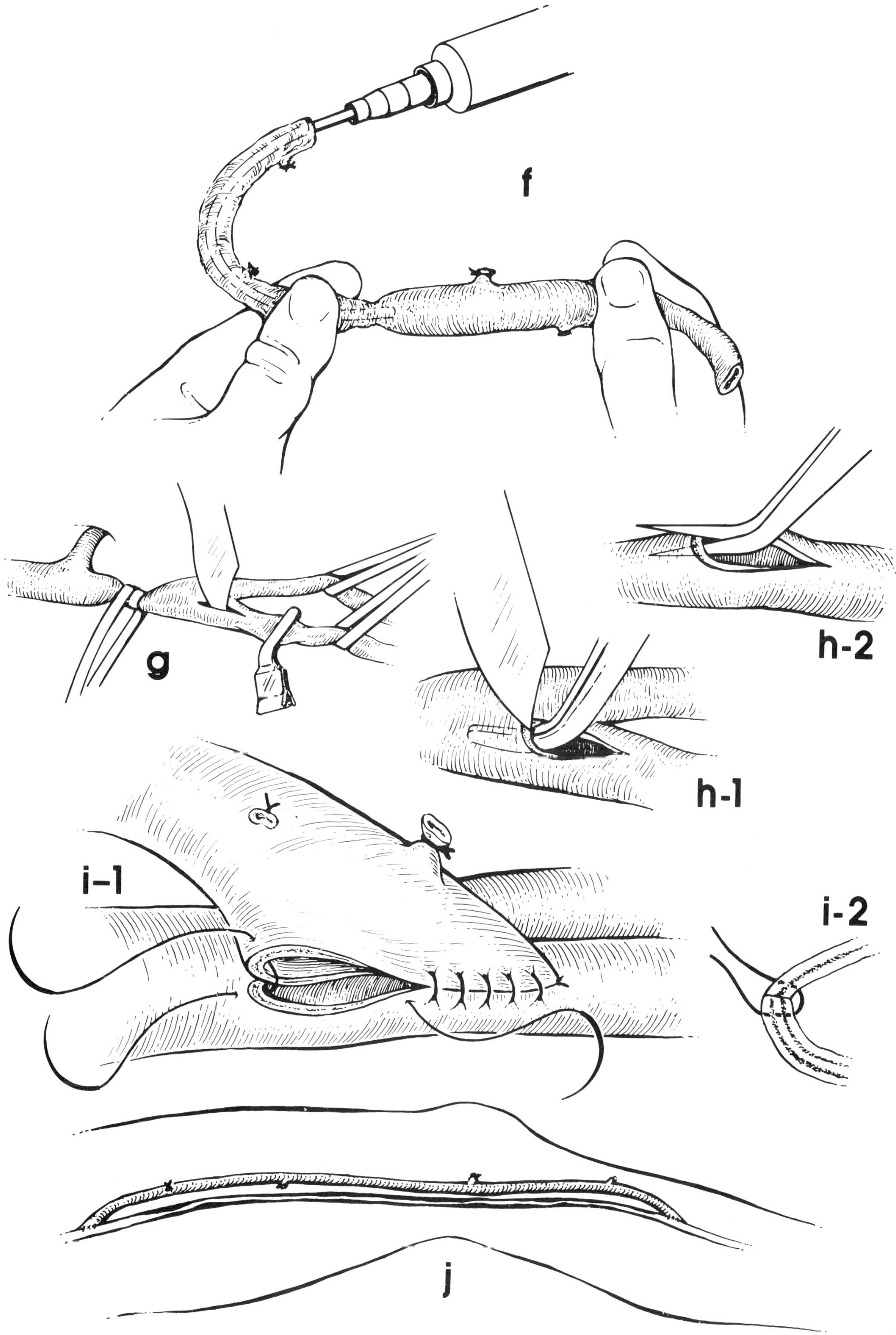
f
g
h-2
h-1
i–1
i-2
j

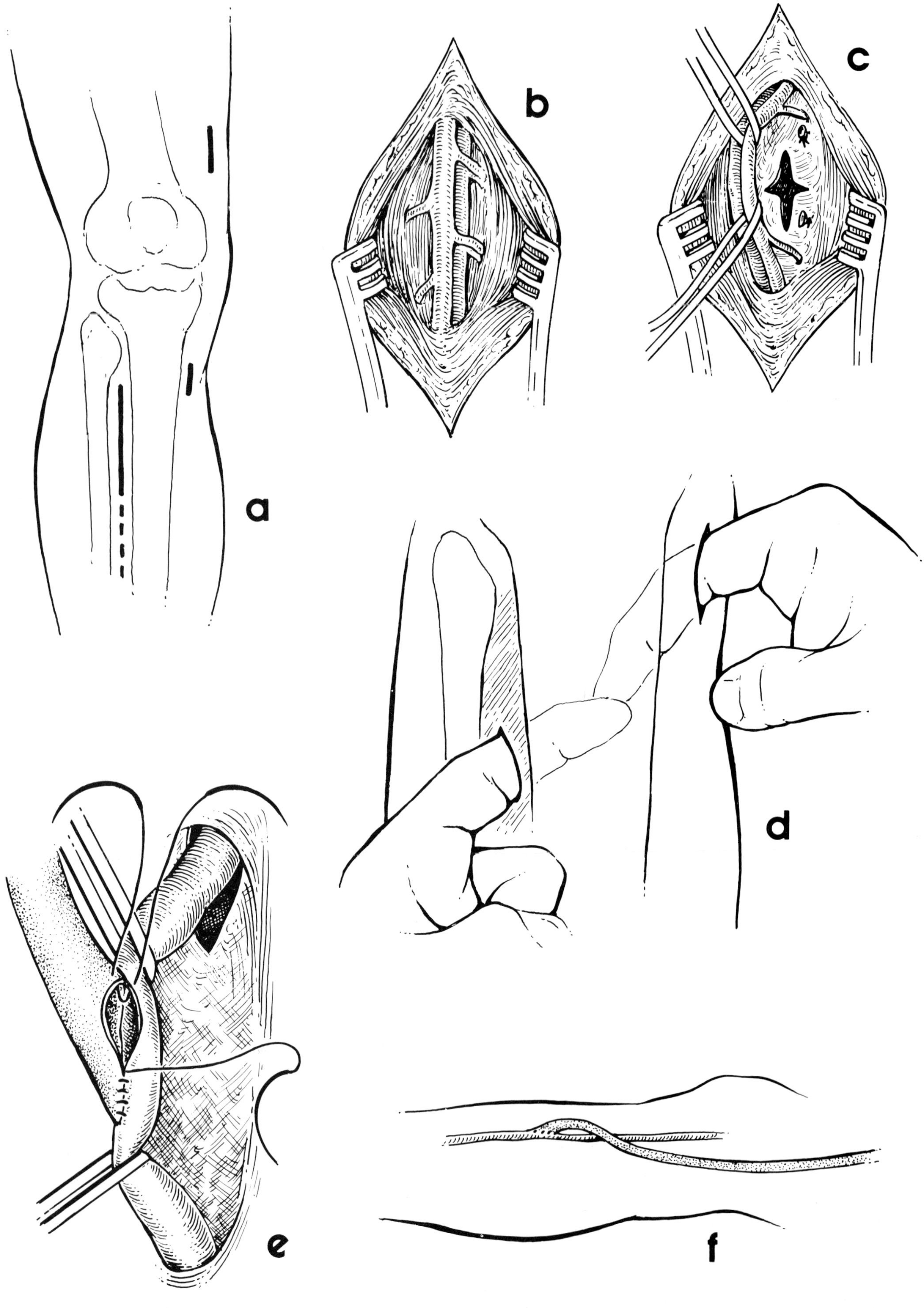
a
b
c
d
e
f

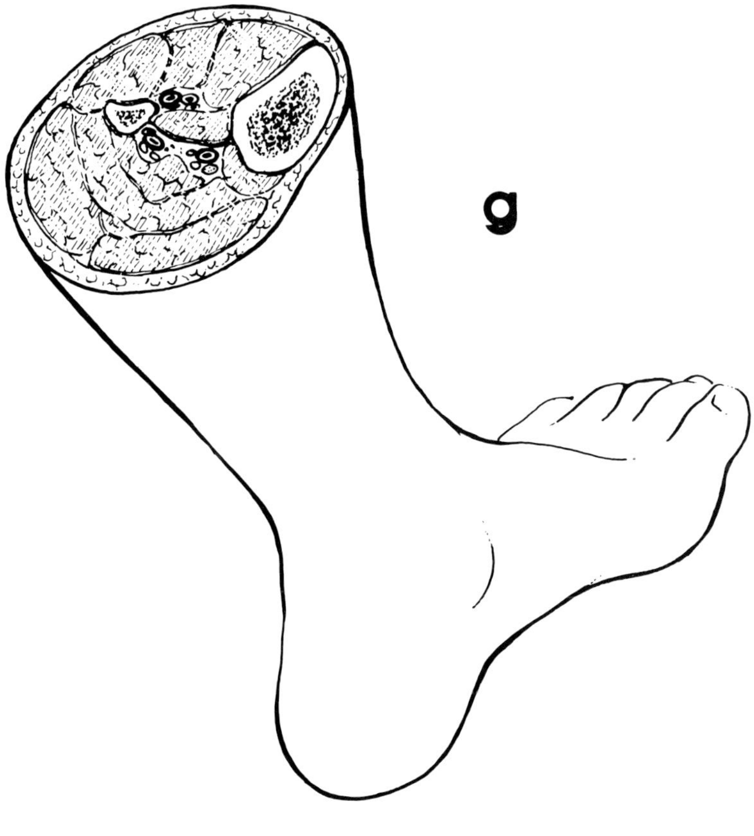

g

Fig. 2 Bypass to the Anterior Tibial Artery in the Upper and Middle Thirds of the Leg.

(A) This requires an anterolateral incision in the leg midway between the tibia and fibula over the appropriate segment of patent artery. Additional small medial incisions are also required for tunneling.

(B) The anterior incision is carried through the deep fascia and the fibers of the anterior tibial muscle and the long extensors of the toes are separated to reveal the neurovascular bundle. Mobilization of accompanying veins with division of branches allows visualization of the anterior tibial artery which can then be carefully mobilized as already described.

(C) After the artery is freed, it is elevated and retracted along with the accompanying veins by silastic loops. This permits further posterior dissection, which allows the interosseous membrane to be visualized and incised in a cruciate fashion.

(D) Careful blunt finger dissection from this anterior approach *and* from the popliteal fossa via the medial incision facilitates creation of a tunnel without injuring the numerous veins in the area. By elevating the anterior tibial artery, a meticulous distal anastomosis can be constructed.

(E) Shows this in progress with a polytetraflouroethylene graft. Other operative anastomotic details are similar to those already described.

(F) The resulting graft in place. The anterior tibial artery can also be approached by a lateral incision with fibulectomy, but we believe this approach to be bloodier and more time-consuming than the one we have described. Moreover, the lateral approach does not offer any better exposure of this vessel, and we do not recommend it.

(G) The position of the three major arteries with relationship to the bones and muscles of the mid-leg.

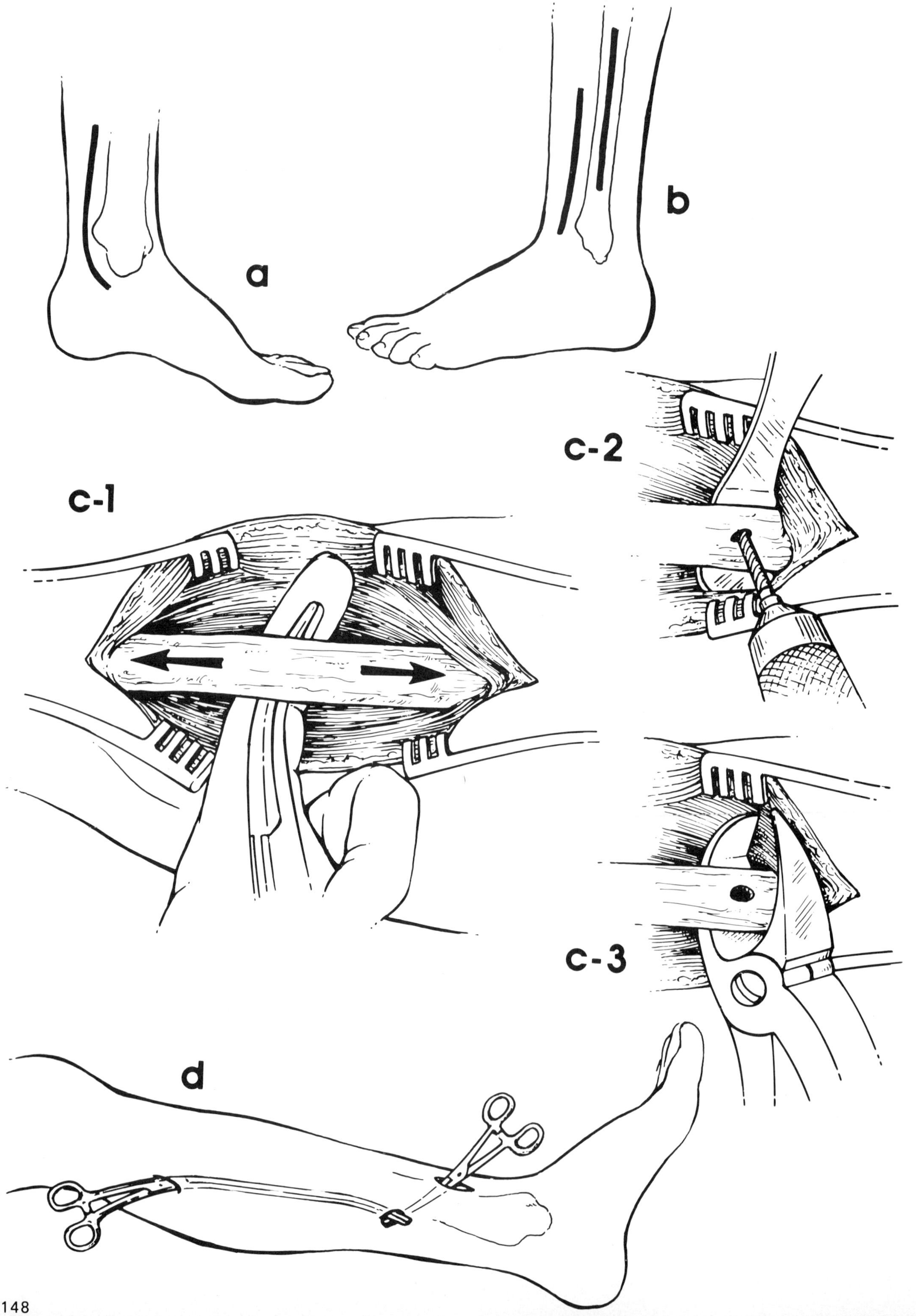
a
b
c-2
c-1
c-3
d

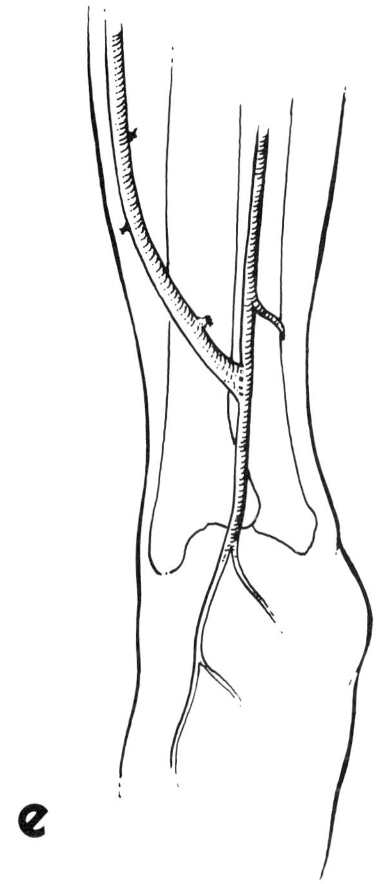

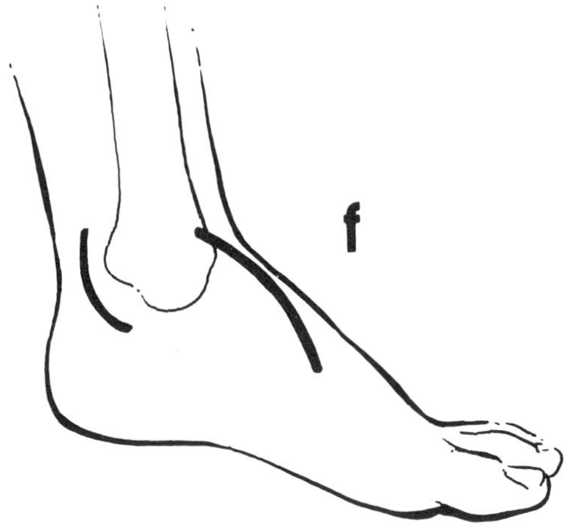

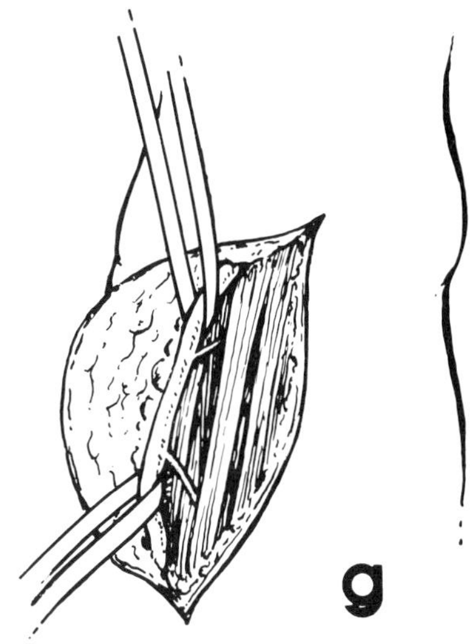

Fig. 3. Bypasses to the Distal Third of the Leg and the Foot. Bypasses to the anterior tibial, posterior tibial, or peroneal arteries in the distal leg can be performed by techniques similar to those already described, with the exception of certain features illustrated here.

(A) The distal posterior tibial artery can be approached by an incision along the posterior edge of the tibia. By deepening this incision along the tibialis posterior muscle and the posterior surface of the tibia, the distal peroneal artery can also be located and isolated just medial to the medial edge of the fibula. By dividing restraining fascia and fibers of the flexor hallucis longus muscle, it is possible to free this artery and elevate it into the wound so that a careful anastomosis can be constructed. However, in most patients, particularly those with a stout calf and ankle, this vessel is best approached by a lateral incision with excision of the fibula (Fig. 1B).

(C) This is accomplished by freeing a long segment of fibula from its muscle attachments using a combination of blunt and sharp dissection. Particular care should be taken in the dissection along the medial edge of the bone, since the peroneal vessels are just deep to this edge and are easily injured by instruments. Once a finger has been passed around the fibula, this free edge of bone can be further developed by pushing a right-angled clamp forcefully inferiorly and superiorly. A right-angled retractor can then be passed behind the bone and a hole drilled in it. Then the fibula can be easily and cleanly divided with a rib shears. The peroneal artery can then be dissected free from surrounding veins so that it can be used for construction of a distal anastomosis. Gentle blunt finger dissection is required to develop a tunnel from this lateral wound to the lower popliteal fossa. Great care is taken to avoid injury to the numerous veins in the area. From there, the tunneling to the femoral artery wound is performed in the previously described fashion. Because it is the least accessible of the three leg arteries and normally has the poorest connections with the arteries of the foot, we recommend use of the peroneal artery as a distal implantation site only when the anterior and posterior tibial arteries are not suitable for use.

(D) The tunnel from the distal posterior tibial artery to the popliteal fossa is made just deep to the deep fascia. This is best accomplished with a long, gently curved clamp. The distal anterior tibial artery is approached by an anterior incision midway between the tibia and fibula (B).

(D) For bypasses to this vessel, a tunnel is made from the distal popliteal fossa, deep to the deep fascia, to a point 5 to 7 cm above the medial malleolus. This is best accomplished with a large, gently curved clamp.

(E) From this point, the tunnel is made subcutaneously in a gentle curve across the tibia and adjacent tendons to reach the anterior tibial wound. The underlying tendons are those of the anterior tibial muscle and the long extensors of the toes. The tunnels are marked with umbilical tapes for subsequent identification. After completion of the distal anastomosis and drawing the graft through these tunnels, any tendons that distort or compress the graft in its course around the tibia are divided. This is usually required in the very low anterior tibial bypasses. When no more proximal procedure is possible, bypasses to the ankle region or foot can be used to salvage limbs.[2,5] The dorsalis pedis artery can be easily approached via an incision on the dorsum of the foot.

(F) We place this incision laterally, curve it and raise a flap so that the incision will not be directly over the anastomosis. If this artery must be approached at the ankle, it is necessary to divide the extensor retinaculum. Otherwise the operation is performed as already described for the distal anterior tibial bypass. The posterior tibial artery can be approached down to a point a few centimeters below the medial malleolus. Below this level the artery plunges laterally, and we have not found it suitable for anastomosis. All other details of this procedure are similar to those already described for posterior tibial bypasses in the lower leg.

After completion of the distal anastomosis, all hemostatic elements are removed, and the graft and recipient artery are flushed gently with heparinized normal saline. Large leaks are visualized and carefully fixed, usually by adventitial sutures; small or moderate leaks are ignored and stop spontaneously.

The saline filled graft is then drawn through the previously fashioned tunnels by using a large clamp or by placing a plastic tube (Argyle Thoracic Catheter Container) through the tunnel, cutting off the end, and then drawing the graft through the tube using a bronchoscopy grasping forceps. Care is taken to prevent rotation of the graft within the tunnel and to avoid redundancy, excessive tension, or sharp angulation.

The segment of artery to be used for the proximal anastomosis is then isolated between gently applied vascular clamps, again using the minimum amount of force and distortion consistent with a bloodless operative field so as to minimize clamp injury. Proximal anastomoses are generally begun by placement of a double-armed distal heel stitch. Each arm of this is run proximally to the midpoint of the anastomosis. The proximal apical suture is then placed and tied, and each arm of this is run to *the midpoint* of the anastomosis and tied. Since the vein component in this anastomosis may be small, care is taken to make the suture bites in the vein small, catching equal portions of all layers.

After completion of both anastomoses and removal of all occluding clamps, heparin is neutralized by protamine, and meticulous hemostasis is obtained from the anastomoses and all other wounds. Usually this requires considerable patience, particularly for anastomoses in which polytetraflouorethylene grafts are employed. Intraoperative angiography is performed if indicated, and all wounds are closed using meticulous plastic techniques. Dressings are applied, and any necrotic or infected tissue in the foot is widely debrided. This may require removal of one or more toes or a partial or total transmetatarsal amputation. Generally these debridements are best left open. Although we continue our patients on aspirin (0.6 g/day) and dipyridamole (50 mg/day) postoperatively, there is no firm evidence in humans that this is helpful. No other anticoagulants are used postoperatively.

REFERENCES

1. Veith FJ, Moss CM, Fell SC, Montefusco CM, Rhodes BA, Haimovici H: Comparison of expanded polytetrafluoroethylene and autologous saphenous vein grafts in high-risk arterial reconstructions for limb salvage. Surg Gynecol Obstet 147:749, 1978
2. Veith FJ, Moss CM, Fell SC, Daly V, Haimovici H: New approaches to limb salvage by extended extra-anatomic bypasses and prosthetic reconstructions to foot arteries. Surgery, 84:764, 1978
3. Reichle FA, Tyson RR: Bypasses to tibial or popliteal arteries in severely ischemic lower extremities: Comparison of long-term results in 233 patients. Ann Surg 176:315, 1972
4. Veith FJ, Gupta SK, Daly VD: Femoropopliteal bypass to the isolated popliteal segment: Is polytetrafluoroethylene graft acceptable? Surgery (in press)
5. Gupta SK, Veith FJ: Three year experience with expanded polytetrafluoroethylene (PTFE) arterial grafts for limb salvage. Am J Surg (in press)

Sequential Bypass Grafting

William R. Flinn, D. Preston Flanigan,
John J. Bergan, James S.T. Yao

Femoropopliteal bypass grafting has been used successfully in the treatment of lower-limb ischemia. However, many investigators have noted reduced graft patency when significant distal outflow disease is present. Mannick, Jackson, and Coffman[1] have reported excellent graft patency in saphenous vein bypass grafting to a so-called isolated popliteal segment. But such a graft relies on the availability of collateral channels to increase perfusion of the foot and measurable hemodynamic improvement is often slight. To further enhance the outflow from a femoropopliteal bypass, DeLaurentis and Friedman[2] first suggested a "jump" graft from the popliteal artery to a tibial artery and have subsequently reported good results with this technique. Bliss and Fonseka[3] similarly described the "hitch-hike" graft and reported encouraging results. Other researchers[4,5] have documented significantly increased flow through sequential grafts in the lower extremity. Our recent experience of sequential grafting has supported the value of this procedure for limb salvage procedures.[6]

In addition to the actual bypass technique, intraoperative arteriography as described below is of crucial importance to the overall planning of sequential grafting. Angiography, including its application in prebypass and postbypass stages, allows accurate and successful decision-making.

INTRAOPERATIVE ARTERIOGRAPHY

A careful review of the preoperative lower extremity angiogram is essential to select appropriately patients who may be candidates for sequential bypass grafting. Characteristically, these patients will have an occlusion of the superficial femoral artery with reconstitution of the popliteal artery somewhere along its course. From this popliteal segment, unnamed collaterals may arise. More distally, there will be reconstitution of an anterior tibial, posterior tibial, or peroneal artery. If one or more normal or minimally diseased tibial vessels originate directly from the popliteal artery, then sequential grafting is not recommended, since it is unlikely that any pressure gradient will exist between the popliteal and tibial arteries. In such circumstances, femoral-popliteal bypass alone would be effective. Another angiographic configuration that may be seen is a single, slightly diseased tibial artery in continuity with the popliteal segment. However, a different tibial vessel reconstitutes distally and appears normal or near normal to the foot. In such a case, sequential grafting may be elected to provide more comprehensive revascularization of the extremity, provide increased outflow for the graft, and presumably increase the likelihood of patency.

Often, it will be difficult to visualize with anatomic certainty the distal popliteal and tibial vessels on the preoperative arteriogram. This is especially true in cases where it has been necessary to perform translumbar aortography. In this situation, a reliable assessment of infrageniculate arterial anatomy can be obtained only by performance of intraoperative prebypass arteriography using the following technique.

SURGICAL PROCEDURE

The common femoral artery is isolated through a standard groin incision. A standard x-ray cassette (20 x 24 inches) in a disposable sterile cover is positioned obliquely (corner-to-corner) under the leg and foot (Fig. 1). In most patients, it will be possible to visualize an area from the distal popliteal fossa to and including the foot. The latter is of importance so that the pedal arch anatomy will be seen. A 16-gauge intravenous cannula is then introduced into the common femoral artery, and the artery is crossclamped proximally. Approximately 50 cc of contrast material (Renografin 60) is injected rapidly. The clamp across the common femoral artery is then released, and after delay of 10 to 15 seconds the single x-ray exposure is made.

Using this technique, it should be possible to delineate clearly the outflow from an isolated popliteal segment and to identify patent distal tibial or peroneal arteries and their arborizations. It has been our experience that, when this technique is used and no distal named vessels are identified, the likelihood of successful distal reconstruction of any kind is extremely small. In such cases, this technique may be advantageous since no distal incisions have been made that might be slow to heal or interfere with future amputation sites.

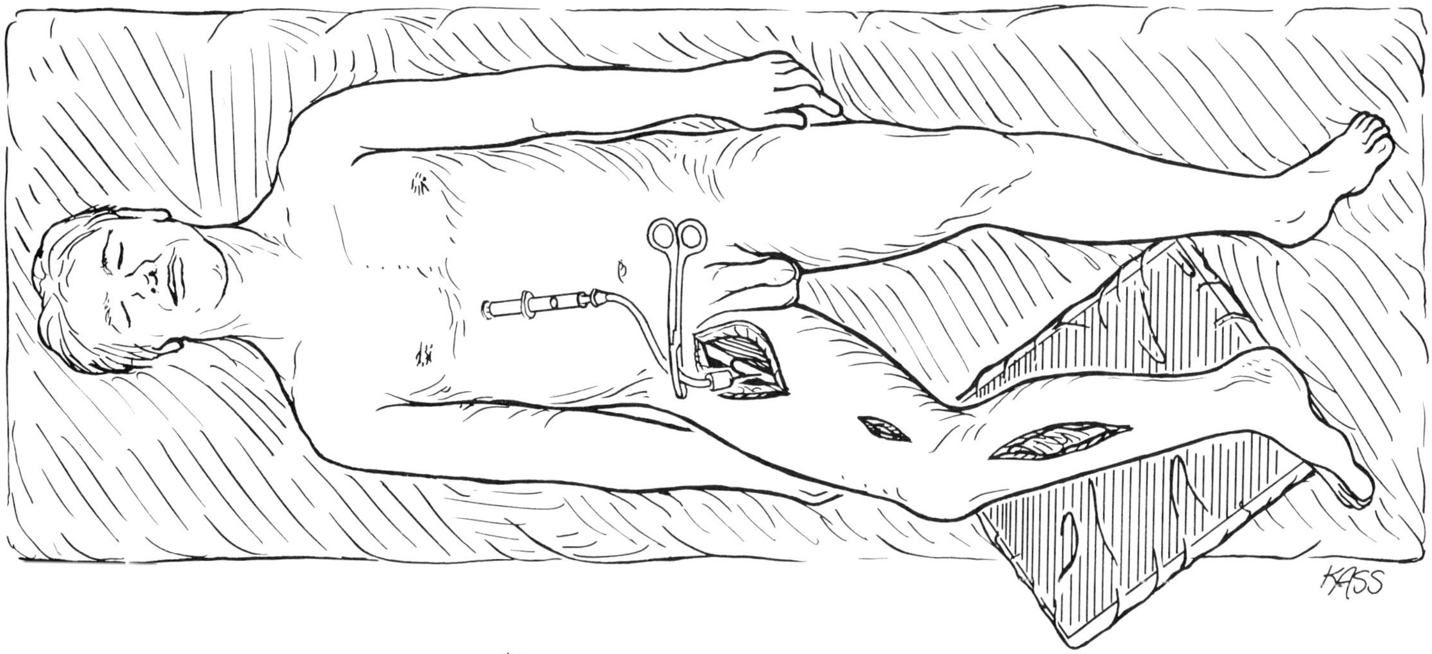

Fig. 1. Intraoperative prebypass angiography may aid evaluation of distal arterial anatomy. A similar technique of cassette placement is used after bypass to confirm satisfactory technical results.

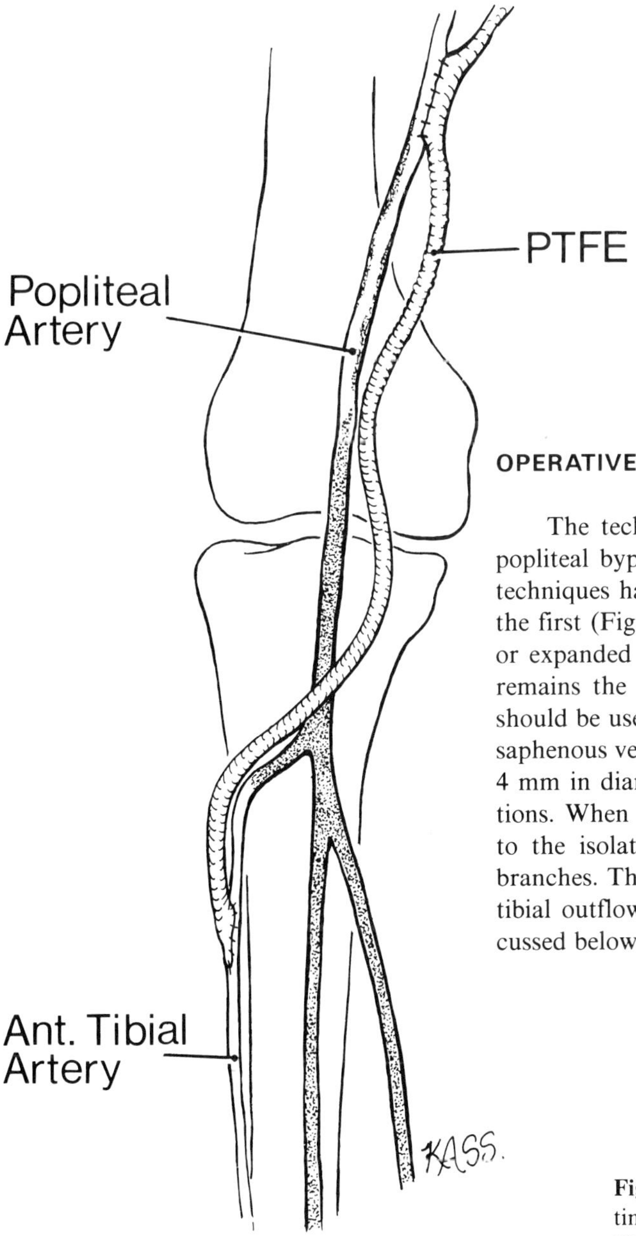

OPERATIVE TECHNIQUES

The technique of femoral-sequential grafting combines classical femoral-popliteal bypass with newer approaches to the distal tibial vessels. Two basic techniques have proved useful in the construction of these sequential grafts. In the first (Fig. 2), a continuous graft is used. Either autogenous saphenous vein or expanded polytetrafluoroethylene (PTFE) may be selected. Saphenous vein remains the graft material of choice in all lower-limb revascularizations and should be used whenever it is adequate. Expanded PTFE is used only when the saphenous vein is inadequate or unavailable. The use of saphenous vein less than 4 mm in diameter when gently dilated is probably unwise in these reconstructions. When the continuous graft technique is used, a side-to-side anastomosis to the isolated popliteal segment provides revascularization of its collateral branches. The graft then continues distally to an end-to-side anastomosis to the tibial outflow vessel of choice. Further specifics of surgical technique are discussed below.

Fig. 2. Technique for construction of the continuous sequential bypass graft, in this case, PTFE.

The second basic technique is to utilize a composite graft of autogenous saphenous vein and PTFE (Fig. 3). Almost all patients who have not had their saphenous veins removed have a proximal segment of vein of adequate size and length to be potentially useful in this composite configuration. Bypass from the common femoral to the popliteal segment is performed in the standard fashion with PTFE, and then the saphenous segment is continued distally as a jump graft from the distal portion of the PTFE. Thus, the distal tibial anastomosis is constructed with the reversed saphenous segment. This is technically much easier with vein than with prosthetic material.

As previously noted, a longitudinal groin incision is used to expose the common, superficial, and profunda femoris arteries. This incision can be carried medially and longitudinally to expose the proximal portion of the saphenous vein. A medial thigh incision performed longitudinally just above the knee is then used both to harvest the distal portion of the above-knee saphenous vein if it is suitable for grafting and to enter the popliteal fossa. The deep fascia of the thigh just anterior to the sartorius muscle is incised throughout the length of this incision. This will facilitate exposure of the superior portion of the popliteal artery and allow creation of anatomic tunnels (Fig. 4).

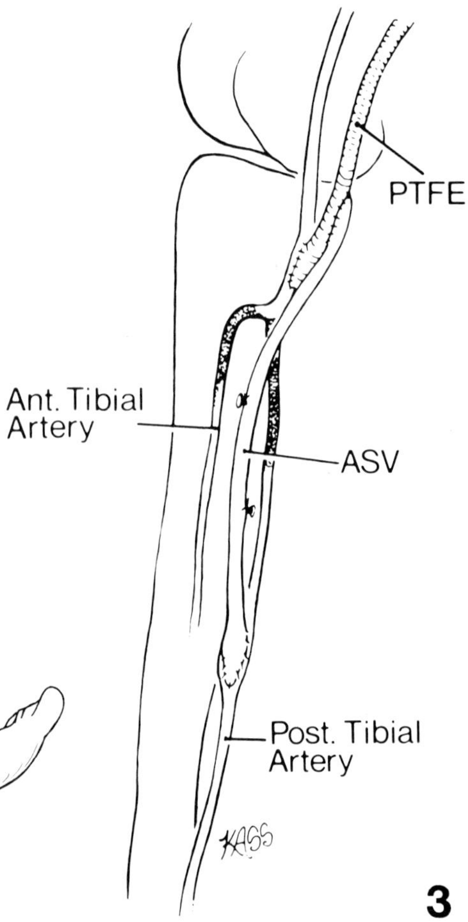

Fig. 3. Technique for construction of the composite sequential graft.

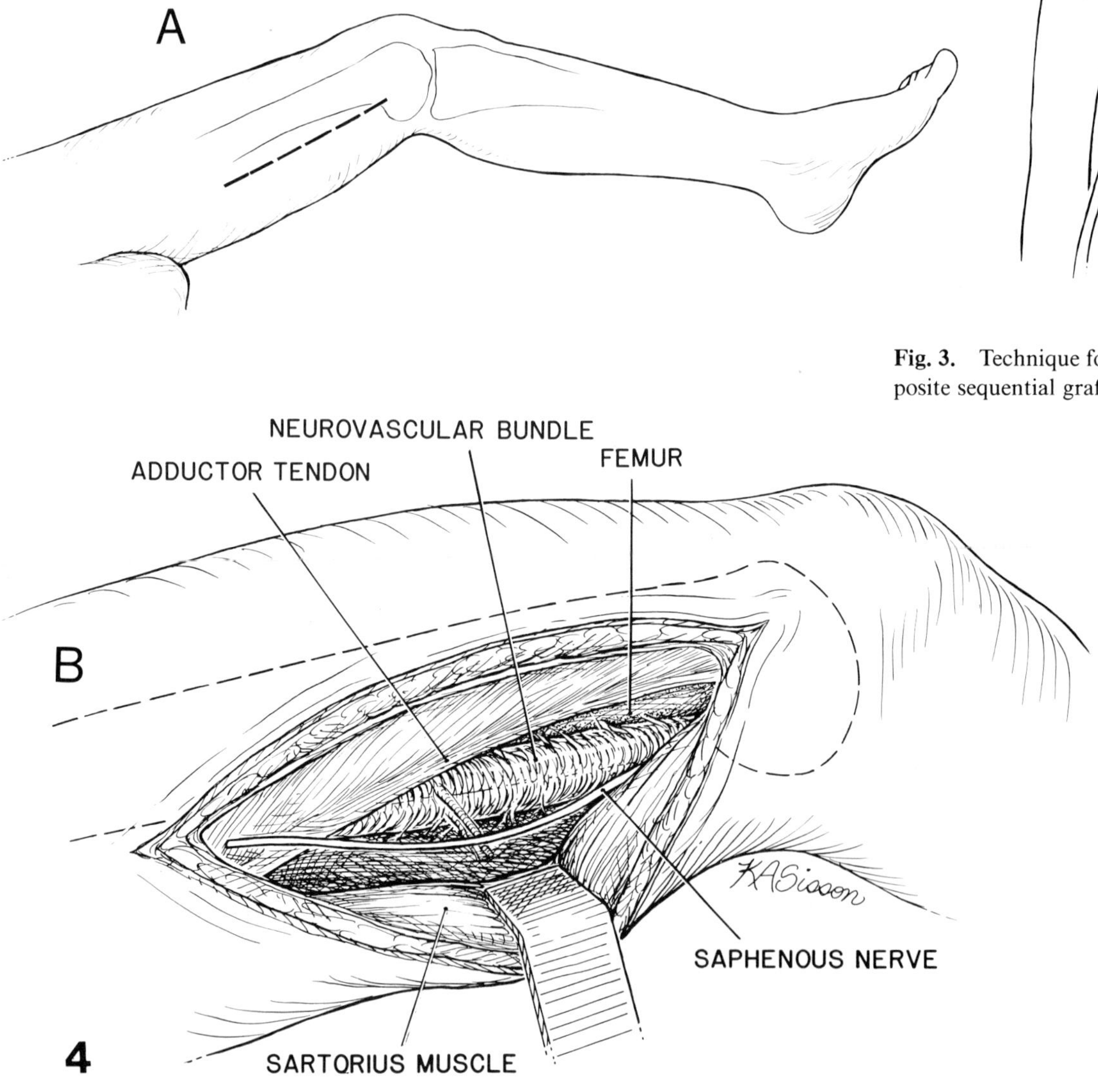

4

Fig. 4. Incision of the deep fascia of the thigh just anterior to the sartorius muscle facilitates exposure of the superior portion of the popliteal artery and allows creation of anatomic tunnels.

An anteromedial calf skin incision just posterior to the tibial ridge below the knee is used to expose the most distal portion of the saphenous vein as well as the distal popliteal artery and its branches. By incising the deep or soleal fascia along the tibia, the distal popliteal fossa may be entered (Fig. 5). If this medial calf wound is extended more distally, it can be used for exposure of both the posterior tibial and peroneal arteries in the distal calf. By dividing sharply the medial soleus origin off the tibia, the posterior tibial artery can be identified running in close association with the large posterior tibial nerve and paired tibial veins (Fig. 6). If the musculofascial dissection is deepened laterally beneath the fibula, the peroneal artery will be identified running parallel to the posterior tibial and rarely more than 2 to 3 cm away. Using this medial exposure, it has been possible to perform bypass grafting to the peroneal artery distally to just above its bifurcation into the anterior and posterior communicating branches, without the attendant fibulectomy that has been described with lateral approaches to this vessel.

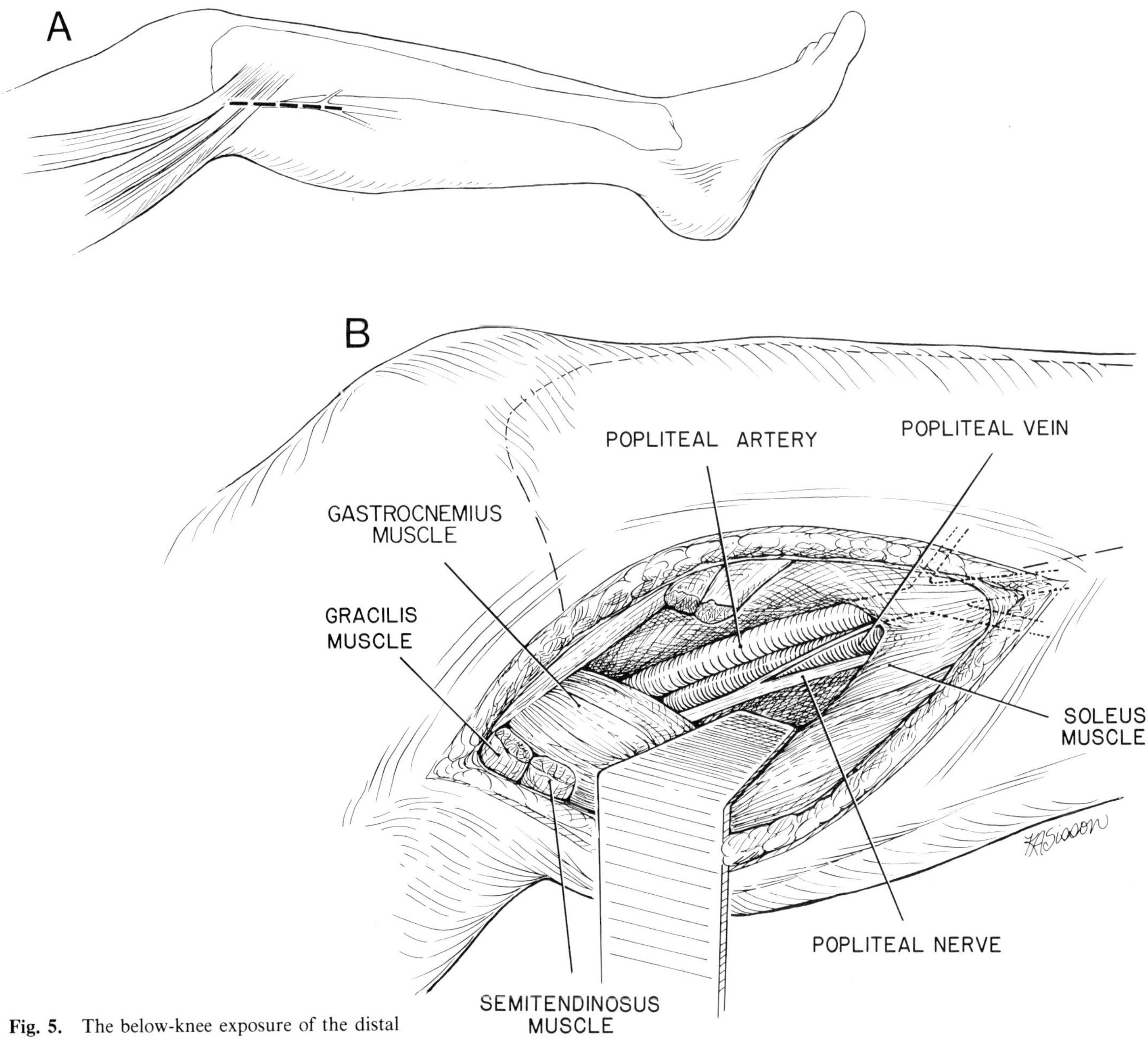

Fig. 5. The below-knee exposure of the distal popliteal artery facilitates anastomosis to a patent isolated segment in this area or provides more distal exposure of the tibioperoneal trunk.

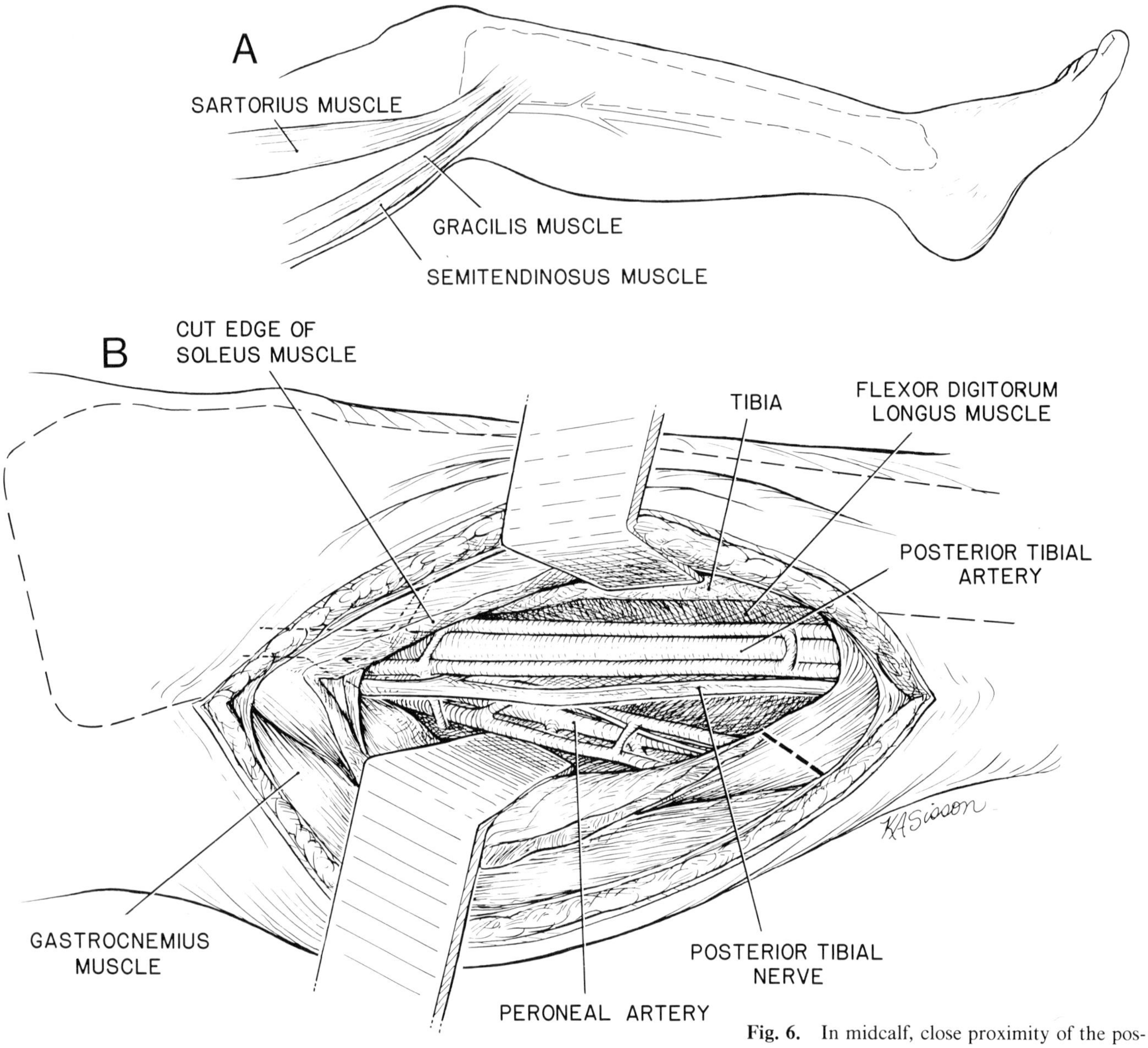

Fig. 6. In midcalf, close proximity of the posterior tibial and peroneal arteries is striking. Both vessels are readily exposed through a medial approach.

The anterior tibial artery is exposed through a longitudinal skin incision in the midportion of the anterior compartment, which is usually about two fingerbreadths lateral to the tibial ridge (Fig. 7). After opening the deep fascia of the compartment about 2 to 3 cm above and below the limits of the skin incision, the muscle bellies of the tibialis anterior and extensor digitorum communis are separated with a self-retaining retractor. The anterior tibial artery and its paired vein and nerve will be easily identified running along the interosseous membrane in this plane.

Once the tibial outflow vessel chosen for distal grafting is identified, dissection is carried distally along the artery to an area that is free of or minimally involved with obvious atheromatous changes. Complete exposure proximally and especially distally is essential to ensure that no significant occlusive disease exists in an area just beyond the insertion of the distal anastomosis.

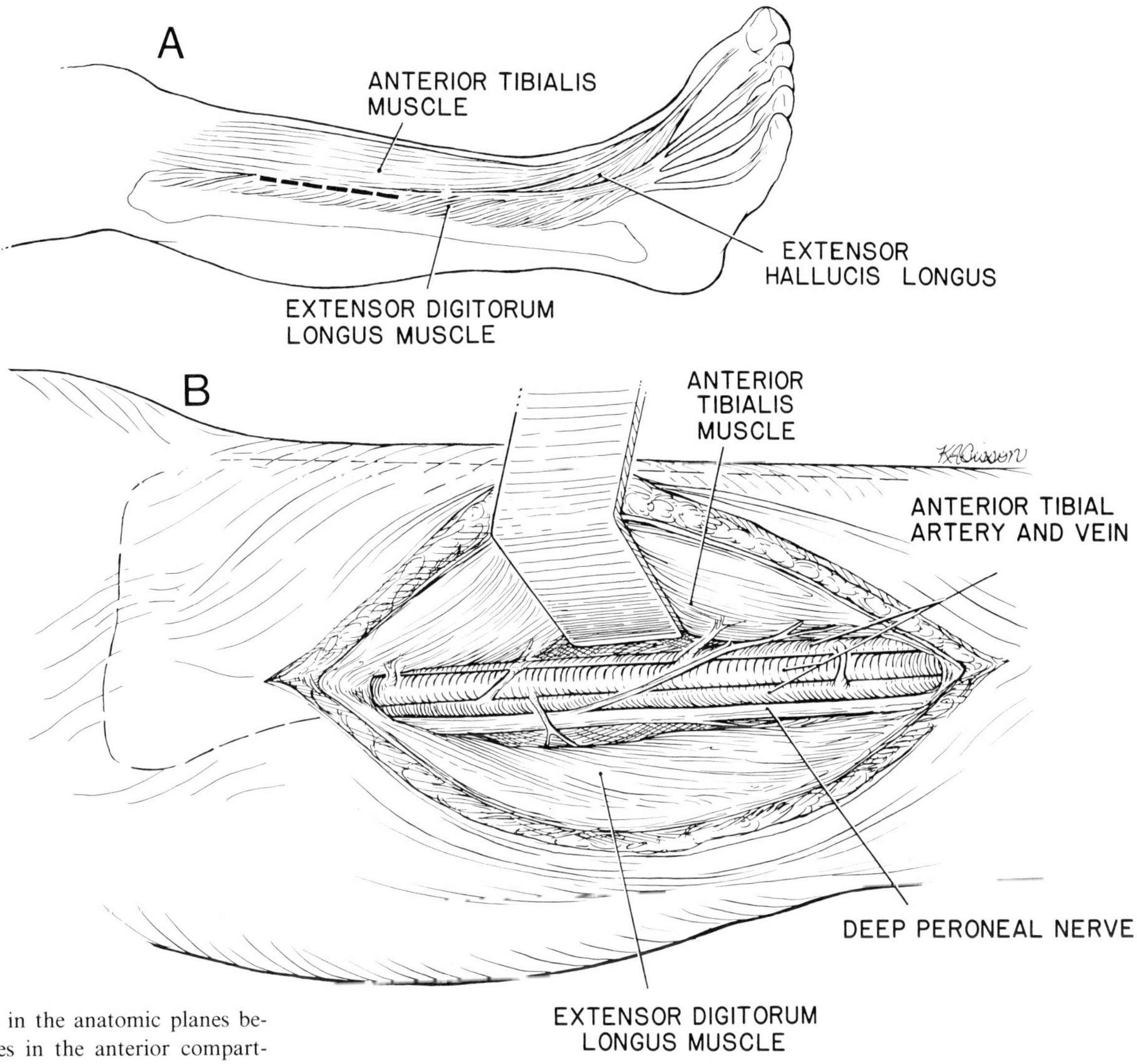

Fig. 7. Dissection in the anatomic planes between muscle bellies in the anterior compartment allows almost completely atraumatic exposure of the anterior tibial artery.

Proximal and distal control of the artery is obtained with small silastic slings (Vessel-Loops) that can be double-looped into the classic Potts' tie to prevent backflow during construction of the anastomosis. Individual small branches of the tibial artery are preserved as much as possible to insure maximum outflow. Control of these branches can usually be accomplished with smaller vessel loops held by the weight of a small mosquito hemostat. This provides control of back-bleeding without traumatizing the intima or shearing off the branches as looped sutures might.

When the distal artery has been chosen and a suitable area identified and dissected for the distal anastomosis, the graft material is chosen and passed through the anatomic tunnels. A subsartorial tunnel is created between the groin incision and the medial thigh wound. This is continued through the popliteal fossa between the heads of the gastrocnemius muscle and distally through the medial calf dissection to the posterior tibial or peroneal artery. If the anterior tibial artery is chosen as the distal outflow vessel, then a tunnel from the distal popliteal fossa to the anterior compartment is made by bluntly enlarging the v-shaped orifice normally present in the upper margin of the interosseous membrane. The tunnel continues between the muscle bellies through the anterior compartment to the level chosen for anastomosis.

Once the tunnel is completed and there is no evidence of bleeding, the patient is systemically anticoagulated with 5000 to 7500 units of heparin.

If two operating teams are available, it is desirable to perform the distal tibial anastomosis and the proximal common femoral anastomosis simultaneously. If this is not possible, the distal anastomosis is performed first, since it is the most critical and most technically demanding. The mid-leg popliteal anastomosis is performed last, because it is the least critical aspect of the reconstruction and because in some cases the atheromatous involvement of this vessel may make it unsuitable for anastomosis despite angiographic appearance of patency.

Examination, preparation, and anastomosis to the distal tibial artery are generally performed with loupe magnification. A longitudinal arteriotomy is performed for a distance of 2 to 2.5 cm. After careful inspection of the proposed anastomotic site to document the absence of significant disease, a No. 3 Fogarty catheter is passed distally to insure that no major atheromatous occlusion exists between the arteriotomy and the ankle. No attempt is made to fill the balloon on the catheter as this may cause intimal damage. The passage is simply to confirm the absence of occult distal disease. Coronary artery dilators are passed distally to size the vessel rather than to dilate it as, again, forceful dilation may cause intimal damage and resultant increased thrombogenicity. The size of the outflow vessel is recorded and, prior to the completion of the anastomosis, the same-size dilator is passed through the hood of the anastomosis to ensure that no narrowing of the outflow tract has occurred. After sizing, the distal vessel is irrigated with heparinized saline through a No. 16 or No. 18 intravenous cannula.

An arteriotomy 2.0 to 2.5 cm in length is made, and a similar-size graft hood is constructed. For Gore-tex grafts, the hood can be fashioned easily by placing a curved clamp on the graft. The excess graft material is cut with a surgical knife (Fig. 8). A 7–0 polypropylene double-armed suture is used. Initially, the heel of the anastomosis is tied in place to the artery. One half of the posterior row of sutures is then placed in a continuous fashion, and this suture is held with a rubber-shod mosquito hemostat while one half of the anterior sutures are placed. The posterior row is then again continued around the toe of the anastomosis. Care is taken to sew individual bites of graft and then artery, so that each arterial bite is taken full-thickness and under direct vision. After the suture line is completed around the toe, the appropriate coronary dilator is passed to ensure adequate luminal diameter as mentioned above. The anastomosis is then completed along the anterior wall in full view of the operating surgeon.

After completion of the distal tibial and proximal common femoral anastomoses, attention is turned to the midleg sequential anastomosis. Passage of the graft through previously described anatomical tunnels allows it to be approximated easily to the popliteal artery without undue kinking in the medial approach, either above or below the knee. If a segmental or composite sequential graft technique is used, then all anastomoses are performed in an end-to-side fashion. This is technically easier than fashioning a composite anastomosis at the popliteal level and allows for standardization of the anastomotic orifice in each case.

Fig. 8. Application of a curved clamp facilitates cutting of the PTFE graft.

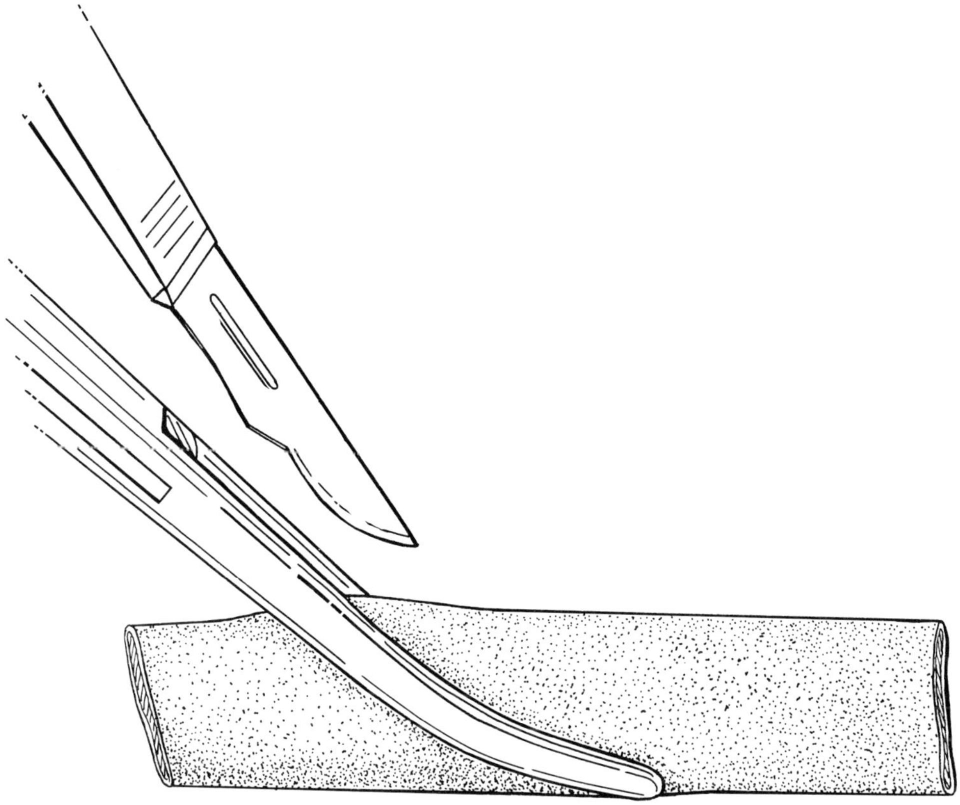

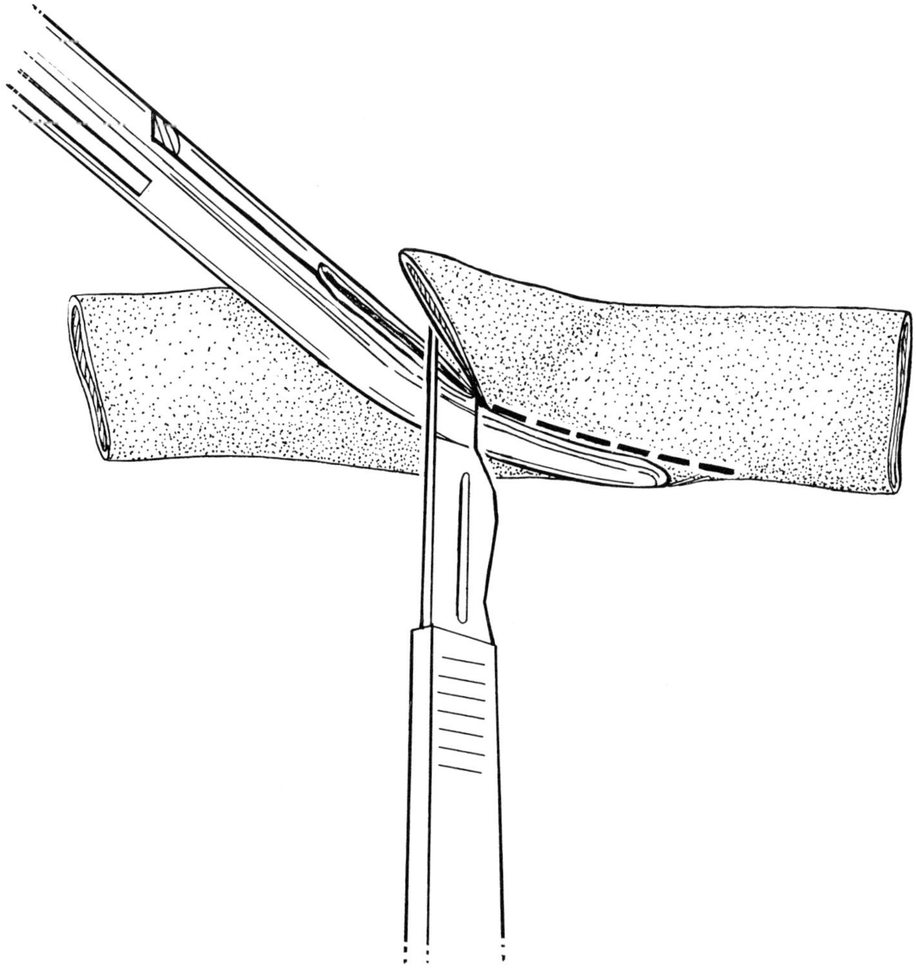

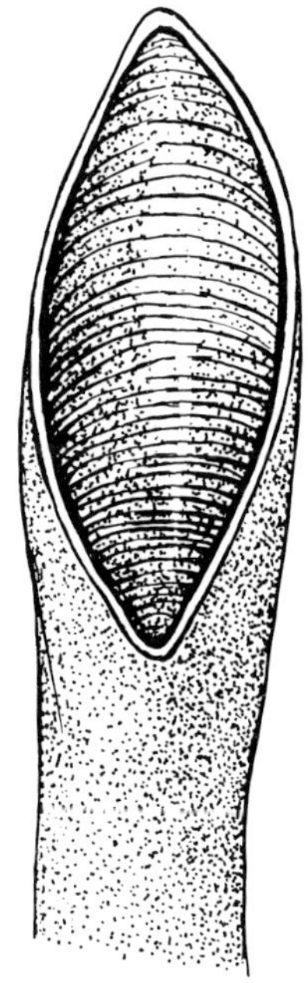

If sequential grafting is performed with a continuous graft of PTFE or autogenous saphenous vein, the popliteal anastomosis is performed side-to-side. By palpation of the artery, the least diseased portion of the popliteal segment that is accessible is chosen for the anastomosis. An arteriotomy 2 to 2.5 cm long is performed, and patency of the segment is confirmed by gentle passage of a coronary artery dilator or No. 3 Fogarty catheter. No attempt is made to endarterectomize the popliteal segment. A corresponding opening is made in the graft, and a small ellipse of vein or PTFE is removed in this area. The anastomosis is begun with a double-armed 6–0 polypropylene suture by tying the middle of the posterior wall of artery and graft (Fig. 9). One arm of the suture is then used to sew the distal portion of the posterior row until the distal corner is rounded. The proximal portion of the posterior row is then sutured with the remaining arm and continued around the proximal corner and down the anterior row. The anastomosis is completed along the anterior wall, and the two sutures are tied together. With the anastomosis of the described length and with the relative rigidity of the popliteal segment, there is really no danger of purse stringing.

During the restoration of distal flow, the graft is first flushed to the retrograde and then to the antegrade portion of the popliteal segment. Finally, flow is restored to the distal graft segment and the tibial outflow vessel. If autogenous saphenous vein has been used as a continuous sequential graft or as the distal segment of a composite sequential bypass, flow rate through the graft can be measured using an electromagnetic flowmeter. An attempt should be made to record flow measurements first with the popliteal anastomosis occluded and then with it opened, to ascertain its effect on overall limb blood flow. Edwards, Gerity, and Larkin[4] have described increased flow in sequential grafts after opening this anastomosis. This may seem somewhat cumbersome when a side-to-side popliteal anastomosis has been performed, but it can be accomplished simply by temporarily occluding the popliteal artery above and below the anastomosis with arterial tissue forceps. This will facilitate accurate measurement without distorting the vein graft or traumatizing the popliteal segment.

Intraoperative arteriography is performed at the conclusion of the procedure. Direct puncture of the graft is performed, and a 20-gauge intravenous cannula is advanced into the lumen just below the common femoral anastomosis. The graft is crossclamped proximally and contrast material injected. Usually, it is necessary to perform two separate exposures to examine the technical adequacy of the two anastomoses as well as to delineate clearly the anatomy of the distal tibial runoff vessel and the pedal collateral circulation. The x-ray cassettes are wrapped in sterile covers and positioned appropriately under the leg as described previously for prebypass arteriography. Generally, the first exposure is performed to delineate the knee area and the proximal anastomosis, and a second exposure is used for the distal anastomosis and the foot. Because of the diversion of some of the contrast material through the proximal anastomosis, visualization of the pedal circulation is facilitated by release of the proximal occluding clamp on the graft after a 3- to 5-second delay after the contrast has been injected. Once the intraoperative arteriogram has demonstrated satisfactory technical results, closure of the wound is effected in the usual manner using Dexon sutures for fascia and subcuticular closure for the skin.

Fig. 9. Technique for performing side-to-side anastomosis in continuous sequential graft. Beginning in the midposterior wall allows precise placement of full thickness arterial bites to minimize leakage from this less-accessible area. Completion anteriorly facilitates back-bleeding and flushing of the anastomosis under direct vision.

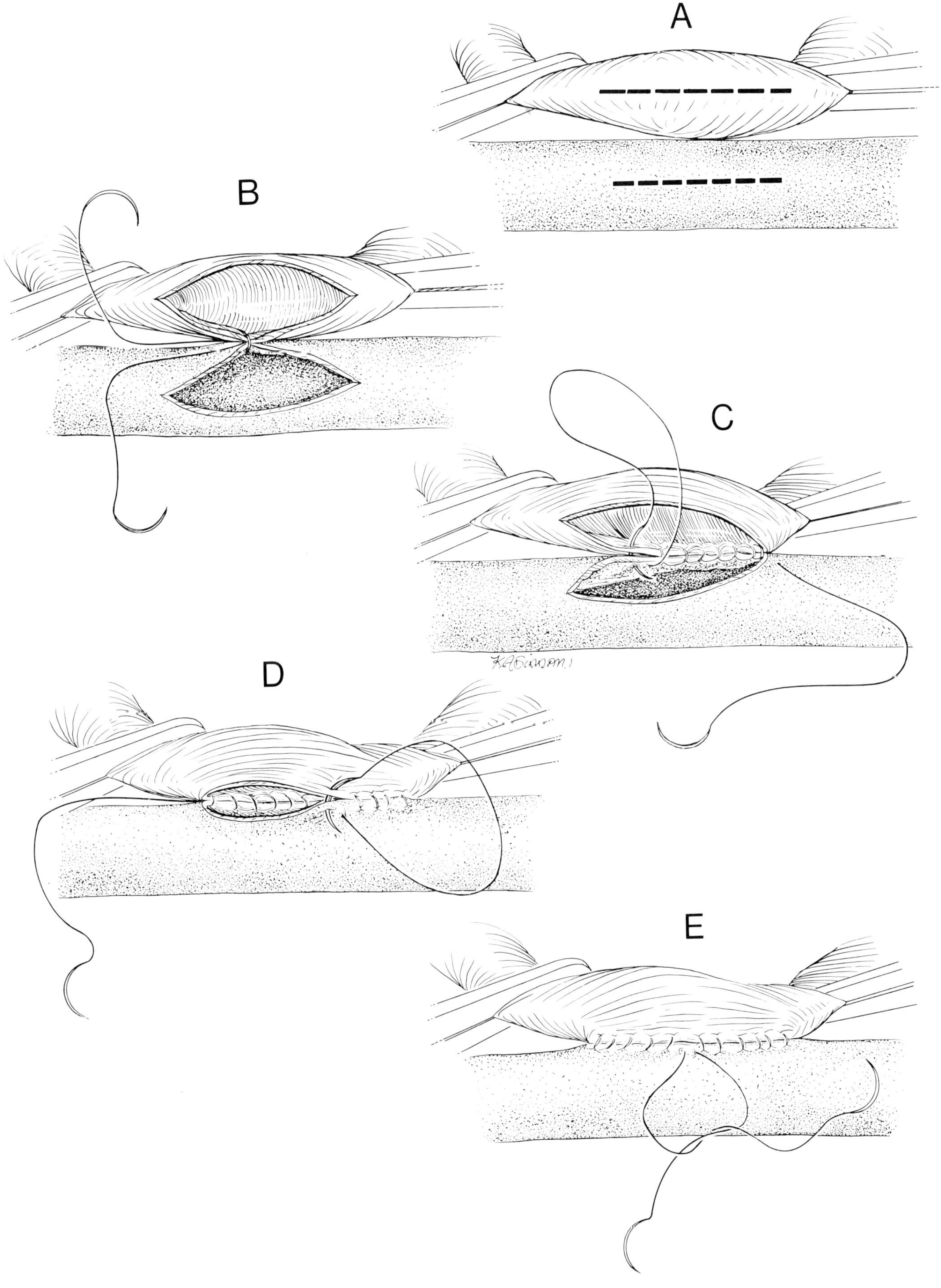
A
B
C
D
E

COMMENTS

Sequential femoropopliteal-tibial bypass is a useful technique for relief of severe ischemia in patients with complex, multisegmental atherosclerotic arterial occlusions in the lower extremity. Increased outflow tracts may provide more comprehensive limb revascularization than increased flow through a single graft. This technique may allow successful use of a segment of saphenous vein in a composite configuration when the entire vein, for one reason or another, would not be of sufficient length as a continuous graft. This technique also has the advantage of having flexible vein pass behind the knee joint. Also, electromagnetic flowmeter measurements may be made. Initial experience with composite sequential grafts has been gratifying.[6] In our experience, even with distal occlusion of the sequential graft, perfusion of the foot has been preserved by the remaining proximal limb of the graft. Consequently, an increased rate of limb salvage may be achieved with this technique.

REFERENCES

1. Mannick JA, Jackson BT, Coffman JD: Success of bypass vein grafts in patients with isolated popliteal artery segments. Surgery 61:17, 1967
2. DeLaurentis DA, Friedman P: Arterial reconstruction about and below the knee: Another look. Am J Surg 121:392, 1971
3. Bliss BP, Fonseka N: "Hitch-hike" grafts for limb salvage in peripheral arterial disease. Br J Surg 63:562, 1976
4. Edwards WS, Gerity E, Larkin J: Multiple sequential femoral tibial grafting for severe ischemia. Surgery 80:722, 1976
5. Jarrett F, Berkhoff HA, Crummy AB: Sequential femoral-tibial bypass grafting for limb salvage. Ann Surg 188:685, 1978
6. Flinn WR, Flanigan DP, Verta MJ Jr, Bergan JJ, Yao JST: Sequential femoral-tibial bypass for severe limb ischemia. Surgery 88:357, 1980

Composite Arterial Grafting

Jonathan B. Towne

The saphenous vein remains the benchmark for lower extremity arterial grafting, having withstood the test of time for both femoral-popliteal and femoral-tibial bypasses. Satisfactory 5- and 10-year patency rates have documented the durability of this conduit. However, in approximately twenty percent of patients, the saphenous vein is either inadequate or not present. Previous stripping and ligation, varicose degeneration of the vein, diameter less than 4 mm, duplication of a segment of the vein resulting in two channels of marginal size, and areas of fibrous thickening from previous superficial phlebitis render the saphenous vein unuseable for peripheral arterial grafting. The surgeon in this situation has two choices: use of artificial conduits such as knitted Dacron or polytetraflur-oethylene (PTFE), or composite grafting. Composite grafting in its commonest form utilizes autogenous vein to cross the knee and for the distal anastomosis and artificial graft proximal to the knee. A less commonly used form of composite grafting is the combination of a short segment of reversed autogenous vein with thromboendarterectomy and/or patch angioplasty of the femoral system. Other uses of composite grafting in vascular surgery include patch angioplasty of the profunda femoris artery with autogenous tissue performed in conjunction with aortofemoral bypass, and the use of autogenous tissue for the extra-anatomic bypass of arterial sepsis. Autogenous vein has many characteristics that make it ideal as an arterial substitute. Its endothelium resists thromboses in low-flow bypasses such as distal popliteal and tibial grafts. It is flexible and tolerates bending at the knee joint quite well. Also because it is autogenous tissue, it resists infection better than nonviable artificial grafts.

COMPOSITE VEIN ARTIFICIAL GRAFT

The combination of autogenous vein and artificial graft is a valuable technique when there is not sufficient saphenous vein to perform a femoral-distal bypass. This technique, which was popularized by Linton and Wirthlin,[1] usually utilizes 6- or 8-mm knitted Dacron or 6.5 × 4.5 mm polytetrafluroethylene (PTFE) for the proximal portion. Usually there is sufficient vein of at least 4 mm in diameter to extend across the knee joint to the distal anastomosis. In patients who have had previous stripping and ligation of the saphenous vein or have had a previous saphenous femoral-distal bypass, a segment of arm vein, usually the cephalic, is a satisfactory alternate. Because arm veins are not subjected to the hydrostatic pressure that the saphenous system encounters, they are thin-walled and must be delicately dissected to avoid injury. A continuous incision rather than multiple interrupted incisions is recommended for vein harvest. The largest vein in the forearm is identified just distal to the wrist and dissected proximally, choosing the larger diameter channel at all branch points. The branches are ligated with 3–0 nonabsorbable suture adjacent to the vein graft and occluded distally with metallic clips. Because of the fragility of the arm veins, special care must be taken to avoid compromising the venous lumen with the ligature, as illustrated by Campbell and associates.[2] The cephalic vein is most commonly used, but on occasion the basilic vein is a better graft.

It is ideal to place the vein–artificial graft anastomosis so that it can be visualized through the incision at the adductor hiatus made to tunnel the graft from the popliteal fossa, so that when flow is restored the anastomosis can be checked for suture-line bleeding. The distal anastomosis is done first in the usual end-to-side fashion. We utilize the pneumatic tourniquet to avoid the application of vascular clamps on the popliteal and tibial arteries.[3] This aids in the performance of the anastomosis by not having clamps in the way and avoiding trauma to the vessels. The most important aspect of composite grafting is the performance of the vein-to-graft anastomosis. This should be a gradual tapering transition from the prosthesis to the vein to reduce the tendency for tubulent flow, which occurs with abrupt changes in graft diameter, and to compensate for compliance mismatch between the two conduits. We do not use a stent in construction of this anastomosis as recommended by Linton;[4] however, we calibrate the anastomosis with a 4-mm coronary artery dilator prior to completion of the anastomosis. Both the vein graft and the artificial graft are cut on a bevel, so that the anastomosis is approximately 4 to 5 cm long (Fig. 1). The tip of each graft is cut transversely so that it is blunt and approximately 2.5 mm wide. The anastomosis is begun by placing a stitch in the tip of the prosthesis, suturing it into the crotch-like defect in the saphenous vein. The anastomosis is constructed with a continuous running suture beginning at the anchoring suture and extending one-third the distance down each side. Attention is then directed to the opposite end, where the anastomosis is similarly constructed. Care must be taken not to place the suture so tightly that the vein is stretched as a drumhead over the artificial graft. The bites in the vein have to be approximately 1 mm deep and 1 mm apart. The anastomosis is then completed in the standard fashion.

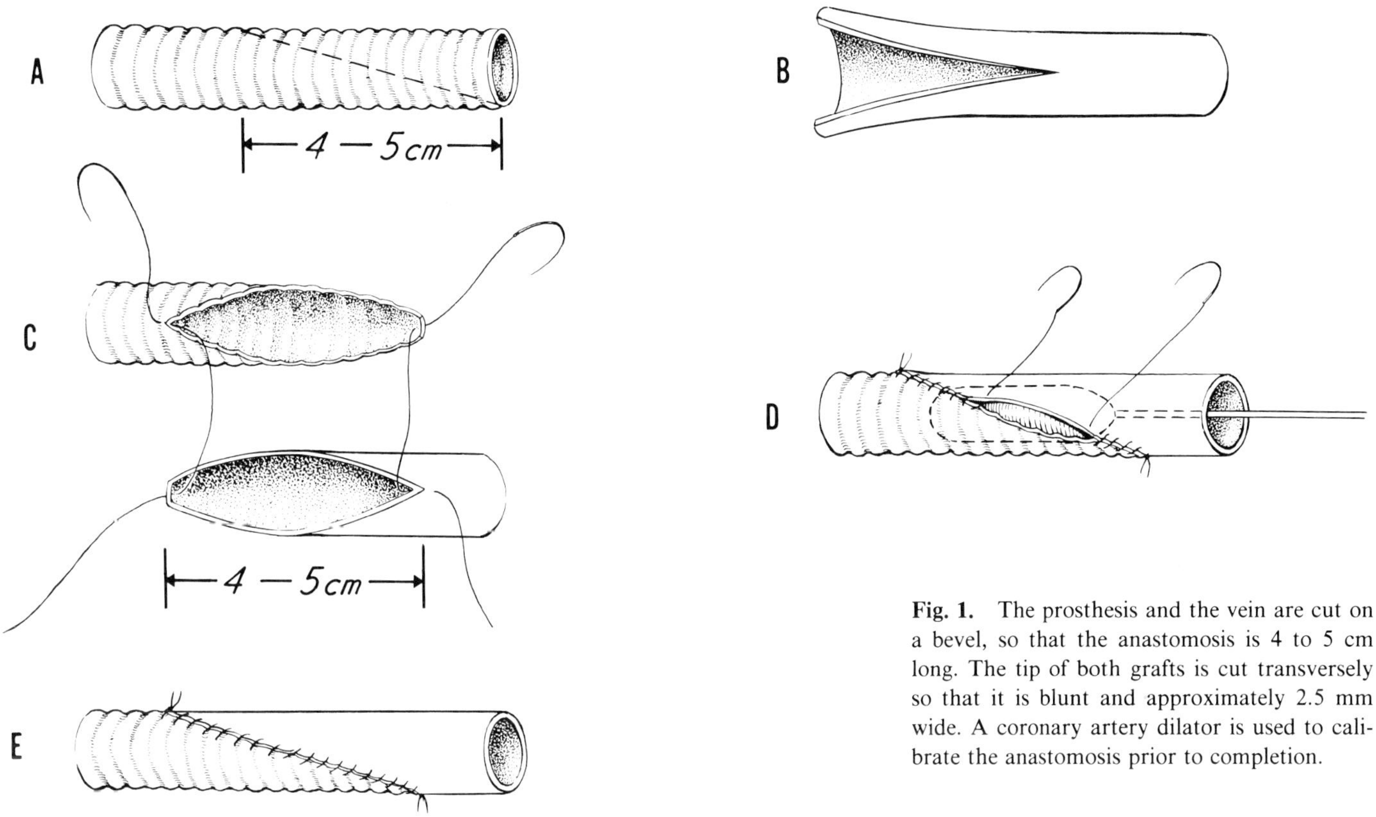

Fig. 1. The prosthesis and the vein are cut on a bevel, so that the anastomosis is 4 to 5 cm long. The tip of both grafts is cut transversely so that it is blunt and approximately 2.5 mm wide. A coronary artery dilator is used to calibrate the anastomosis prior to completion.

Following completion of the distal anastomosis, a small bulldog clamp is placed across the distal vein graft. When the composite anastomosis is completed, the vein graft is distended with heparinized Ringer's solution. This again allows examination of the anastomosis, and more importantly aids in avoiding twisting the graft while placing the graft in the subfascial tunnel (Fig. 2). The proximal anastomosis is usually performed at the common femoral artery. On occasion, thromboendarterectomy of the common femoral with an orifice profundaplasty is required. In this situation, the artificial graft will serve as a patch angioplasty of the common femoral artery. The anastomosis is performed with a 5–0 suture. Following completion of the proximal anastomosis, a vascular clamp is placed across the proximal graft and blood flow is restored in the common femoral artery while the vascular graft remains clamped. This allows correction of any suture line defects in the proximal anastomosis prior to establishing flow in the graft. If at all possible, we try to avoid clamping the graft for any reason following restoration of blood flow to the lower leg. Following restoration of flow, an operative angiogram is obtained. This is of particular importance in composite arterial grafting because there are three anastomoses and the vein-graft anastomosis can be the site of a twist in the graft (Figs. 3–4).

The choice of the arterial conduit is either 6- or 8-mm knitted Dacron graft or 6.5-mm to 4.5-mm tapered PTFE graft. PTFE is more convenient to use because of its taper and because it does not require preclotting. Since extensive experience with PTFE is just approaching 3 years, reliable long-term data regarding its durability are not available at this time.

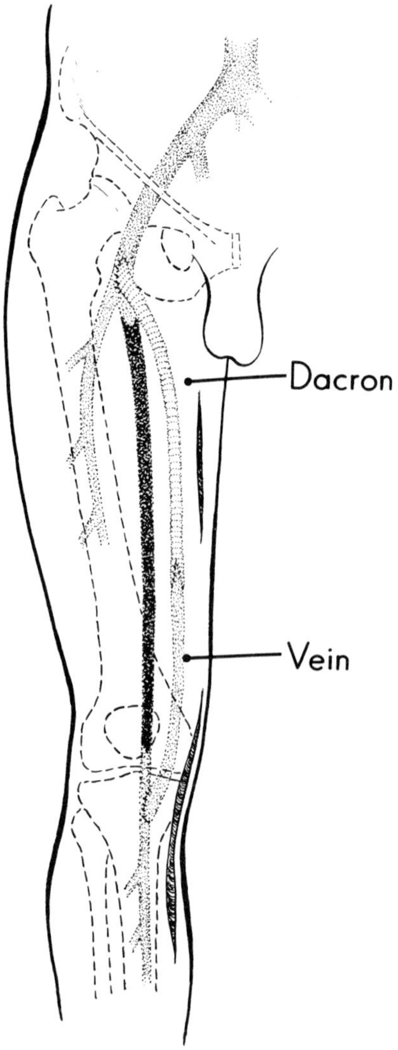

Fig. 2. The graft is placed in a subfascial tunnel. The proximal anastomosis is performed at the common femoral artery.

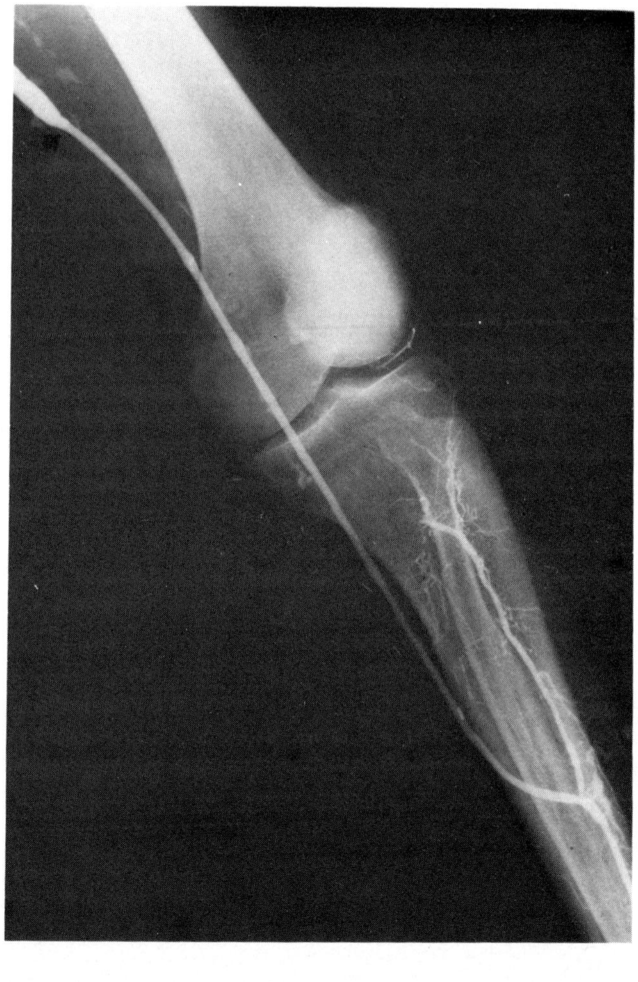

Fig. 3. Composite femoral-tibial graft of bovine and autogenous vein. The anastomosis has a smooth taper without evidence of twists.

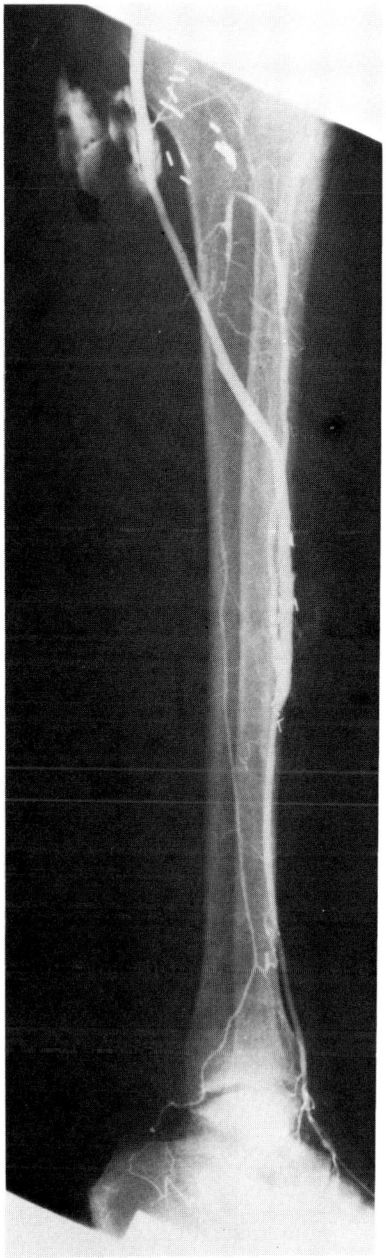

Fig. 4. Composite femoral tibial bypass of PTFE and autogenous vein. The arrow marks the site of the composite anastomosis. There was not sufficient autogenous vein to extend proximal to the knee joint as is desirable. The extravasation is from the composite anastomosis, which stopped spontaneously.

Several modifications of this technique of composite grafting have been proposed. In an attempt to avoid twisting or kinking of the composite anastomosis, DeLaurentis and Friedman[5] have proposed performing a femoral proximal popliteal bypass using an 8-mm Dacron tube, performing, if necessary, a thromboendarterectomy on the proximal popliteal artery. A short segment of autogenous vein is then used to perform a separate popliteal-to-tibial or distal popliteal bypass (Fig. 5A). This eliminates the need for the composite anastomosis; however, it does require the construction of an additional anastomosis. Another modification suggested by Lord and colleagues[6] was to perform the composite anastomosis end-to-side rather than end-to-end. This is done by ligating the vein approximately 3 cm proximal to the composite anastomosis (Fig. 5B). A long end-to-side graft to saphenous vein anastomosis is constructed measuring 20 to 25 mm in length. Following completion of the anastomosis, a suture is then used to encircle the vein at the proximal end of the anastomosis to obliterate the cul-de-sac between the proximal anastomosis and the suture used to ligate the vein. This avoids thrombus formation, which could possibly extend into the anastomosis and embolize distally. The composite anastomosis is then anchored to the fascia by suturing the obliterated proximal portion of the vein graft to the adductor fascia, which prevents twisting of the anastomosis. I have not found either of these measures necessary if care is given to the tunneling of the graft and if operative angiograms are obtained.

A reliable technique for insuring that twisting has not occurred during passage of the graft through the tunnel is to intermittently pulse 3 to 4 ml of heparinized Ringer's solution into the arterial conduit at its proximal end. If the pressure wave can easily be felt throughout the length of the graft and at the distal anastomosis, the graft is in proper position without twists.

Thromboendarterectomy of the superficial femoral artery with vein bypass from the distal superficial femoral artery to the distal popliteal or tibial vessels is useful in exceptional circumstances. Variations of this technique include the semiclosed endarterectomy as recommended by Bartos et al[7] and the long proximal patch angioplasty of the entire superficial femoral artery as described by Linton et al.[8] The former is unreliable and the latter is tedious and time-consuming and associated with poor long-term patency rates. These techniques should therefore be limited to specific circumstances and not routinely employed.

USE OF COMPOSITE GRAFTS IN ARTERIAL SEPSIS

One of the most difficult problems in vascular surgery is the treatment of vascular infection in the femoral triangle. Most commonly, this is the result of infection in the distal limb of an aortofemoral bypass, the proximal portion of a femoral distal bypass, or the prolonged use of balloon pumping. Surgical care has two objectives. The first is the eradication of infection, which in most instances requires excision of the infected graft and debridement of the host vessel with suture ligation of all femoral artery branches or vein patch angioplasty to close the defect in the femoral artery. The second and more technically challenging objective is to maintain limb viability with extra-anatomical bypass grafts. When adequate length of autogenous vein is not available, composite arterial grafting is a useful technique for rerouting blood around an infected groin. Because of its inherent ability to resist infection, autogenous vein is used for the distal anastomosis and that portion of the graft passing adjacent to the infected area. The medial crossover femoral–femoral graft can be used when sepsis is limited to one groin and there is not significant obstructive disease in the contralateral iliac system. If there has been no exsanguinating hemorrhage which makes immediate vascular control a life-saving measure, the extra-anatomical bypass is inserted first, followed 2 days later by the excisional debridement of the infected region. This 48-hour interval allows for adequate sealing of the bypass incisions.

The patient is placed supine on the operating table. Adhesive plastic drapes are used to exclude the infected femoral triangle from the operative field, and the patient is then prepped and draped in the usual manner. If the distal superficial femoral artery is patent, the medial incision is made in mid-thigh, exposing the distal superficial femoral artery in its subsartorial canal (Fig. 6). If the superficial femoral artery is occluded, the proximal popliteal artery is exposed at the adductor hiatus. A small transverse incision is made in the skin at the inferior border of the symphysis pubis and subcutaneous tunnel is made passing adjacent to the scrotum in men and labia in women, along the most medial aspect of the thigh. Saphenous vein or cephalic vein is harvested and used for the distal anastomosis. The vein has to be long enough to extend from the distal anastomosis to the medial aspect of the pubic tubercle, so that autogenous vein is the graft material adjacent to the infected groin. A composite anastomosis 4 to 5 cm long is then constructed, using monofilament suture. The prosthetic end of the composite graft is then tunneled across the pubis to the contralateral external iliac or femoral artery.

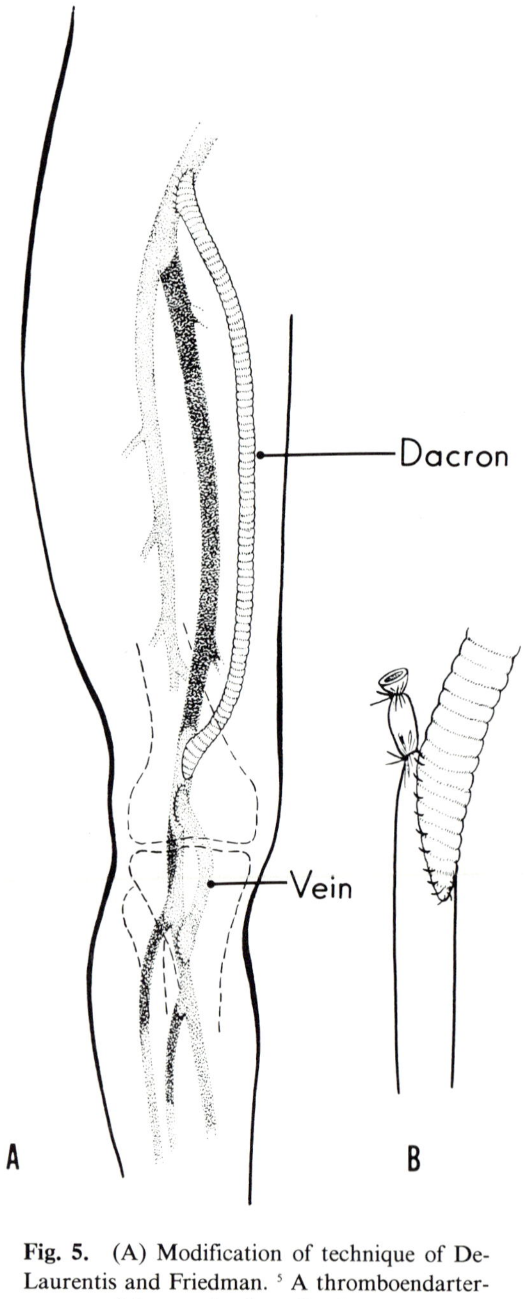

Fig. 5. (A) Modification of technique of DeLaurentis and Friedman.[5] A thromboendarterectomy of the proximal popliteal artery is often necessary.
(B) Modification of technique of Lord et al. It is important to ligate the vein at the proximal end of the anastomosis to obliterate the cul-de-sac between the proximal anastomosis and the suture used to ligate the vein.

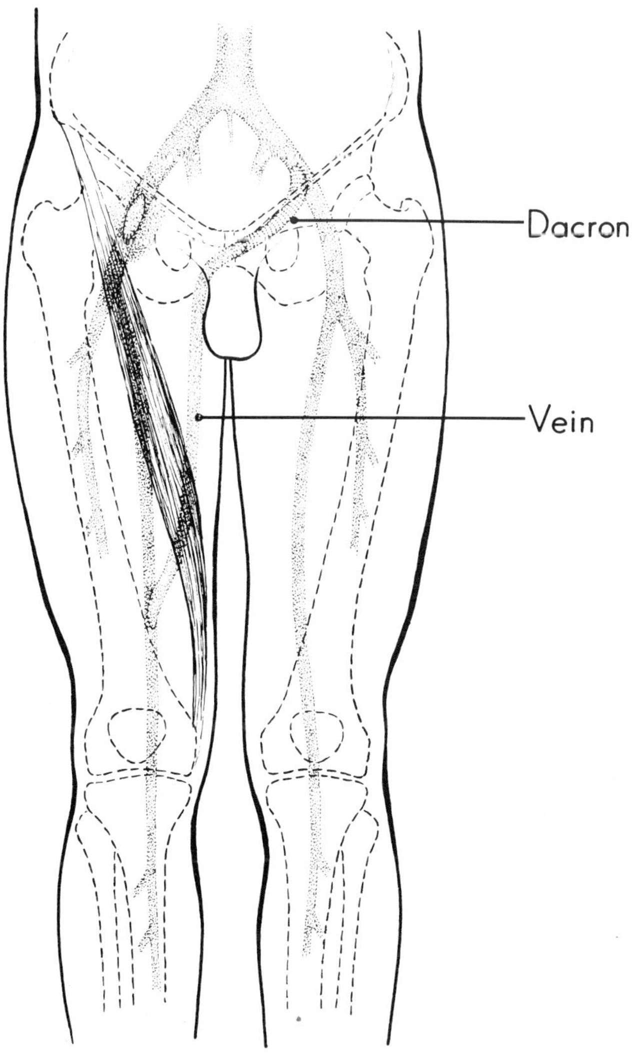

Fig. 6. Medial crossover femoral–femoral graft. It is important to make the subcutaneous tunnel inferior to the symphysis pubis and adjacent to the scrotum in men and labia in women.

When the contralateral iliac femoral system cannot be used as a source of blood supply because of bilateral infection or occlusive disease, a composite axillary-femoral graft can be carried to the middle third of the profunda femoris artery or to the distal femoral popliteal segment if it is patent (Fig. 7). The profunda femoris artery is exposed through a lateral approach. The patient is placed on the operating table and the infected groin is excluded with plastic adhesive drapes. The incision is made at the junction of the proximal and middle third of the thigh, parallel and lateral to the sartorius and adjacent to the lateral border of the rectus femoris muscle. A plane of dissection is then developed medially beneath rectus femoris muscle but superficial to the vastus medialis muscle to the adductor longus muscle. The fibers of the adductor longus muscle are spread revealing the middle third of the profunda femoris artery. The tunnel is then developed proximally from this point. In some patients, it is possible to pass just medial to the anterior superior iliac spine without contamination from the infected field. However, in other cases where this is not possible, we cut a notch in the wing of the ileum for the graft, allowing the course of the graft to be more lateral. An 8-mm Dacron graft is used to construct the usual end-to-side anastomosis to the axillary artery. The graft is tunneled beneath the pectoralis major muscle along the anterior axillary line to the groin. Autogenous vein is harvested so that there is sufficient graft to extend from the distal anastomosis in the mid-profunda artery proximal to the anterior superior iliac spine. The composite anastomosis is constructed as previously outlined. The wound is then closed, and, if possible, the infected graft is removed 2 days later. In performing these secondary procedures for arterial sepsis, it is important that accurate and precise bacteriology be obtained and that the patient be on adequate levels of the appropriate antibiotic preoperatively. These techniques have been used in several cases without any incidence of secondary infection of the bypass graft.

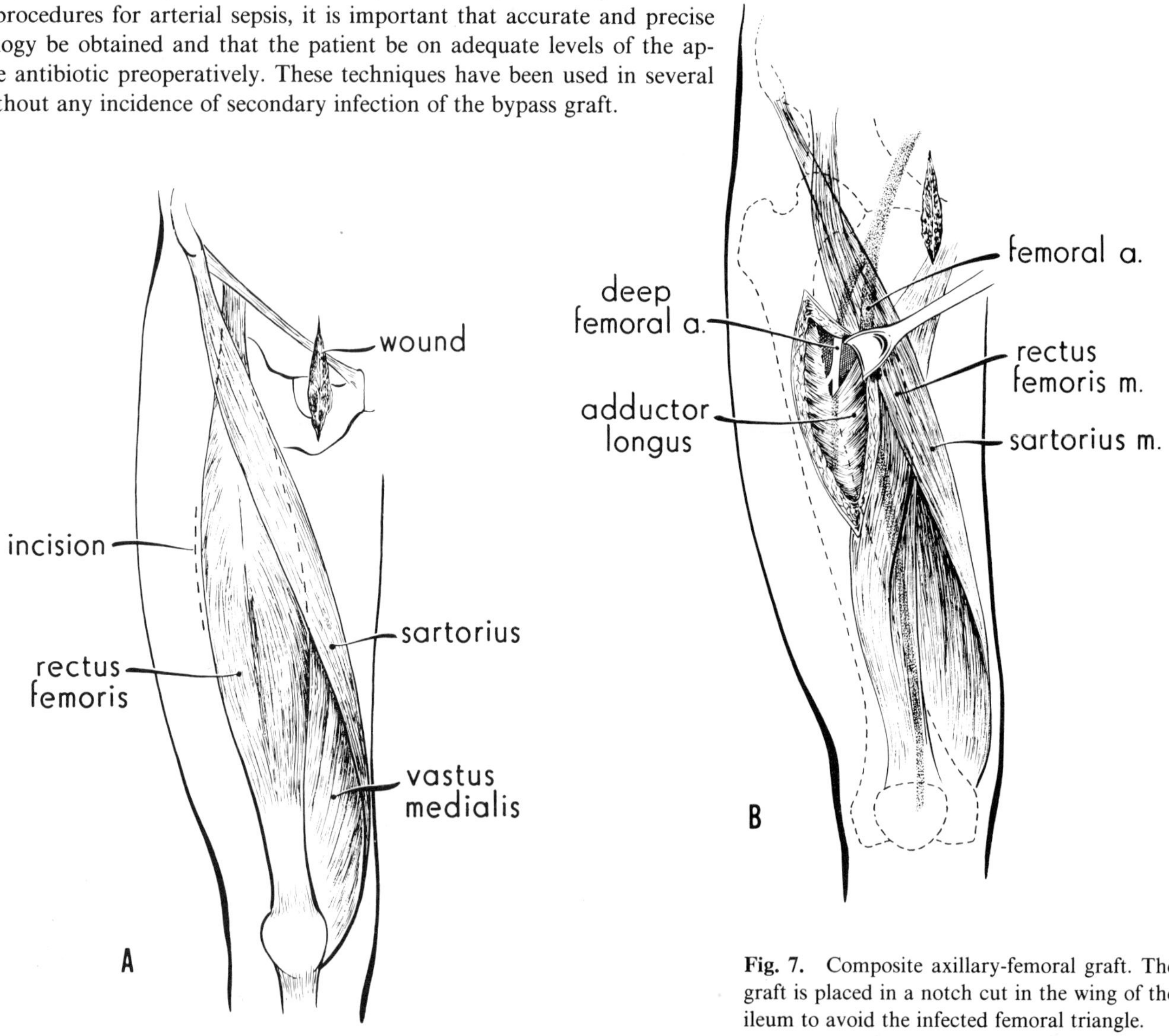

Fig. 7. Composite axillary-femoral graft. The graft is placed in a notch cut in the wing of the ileum to avoid the infected femoral triangle.

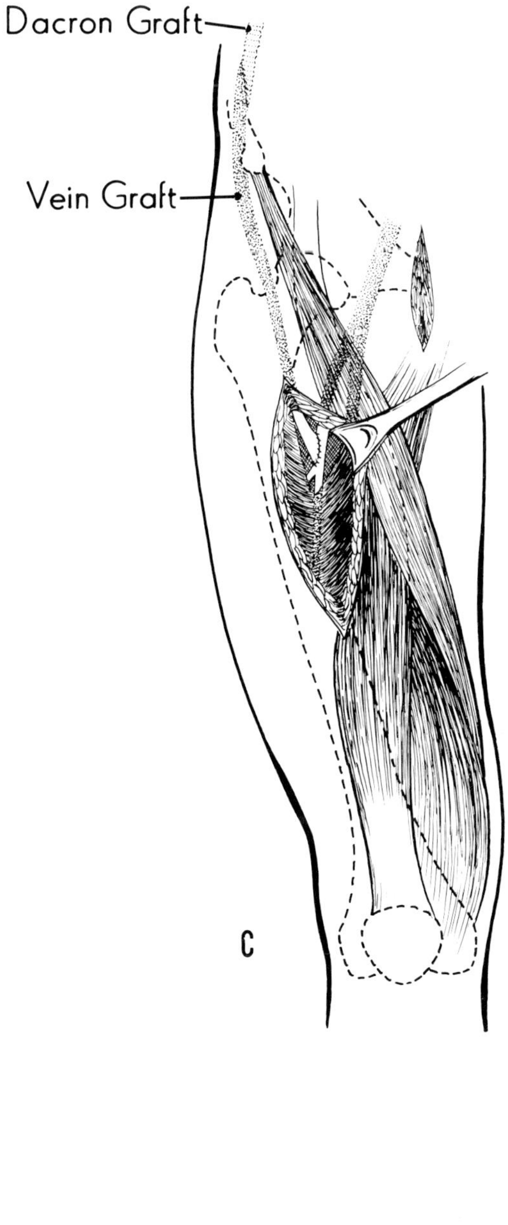

C

USE OF COMPOSITE GRAFTS IN AORTOFEMORAL BYPASSES

Another use of composite arterial grafting is the performance of profundaplasty in conjunction with aortofemoral bypass. In patients who require profundaplasty as an adjunct to an aortofemoral bypass, the superficial femoral artery is invariably occluded. On occasion, the profundaplasty must be extended 8 to 10 cm distally to insure sufficient runoff to maintain patency of the aortofemoral graft and ultimate viability of the lower extremity. In these situations, we have preferred a composite graft using a segment of superficial femoral artery (Fig. 8). The superficial femoral artery is excised and incised in its long dimension, with removal of the occluding atherosclerotic core. The resulting patch material consists of the adventitia and occasionally the media. The patch is tailored to the profunda femoris artery using 5–0 suture in the standard fashion (Fig. 9). The endarterectomized patch is then sutured to the limb of the aortofemoral graft and the common femoral artery. The advantage of using the endarterectomized superficial femoral artery as a patch is that it is autogenous tissue that does not leak, does not require preclotting, and it is easy to handle, enabling a more precise profundaplasty to be fashioned.

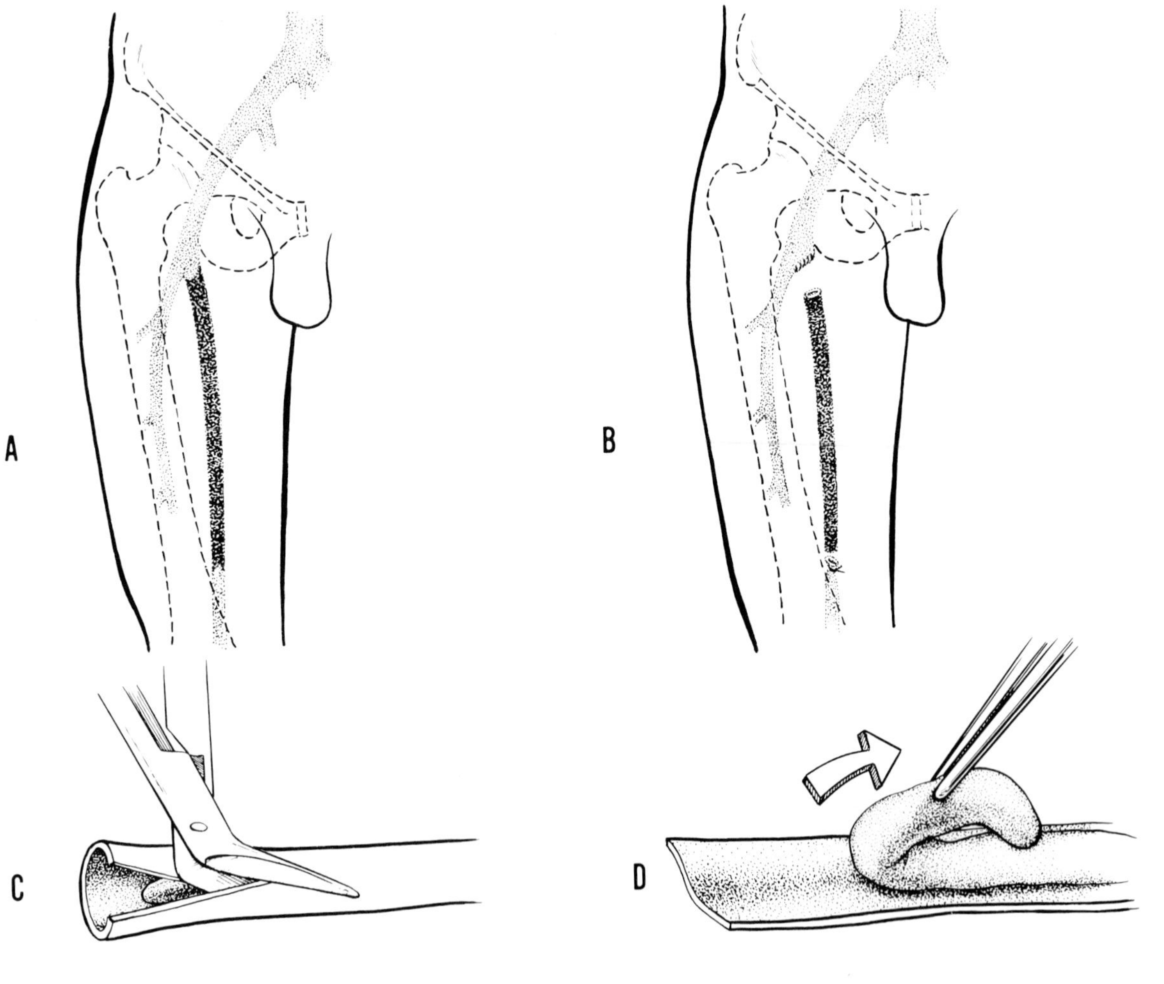

Fig. 8. The occluded superficial femoral artery is harvested and incised lengthwise, and an endarterectomy is performed.

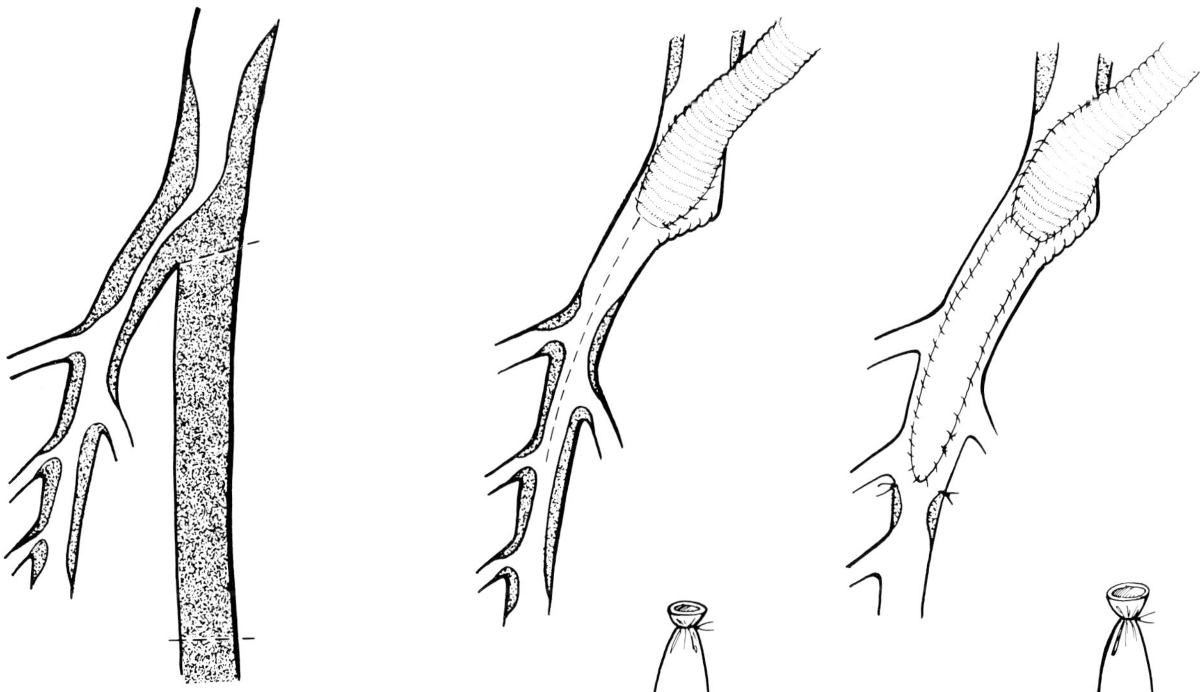

A B C

Fig. 9. Composite profundaplasty. The segment of endarterectomized superficial artery is used to patch the profunda. The distal intima is tacked distally. Proximally the patch is sutured to the limb of the aortofemoral graft.

DISCUSSION

Results of composite arterial grafting are not as good as those of autogenous vein grafts. It is more time-consuming, requiring the construction of at least one extra anastomosis. Despite these inherent disadvantages, satisfactory results can be obtained with composite grafts. The only published long-term study of composite grafts was conducted by Linton and Wirthlin[1] who reported a 5-year patency of 55 percent as compared to 72 percent with autogenous vein grafts. Composite grafts constructed with autogenous veins combined with various forms of thrombectomy, endarterectomy, and patch angioplasty of the superficial femoral system have had dismal patency rates of only 25 percent at 3 years.[8] Only time will tell whether composite vein graft is better than PTFE graft for infrageniculate anastomoses. The construction of an extra anatomosis, as well as the composite anastomosis of two different graft materials, make the prevention of kinks and twists of the graft more difficult. An end-to-end anastomosis using the trianglation technique rather than the long tapered anastomosis was associated with poor patency rates as reported by Dale et al.[9] Therefore, the construction of the composite anastomosis must be precise and must use the long tapered anastomosis advocated by Linton.

Composite grafting for revascularizing the lower extremities in cases of graft sepsis is a very useful but thankfully a seldom-needed technique. Using this technique we have been able to salvage limbs and have not had secondary infection of the bypass graft. In general, composite grafting is a technique that should be used by the vascular surgeon in very selected instances and that, if carefully performed, will yield acceptable results.

REFERENCES

1. Linton RR, Wirthlin LS: Femoropopliteal composite Dacron and autogenous vein bypass grafts. Arch Surg 107:748–753, 1973
2. Campbell R, Hoar CS Jr, Gibbons GW: The use of arm veins in femoral-popliteal bypass grafts. Ann Surg 190:740–742, 1979
3. Bernhard VM, Boren CH, Towne J B: Pneumatic tourniquet as a substitute for vascular clamps in distal bypass surgery. Surgery 80:709–713, 1980
4. Linton RR: Atlas of Vascular Surgery. Philadelphia, WB Saunders Co, 1973, pp 454–463
5. DeLaurentis, DA, Friedman P: Sequential femoropopliteal bypasses: Another approach to the inadequate saphenous vein problem. Surgery 71:400–404, 1972
6. Lord, JW Jr, Sadranagani B, Bajwa G, Rossi G: New technique for construction of composite vein grafts for femoro-distal popliteal bypass in the severely ischemic leg. Ann Surg 181:670–675, 1975.
7. Bartos J, Vancara J, Tersip K: Revascularization of severe ischemic legs. Angiologica 78:226–232, 1970
8. Linton, RR, Wilde WL: Modifications in the technique for femoropopliteal saphenous vein bypass autografts. Surgery 67:234–248, 1970
9. Dale WA, Pridgen WR, Shoulders HH Jr: Failure of composite (Teflon and vein) grafting in small human arteries. Surgery 51:258–262, 1962

Peripheral Arterial Aneurysms

Robert W. Hobson II, Zafar Jamil,
Thomas G. Lynch

Peripheral arterial aneurysms are common in vascular surgical practice. They occur in an aging population and their existence may be confirmed by ultrasound with low morbidity. Atherosclerosis is the most common cause, but aneurysms have been described in virtually all peripheral arteries due to many additional causes including trauma, syphilis, congenital defects, and mycotic involvement of a peripheral artery. These aneurysms become symptomatic by expansion and compression of local neural or other structures, whether or not frank rupture, thrombosis and distal embolization occur. Femoral and popliteal arterial aneurysms may be bilateral or coexistent in the same patient. Cutler and Darling[1] reported 45 patients with femoral arterial aneurysms, 12 of whom had associated popliteal aneurysms, and 23 of whom had associated abdominal aortic aneurysms. The association of abdominal aortic aneurysm with popliteal aneurysm has been documented in approximately one half of patients by Wychulis et al[2] and Evans,[3] particularly in the presence of bilateral popliteal arterial aneurysms.[3] Femoral and popliteal aneurysms are second only to arteriosclerotic occlusive disease as a cause of vascular insufficiency in the lower extremities,[4] and surgical management is commonly required.

Subclavian artery aneurysms are also important. Most are caused by thoracic-outlet compression of the artery by the first rib. Post-stenotic arterial dilitation occurs. Atherosclerosis is also of some etiologic significance.[5]

POPLITEAL ARTERIAL ANEURYSM

Surgical management of popliteal arterial aneurysm includes the classic technique of proximal and distal arterial ligation[6] with or without excision of the aneurysm. Arterial reconstruction is done with autogenous saphenous vein or prosthesis. Although excision of popliteal aneurysms was recommended previously,[7] proximal and distal ligation, evacuation of the thrombus, and suture ligation of arterial branches from within the aneurysm by the technique of "endo-aneurismorrhaphy" similar to that described by Matas[8] is preferred. This technique avoids interruption of adjacent popliteal veins, which are frequently adherent to the wall of the aneurysm.

The aneurysm may be approached surgically from the medial aspect of the leg with the patient supine or through the popliteal fossa posteriorly with the patient in the prone position. We have generally employed the medial approach as demonstrated in Figure 1. Although the aneurysm may be explored medially and excised after transection of the medial head of the gastrocnemius muscle as well as the tendons of the gracilis, semitendinous, and semimembranous muscles (Fig. 1B–C), we have preferred to perform proximal and distal ligation with bypass grafting using autogenous saphenous vein (Fig. 1A). The operation is performed using systemic heparinization. A Fogarty catheter is passed distally to remove any thrombus if embolization has occurred or if thrombosis of the aneurysm has developed preoperatively. In a few instances, distal tibial bypass has been required for limb salvage in cases of popliteal aneurysmal disease. When the aneurysm is sizeable and the remaining thrombosed aneurysm would create an anatomical problem at the knee, the technique of endo-aneurysmorrhaphy followed by reconstruction of the popliteal artery is preferred. Using this technique, we have generally excised the redundant portion of the aneurysm avoiding trauma to the adjacent popliteal veins, followed by suture of the remaining aneurysmal sac over the replacement graft (Fig. 1D). In elderly patients, we have not found that division of the medial musculature and tendons causes postoperative disability. Although we approximate the muscular and tendinous portions of the medial head of the gastrocnemius muscle, it is not necessary to reapproximate other tendons.

Fig. 1. Surgical approach to aneurysm from the medial aspect of the leg with the patient supine. Proximal and distal ligation with bypass grafting using autogenous saphenous vein. The aneurysm is excised after transection of the medial head of the gastrocnemius muscle as well as the tendons of the gracilis, semitendinous, and semimembranous muscles.

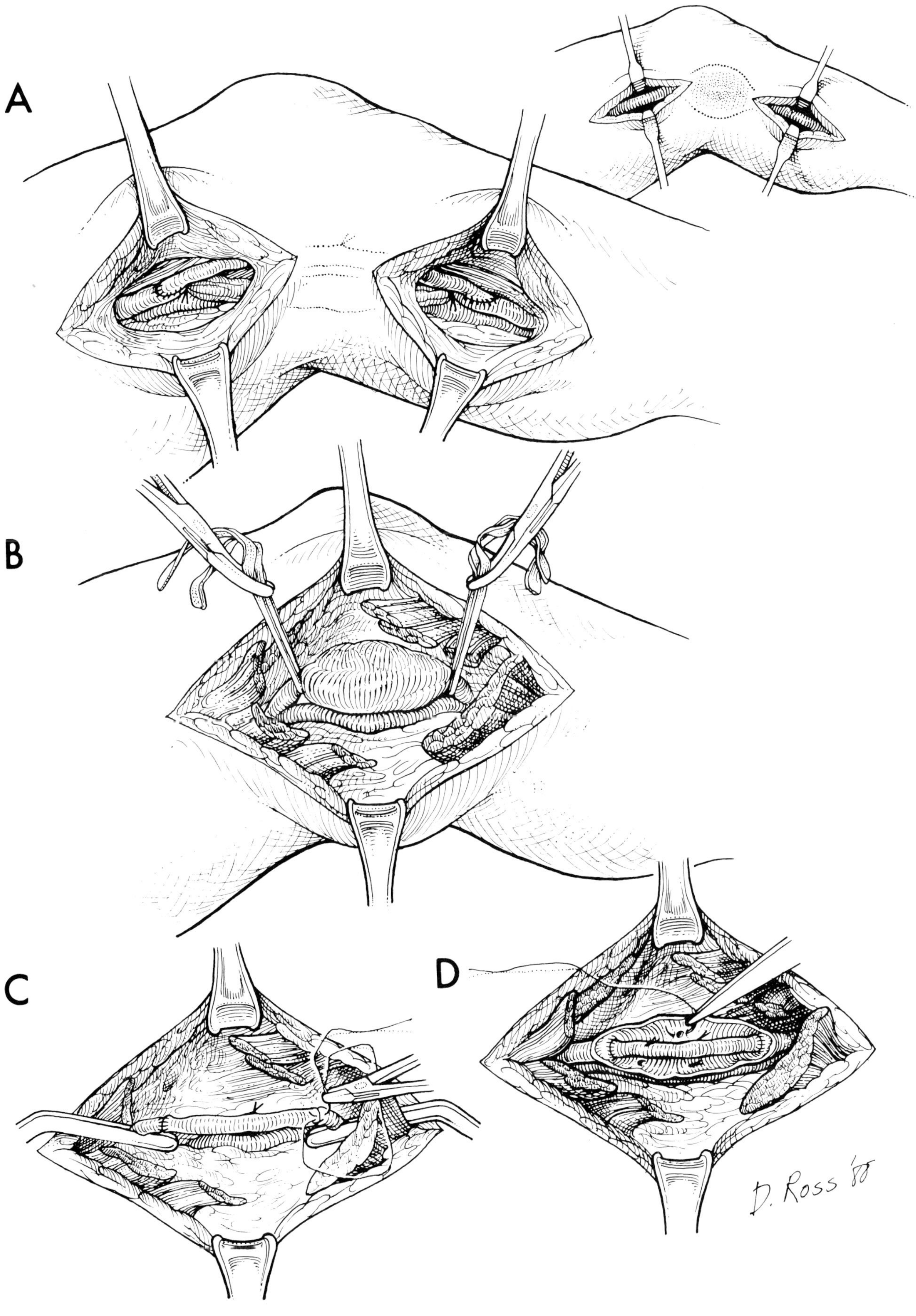
A
B
C
D
D. Ross '88

FEMORAL ARTERIAL ANEURYSM

Surgical management of femoral arterial aneurysms is similar to that of popliteal aneurysms, except that excision of the aneurysm is easier to accomplish and is generally preferred. Restoration of the arterial anatomy by interposition saphenous vein graft or Dacron prosthesis gives equivalent patency results.[1]

Femoral arterial aneurysms may be explored through a linear groin incision (Fig. 2). If the aneurysm is confined to the common femoral artery, proximal control of the artery and distal control of the superficial femoral and profunda femoris arteries are accomplished initially. Using systemic heparinization, excision of the aneurysm is performed, followed by interposition grafting with an autogenous saphenous vein or a Dacron prosthesis. Reconstruction is somewhat more complicated when the aneurysm also involves the proximal profunda femoris artery, as shown in Figure 2A. Under these circumstances, a Dacron prosthesis has been used to reconstruct the common femoral artery. The profunda femoris artery is then sutured directly into the posterior aspect of the Dacron prosthesis, or an additional Dacron prosthesis is utilized to bridge the distance between the newly reconstructed common femoral artery and the profunda femoris bifurcation. If the superficial femoral artery is occluded, direct reconstruction into the profunda femoris artery (Fig. 2B) can be accomplished with or without additional grafting to the reconstituted distal superficial femoral or popliteal arteries.

Fig. 2. Exploration of femoral arterial aneurysm through a linear groin incision.
(A) Aneurysm involving the proximal profunda femoris artery.
(B) Direct reconstruction into the profunda femoris artery.

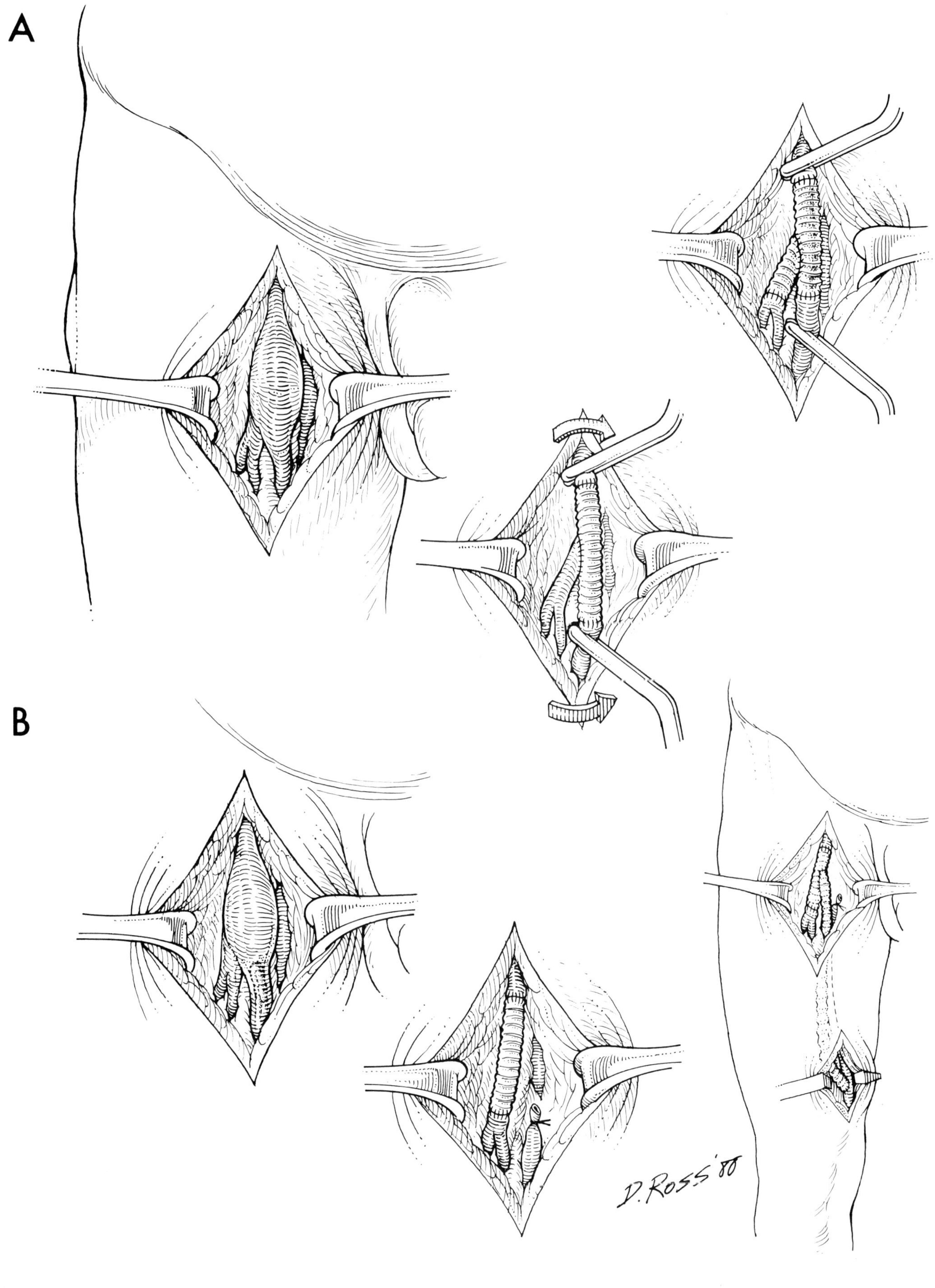
A
B
D. Ross '80

SUBCLAVIAN ARTERY ANEURYSM

The subclavian arterial aneurysm is approached through a supraclavicular incision, as shown in Figure 3. Dependent on the proximal extent of the aneurysm, this may or may not be accompanied by resection of the medial clavicle or, in some instances median sternotomy for proximal control of the subclavian artery.[5] The incision is carried through the platysma muscle with division of the clavicular head of the sternocleidomastoid muscle. Medially, the dissection is carried to the jugular vein. The phrenic nerve is identified crossing the anteromedial aspect of the anterior scalene muscle and is gently retracted medially. Division of the anterior scalene muscle then allows access to the aneurysm and the subclavian artery. Once the subclavian artery has been surrounded with vascular tapes proximally and distally, the patient is systemically heparinized and vascular clamps are applied. Care is taken to avoid traction laterally on the brachial plexus. If the subclavian artery is sufficiently redundant, primary anastomosis can be accomplished. Otherwise, use of an interposition saphenous vein graft or Dacron prosthesis is equally acceptable.

Should the aneurysm be associated with thoracic-outlet syndrome, the above procedure is usually preceeded by first-rib resection, which we have generally performed through a transaxillary approach, with the patient in a semilateral position as described by Roos.[9] However, we would then recommend the above approach to the subclavian arterial aneurysm rather than the axillary incision.

Fig. 3. Approach to subclavian arterial aneurysm through a supraclavicular incision.

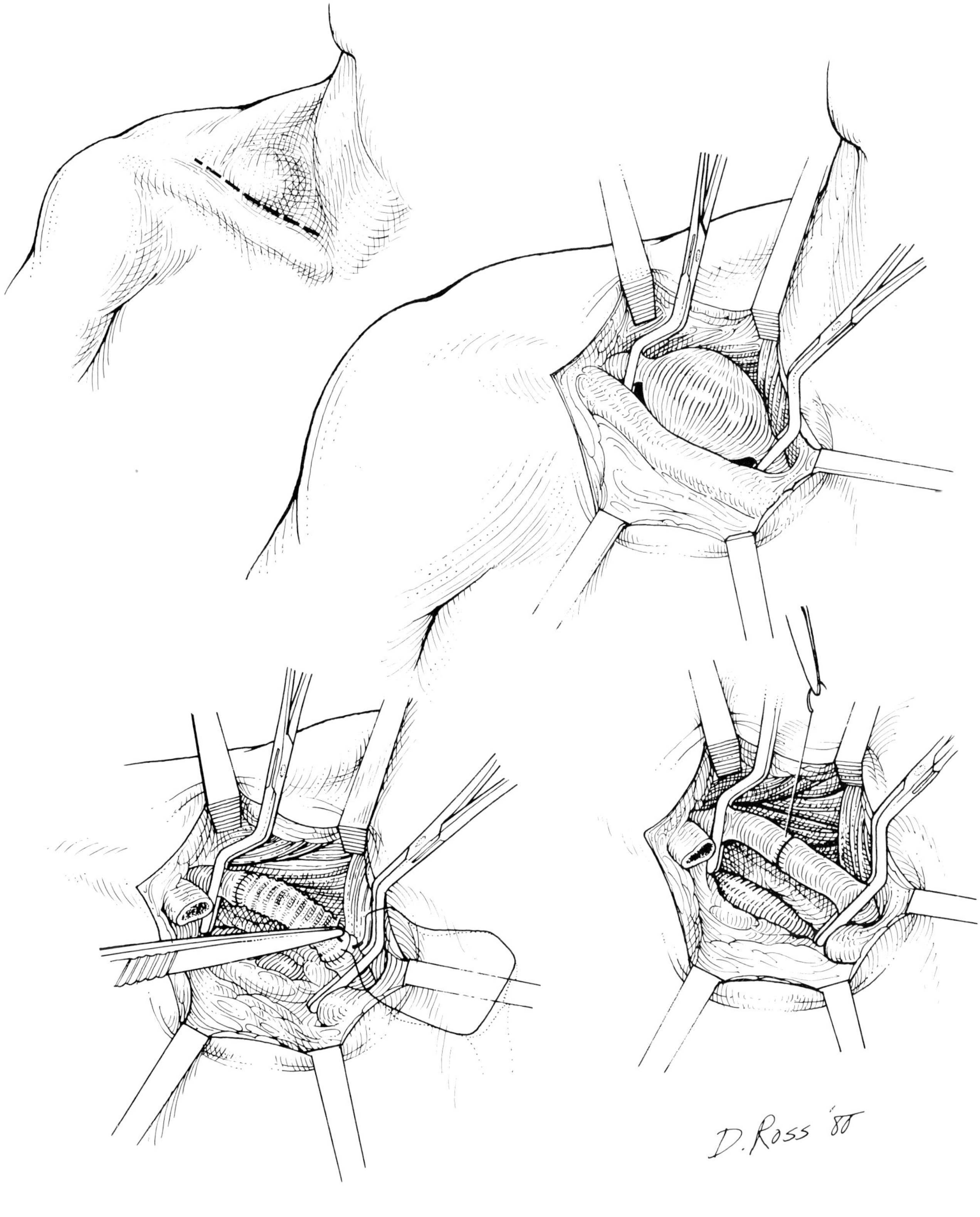
D. Ross '80

REFERENCES

1. Cutler BS, Darling RC: Surgical management of arteriosclerotic femoral aneurysms. Surgery 74:764, 1973
2. Wychulis A, Spittel JA, Wallace RB: Popliteal aneurysms. Surgery 68:942, 1970
3. Evans WE: Popliteal aneurysms. Vasc Surg 10:86, 1976
4. Crawford ES, Edwards WH, DeBakey ME, Cooley DA, Morris GC: Peripheral arteriosclerotic aneurysms. J Am Geriatr Soc 9:1, 1961
5. Hobson RW, Sarkaris J, O'Donnell JA, Neville WE: Atherosclerotic aneurysms of the subclavian artery. Surgery 85:368, 1979
6. Home E: An account of Mr. Hunter's Method of performing the operation for popliteal aneurysm. London Med J 7:391, 1786
7. Linton RR: The arteriosclerotic popliteal aneurysm. Surgery 26:41, 1949
8. Matas R: Endo-aneurysmorrhaphy. Surg Gynecol Obstet 30:456, 1920
9. Roos DB: Transaxillary approach for the first rib resection to relieve thoracic outlet syndrome. Ann Surg 163:354, 1966

Profunda Femoris Reconstruction With and Without Distal Bypass

R.M. Greenhalgh

with illustrations by Stewart Ganley

The surgical importance of the profunda femoris artery has been recognized since the early days of arterial reconstructive surgery.[1] In Great Britain, Martin and coworkers[2] described the vein-patch profundaplasty. To perform this procedure in its simplest form, an incision is made in the common femoral artery and into the profunda femoris artery beyond any stenosis. The stenosis is not removed, but by closing the arteriotomy with a vein patch, the stenosis is overcome. This technique can be used with a long patch if the disease is more extensive, but others have preferred the technique known as 'extended deep femoral angioplasty.'[3]

The profunda femoris artery becomes important when the superficial femoral artery is occluded. This latter vessel almost always becomes diseased before the profunda femoris. It is a long, straight vessel with very few branches and has been described as an artery of conduction rather than of supply. The profunda femoris artery, by comparison, has many branches and is a typical artery of supply. Profunda femoris surgery is almost always carried out in the presence of an occluded superficial femoral artery.

Surgery on the profunda femoris artery is most commonly carried out as an adjunct to aortofemoral bypass grafting. In the presence of an occluded superficial femoral artery, the predominant requirement is to deliver high-pressure blood into the profunda femoris, as this is the major run-off vessel. To achieve this, the Dacron limb is often anastomosed in such a way that the heel of the graft is sutured to the common femoral artery and a tongue of Dacron is anastomosed into the profunda femoris artery. In this way, the Dacron anastomosis widens the profunda and produces a profundaplasty.

SELECTION FOR PROFUNDA FEMORIS SURGERY AND DISTAL BYPASS

Before profunda femoris reconstruction with or without distal bypassing can be performed, it is vital to know that the aortoiliac segment is disease-free. Reconstruction of the aortoiliac segment always takes precedence over profunda femoris surgery. Before distal surgery should be contemplated, the adequacy of the aortoiliac segment must be assessed.

A typical patient for this surgery presents with symptoms and signs of lower-limb ischemia and is found to have a strong femoral pulse and absent popliteal and pedal pulses below. In the presence of a significant profunda stenosis, a bruit is frequently heard just below the inguinal ligament over the femoral pulse. The point at which the bruit is loudest corresponds to the stenosis. Noninvasive techniques are frequently employed to assess the adequacy of the aortoiliac segment and also to further localize distal disease. The typical patient would be expected to have a relatively normal Doppler velocity wave form over the common femoral artery. Segmental Doppler systolic pressure measurements can be taken at the distal thigh, calf, and ankle and one side compared with the other. In association with an occlusion of the superficial femoral artery with or without disease in the profunda femoris artery, the distal thigh cuff pressure is reduced. A further fall in pressure below the distal thigh cuff would imply even more distal disease. The standard exercise test is useful for claudicant patients,[4] so that the response after the operation can be compared with the preoperative findings. The test may also be repeated at follow-up visits to check whether the results of the reconstruction are being maintained long-term.

PREPARATION OF THE PATIENT FOR SURGERY

This surgery is usually performed under general anesthetic, although profunda femoris surgery alone can be performed under local anesthetic after suitable local infiltration. An epidural or spinal anesthetic is also a reasonably satisfactory alternative to general anesthesia for distal bypass surgery, although care must be taken that the blood pressure does not fall as a result of this form of anesthesia. General anesthesia is preferable, but the patient's fitness should be properly assessed in the usual way.

Adequate shaving of the patient, including pubic and leg areas as necessary, should be performed at least 24 hours before surgery. It is very helpful to stand the patient up and to mark the long saphenous vein, from below the knee up to the groin, with an indelible pencil. The patient should bathe thoroughly before surgery. It is customary to paint the surgical field with a suitable skin preparation and then to wrap the leg in sterile towels several hours before surgery. One hour before surgery, the patient should receive a suitable premedication.

TECHNIQUE OF PROFUNDA FEMORIS RECONSTRUCTION WITHOUT DISTAL BYPASS

The patient is placed supine on the operating table, with slight downward tilt of the head, which allows slightly better access to the groin. The feet are placed approximately 24 to 30 inches apart on a suitable board and the skin is prepared widely from the knee to well above the inguinal ligament. Careful placing of towels is necessary, and in particular a small towel is placed over the pubic area. It is helpful to use a plastic drape to seal off the towels and to prevent instruments dropping through toward the perineum.

The details of the technique of profunda femoris reconstruction without distal bypassing are shown in Figure 1. The incision is made slightly to the lateral side of the femoral artery from the inguinal ligament downward. By approaching from the lateral side, the lymphatic vessels are avoided, but care must be taken not to damage the femoral nerve. Also by approaching slightly from the lateral side, an easier exposure of the profunda femoris artery is achieved. The incision is continued down to the femoral sheath, which surrounds the femoral artery, vein, and femoral canal. This sheath is incised, and a rubber sling is passed around the common femoral artery below the inguinal ligament. Further dissection continues through the femoral sheath to expose the superficial femoral artery. It is important to free the latter vessel over 3 or 4 inches and

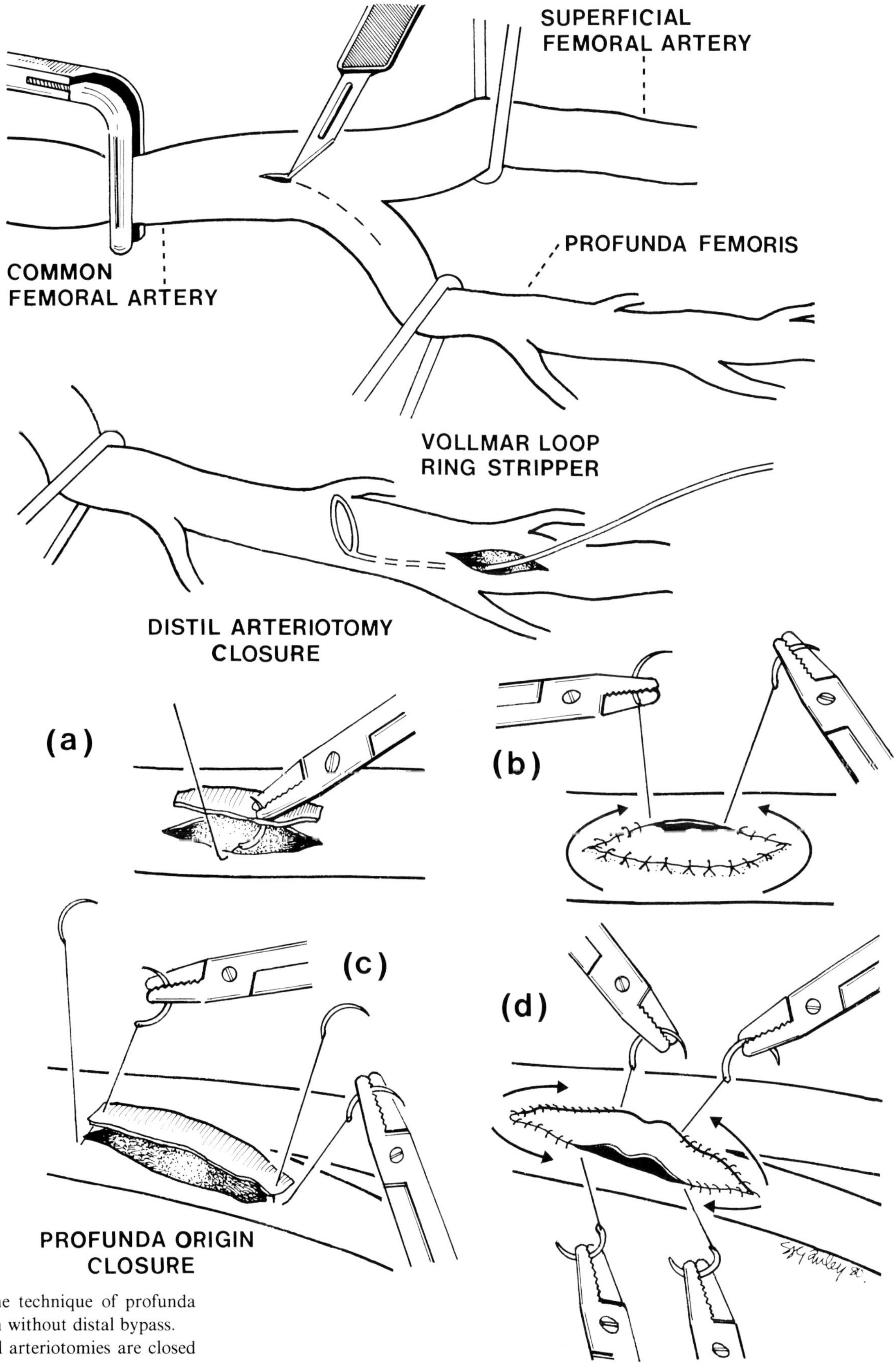

Fig. 1. Details of the technique of profunda femoris reconstruction without distal bypass.
(a, b) The small distal arteriotomies are closed with a vein patch.
(c) Two double-ended prolene sutures are applied at either end of the vein patch to anchor it.
(d) All needles are used to suture the patch from both ends.

to mobilize it totally. This enables a much easier approach to the profunda femoris. Another sling is passed around the superficial femoral artery, and an assistant raises both common femoral and superficial femoral slings. The point where the profunda femoris artery goes off the back of the common femoral is always easy to find because the parent vessel suddenly halves in diameter as it becomes the superficial femoral artery. Behind this point the profunda femoris will arise. With the slings raised, the profunda femoris is approached from the lateral side. A profunda vein almost always passes across the origin of the profunda femoris artery. This must be divided and should be transfixed with, for example, 4–0 prolene. Dissection is carried further down the profunda femoris until branches are seen coming off both sides of it. As arterial branches come off, there is almost invariably a vein passing over the profunda femoris. Small veins can be ligated and larger ones should be transfixed as before.

The profunda femoris should be palpated along the whole of its length, and exposure should continue until a normal-feeling artery is found. The whole length of the profunda femoris artery can be exposed by placing a self-retaining retractor quite deeply and dividing the veins lying in front of the artery until the continuation of the artery itself is about the same size as its branches. At this point, the artery is just in front of the femur. Each of the branches must be controlled with a fine plastic sling.

The patient is now given 5000 units of heparin intravenously. No clamps are applied for 3 minutes after heparin has been given, to allow adequate circulation of the heparin and proper anticoagulation. A soft clamp (the variety with silastic implants are very atraumatic) is now applied to the common femoral artery. Usually no control is required for the superficial femoral artery, which will have no back-bleed. Small bulldog clamps are placed on lateral and medial femoral circumflex vessels.

An incision is made into the common femoral artery with a knife. The arteriotomy is enlarged using angled scissors and carried into the origin of the profunda femoris artery. The back-bleed from this vessel is assessed, and a decision must be taken whether to continue the arteriotomy downwards or, if the disease is extensive, to make separate arteriotomies further down this vessel as shown in Figure 1. For extensive disease from the most distal arteriotomy, the atheroma is raised and a Vollmar ring stripper is inserted to perform semiclosed endarterectomy. The loop is pushed to the upper arteriotomy and the atheroma lifted free in the common femoral. Pieces should be removed from the proximal arteriotomy and washed out of the artery with saline. The common femoral clamp can be released briefly to flush out loose pieces and check the adequacy of the forward squirt.

The distal arteriotomy in the profunda is by far the most important. The angle scissors should be used to open this to guarantee a very good sight of the end-point of endarterectomy, if such has been performed. It is absolutely vital to ensure that no flap of atheroma occurs at this point. If there is any doubt about this, the atheroma is pinned from within outwards, using both needles of a double-ended 6–0 prolene suture. The suture is tied on the outside. Where the disease is fairly limited to the origin, endarterectomy is avoided; by avoiding it, no distal flap can occur. This extended semiclosed endarterectomy method is only used for extremely extensive disease.

The small distal arteriotomies are closed with a vein patch as shown in Figure 1a and b. A double-ended 5–0 or 6–0 prolene suture is selected: the first suture location is shown. Those needles are used to pass around the patch with a continuous suture and to meet at the other side. The patch selected should be slightly square and can be made to fit into the slit arteriotomy. The square end of patch tends to widen the arteriotomy slit at the edges.

The arteriotomy at the origin of the profunda is generally longer, and a slightly different technique is used. A suitable square-ended patch of vein is again selected and two double-ended prolene sutures are applied at either end to anchor the vein patch (Fig. 1c). Suturing takes place from both ends using all needles, (Fig. 1d). When the continuous suturing meets the other needle, the sutures are tied together halfway along each side. Blood is allowed to back-bleed up the profunda to fill the space as the last sutures are being placed. All clamps are removed, and a gauze swab is placed over the suture line for the first few beats. An electromagnetic-flow probe is applied to the common femoral artery, and the flow down the profunda femoris is measured and the wave form examined. The flow should certainly be in excess of 100 ml/min, and it is generally much greater than this. If there is any doubt about the wave form, a peroperative arteriogram should be performed.

TECHNIQUE OF PROFUNDA FEMORIS RECONSTRUCTION WITH DISTAL BYPASS

Conduit for Distal Bypass

Whether the profunda femoris artery is diseased or not, the decision whether or not to combine distal bypass with profunda femoris reconstruction can be very difficult. The decision having been taken to perform distal bypassing, the next decision to be made is on the conduit to be used. There are three main possibilities. The patient's own long saphenous vein is our first choice, provided that this vein is adequate. This autologous vein is approached by continuing the incision from the groin down along the marked saphenous vein. Undermining is avoided, as this tends to lead to necrosis of flaps of skin in an already ischemic leg. A continuous incision is not used, but separate incisions leaving tunnels are perfectly adequate to remove the vein. Retractors are necessary to lift the tunnels, so that the saphenous vein can be dissected free of the subcutaneous tissues.

The saphenous vein is dissected over enough length to enable the appropriate bypass to be performed. Our preference is to approach the vein from below and divide it. A plastic cholangiogram catheter is used to distend the vein, and the vein is tied onto the catheter. The vein is distended with heparin Hartman's solution, but some prefer to distend with blood, claiming that this produces less damage to the vein wall. All branches of the vein are secured with a nonabsorbable suture such as Supolene, although traditionally silk was used. A bulldog clamp is placed on the end of the divided vein, and the vein is distended. Care is taken to remove every last portion of connective tissue from the vein and especially any constricting tissues. If the vein measures less than 4 mm at any point along its length, it should be discarded, in favor of an alternative conduit. If it measures 4 mm or more over the whole of its length, it should prove very adequate. The distended autologous vein is marked with Bonney's blue dots. These are placed approximately every 5 mm and are useful as a guideline to avoid twisting.

The umbilical vein is an alternative conduit to autologous vein. This is stored in a glass tube and mounted upon a glass mandril in a sterile fluid solution. The sterile graft is removed, taken off the mandril, and placed in a receptacle while 6 liters of saline with heparin can be used to pass through the umbilical vein to wash it thoroughly.

Expanded polytetrafluoroethylene is also an alternative to autologous vein. It can be cut to length and sterilized in an autoclave. The preparation of materials is shown diagramatically in Figure 2.

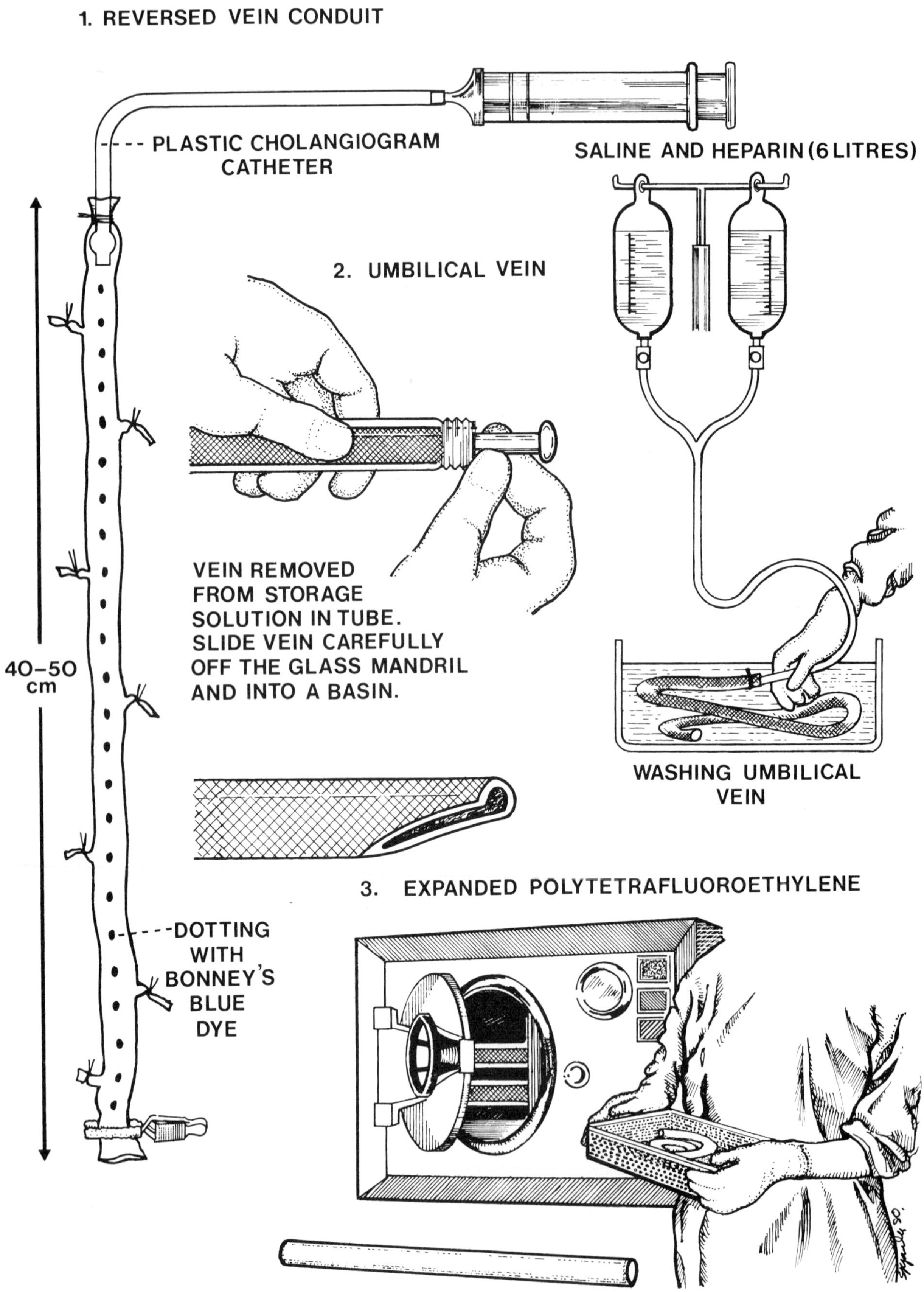

Fig. 2. Preparation of materials for use in distal bypass.

Distal Anastomosis

The leg is placed with the hip laterally rotated and the knee slightly flexed. The leg is held in this position with a wedge placed on the lateral side behind the knee and a rubber ring under the heel.

The distal artery is approached from the medial side with the operator sitting on the opposite side of the table. The line of approach is along the saphenous vein, either above or below the knee joint. The popliteal artery is approached and dissected clear of the popliteal vein and nerves. Plastic slings are passed around the artery, and bulldog clamps with soft rubber covers are used to control the vessel. A longitudinal arteriotomy is made in the popliteal artery, first with a knife and then with angled scissors. Details of the lower-end anastomosis are shown in Figure 3. In the illustration, reverse vein is used. The arteriotomy is measured with a calliper so that the conduit can be cut to exactly the right length obliquely. The portion where the bulldog clamp had been applied for distension of the vein is discarded. No instruments are ever used to occlude a conduit, only the fingers and thumb of an assistant. The first suture is placed at the upper end of the arteriotomy, using a double-ended prolene suture. This draws down the heel of the conduit. These are held with a rubber-shod mosquito clip. The second suture is also a double-ended prolene suture and is placed as shown in Figure 3b. The position chosen is away from the apex of the conduit. One end of the prolene suture is again held in a rubber-shod mosquito clip, and the other end is used to suture continuously around the apex to a similar point on the near side. These sutures are placed with great care so as to avoid narrowing the lumen. A metal grooved dilator is used to check the anastomosis after this portion has been completed, as is shown in Figure 3c. The anastomosis is completed by sewing continuously forward from the heel of the conduit to meet the other suture line on either side, where it is tied.

The clamps are removed and fluid is flushed down the conduit to check that pulsatile flow can be produced in the popliteal artery beyond the conduit. The distended conduit is then passed through a tunnel in the thigh to the groin. There are various ways of producing the tunnel; some prefer to use a tube resembling a sigmoidoscope and pass the conduit through it, but it is often as easy to use a finger to produce a tunnel and to make certain that there are no fibrous strands which could press upon it and constrict it. The conduit can be gently pulled through such a tunnel using a long, curved, artery clip, such as a long Robert's clip. It is better to leave the plastic cannula in an autologous vein up to this point, because the clip can then pull upon the cannula to avoid damage to the conduit. It is important to have the conduit distended at this point to minimise the risk of twisting it in the tunnel. The guideline or dots on the autologous vein also minimise this risk.

Proximal Anastomosis

The upper end of the conduit is sutured in such a way as to produce a profundaplasty. The details are shown in Figure 4. The common femoral, superficial femoral, and profunda femoris arteries are controlled in exactly the same way as previously described. The arteriotomy is made from the common femoral artery and extended into the profunda femoris. If more extensive profunda surgery had proved necessary, it would have to have been performed at an earlier stage in the operation. This is the final anastomosis. The length of the conduit and the right place for anastomosis are determined by straightening the knee joint, so that the anastomosis will not be put under tension when the knee joint extends. The conduit is cut obliquely to the measured length using the calliper. The first suture of double-ended prolene (Fig. 4a) is applied to the heel of the conduit, and the second double-ended prolene suture is used to attach the apex of the conduit to the common femoral artery (Fig. 4b). Continuous suturing is performed as in Figure 4c, beginning from the heel forwards and completing

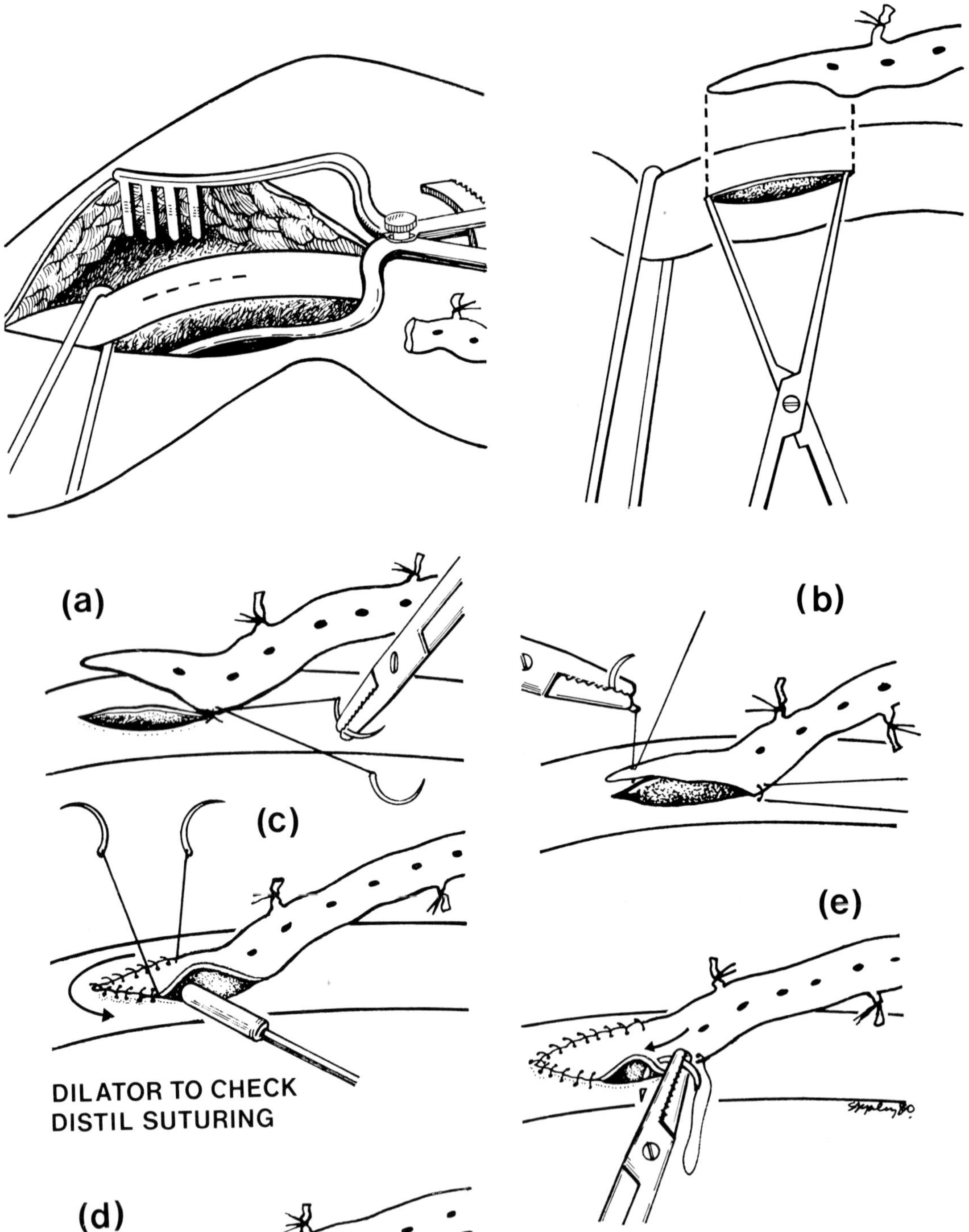

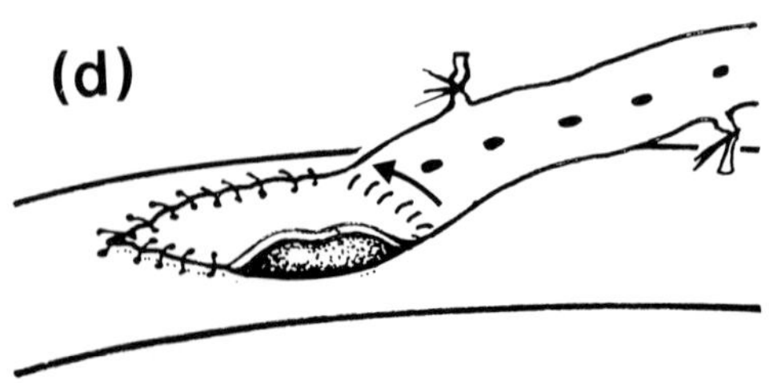

Same technique for all conduits

Fig. 3. Lower-end anastomosis.
(a) The first suture is placed at the upper end of the arteriotomy, using a double-ended proline suture.
(b) Placement of the second suture away from the apex of the conduit. The suture material is double-ended proline.
(c) A coronary artery dilator is used to check the anastomosis.

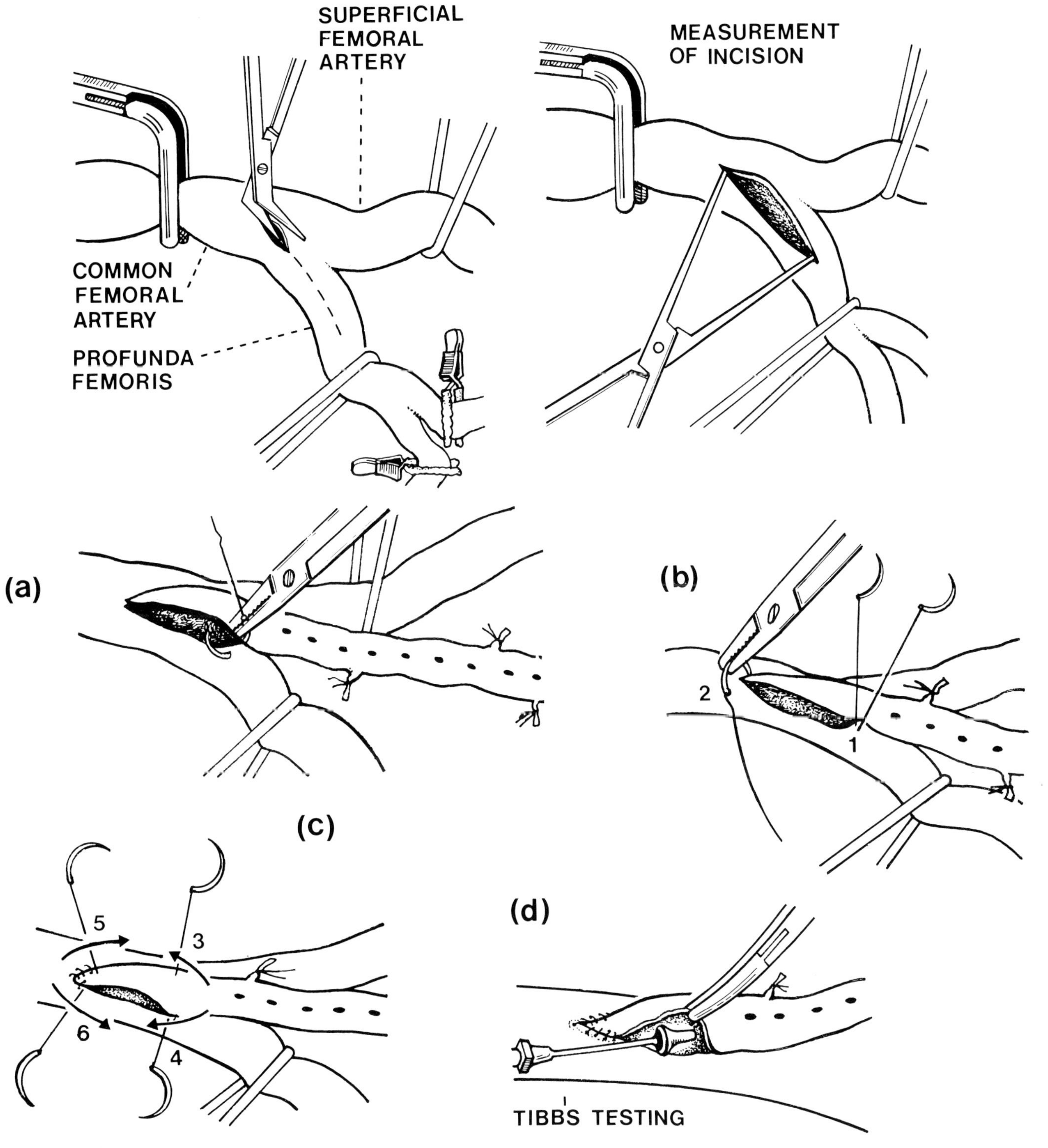

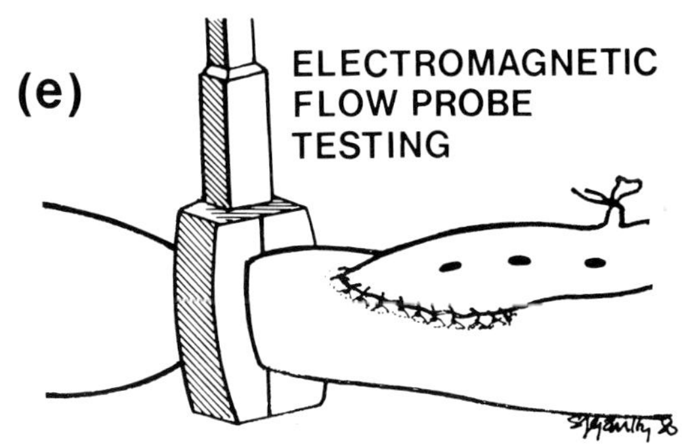

Fig. 4. Suturing of the upper end of the conduit to produce a profundaplasty.
(a) The first suture of double-ended proline is applied to the heel of the conduit.
(b) The second double-ended proline suture attaches the apex of the conduit to the common femoral artery.
(c) Continuous suturing, beginning from the heel forward and completing from the apex backwards.

from the apex backwards. Before the final sutures are placed, a pulsatile squirt is delivered down the autologous vein. An assistant has his or her fingers over the popliteal artery beyond the anastomosis, to see that pulsation is felt. The conduit is never controlled by an instrument; an assistant lightly holds the conduit between finger and thumb. An autologous vein frequently has competent valves, and so there is no back-bleed from it. The common femoral clamp is removed momentarily to check the forward squirt and to remove any debris, before the final continuous sutures are applied.

An electromagnetic flow probe is applied to the common femoral artery. Flow readings are taken with wave-form analysis, first of the whole of the common femoral flow, then with occlusion of the vein bypass with the profunda open, and finally with the conduit open and profunda occluded. A flow in excess of 100 ml/min through a conduit is required to give it an high chance of staying patent and to avoid primary failure. It is important at this stage of the operation that the mean blood pressure is maintained and that after release of the clamps the pressure is monitored from moment to moment to guarantee that it does not fall. If the flow down the conduit is borderline, papaverine hydrochloride is injected into the artery to see if the flow reading is augmented. If it is not, an operative arteriogram is performed, and where necessary the reconstructions are re-explored.

Where umbilical vein or polytetrafluoroethylene is used, it is necessary to cover the whole operation and the postoperative period with a suitable antibiotic. No antibiotic is required for autologous vein. Careful hemostasis is acheived, and a small suction drain is applied near both anastomoses. This is removed usually after 48 hours. The wounds are closed with absorbable sutures in layers. A three-layer closure is necessary in the groin to minimize the risk of hematoma and to ensure proper primary healing. The skin is sutured according to preference, paying careful attention to the proper apposition of the skin edges and to avoidance of any inturning of skin. Sterile dressings that provide a perfect seal around the incisions are applied. Bandaging is not recommended because all constriction should be avoided. The patient should be encouraged to move his or her ankle gently immediately after awakening.

Preference is always given to extended reconstruction of the profunda femoris before distal bypassing. It can often be difficult to decide when a distal bypass should also be performed. The sequence of the operation for a combination of profunda reconstruction and distal bypassing is as follows: After intravenous heparin has been given, the profunda femoris is reconstructed and the distal vein patches are applied as shown in Figure 1. The arteriotomy in the common femoral into the origin of the profunda is left ready for the upper end of the conduit anastomosis. The distal bypass anastomosis is performed next, and this is checked by squirting fluid down the conduit. The last anastomosis to be performed is the conduit to the profunda origin, as a profundaplasty.

REFERENCES

1. Morris GC Jr, Edwards W, Cooley DA, Crawford ES, De Bakey ME: Surgical importance of profunda femoris artery: Analysis of 102 cases with combined aorto-iliac and femoro-popliteal occlusive disease treated by revascularisation of deep femoral artery. Arch Surg 82: 52–57, 1961
2. Martin P, Renwick S, Stephenson C: On the surgery of the profunda femoris artery. Br J Surg 55:539–542, 1968
3. Cotton LT, Roberts VC: Extended deep femoral angioplasty: An alternative to femoro-popliteal bypass. Br J Surg 62: 340–343, 1975
4. Laing SP, Greenhalgh RM: Standard exercise test to assess peripheral arterial disease. Br Med J 2: 13–16, 1980

REOPERATION FOR GRAFT COMPLICATIONS

Aortoenteric Fistulas

Victor M. Bernhard

Fistula formation between the aorta and the lumen of the gastrointestinal tract can occur at any level. However, the vast majority of fistulas arise from a vascular graft or aneurysm in the infrarenal aorta. The third and fourth portions of the duodenum and duodenojejunal flexure are the most common sites for aortic erosion into the intestine due to their anatomic position. However, any segment of the small intestine or colon that becomes directly adhesed to an aneurysm or a graft may become involved.

A fistula is designated as primary when a degenerative process in the aorta, usually an aneurysm, erodes directly into an adjacent loop of bowel. Secondary fistulas develop as a consequence of surgical reconstruction of the aorta and its major branches and are more common.[1] The basic pathologic process is one of progressive pulsatile erosion of a true or false aneurysm or foreign body graft into an adjacent segment of bowel (Fig. 1A–C). Promoting factors such as infection from previous surgery, primary infection in the arterial wall such as mycotic aneurysm, reoperation (which may produce inadvertent injury and contamination from a loop of bowel), and failure to cover an aortic graft with a layer of healthy tissue to separate it from overlying loops of bowel have been demonstrated in the majority of cases.[2]

The classic clinical picture is one of intermittent gastrointestinal bleeding that invariably progresses to exsanguinating hemorrhage. However, when the graft wall erodes into intestine at some distance from the suture line, bleeding occurs through the interstices of the prosthesis, producing guiac-positive stools and anemia, often accompanied by fever.[2,3] This variant is referred to as a paraprosthetic intestinal fistula[3] (Fig. 1D). Regardless of clinical presentation, gastrointestinal bleeding in any patient with previous aortic reconstruction or a pulsatile abdominal mass is due to aortoenteric fistula until proven otherwise and demands prompt laparotomy to confirm the diagnosis and resolve the problem. Preliminary investigations with endoscopy, aortography, barium gastrointestinal study, gallium scans, and CT scans may help establish the diagnosis and reassure the surgeon regarding the proper course of action. However, these studies should be carried out only if the patient is stable and should be accomplished within a few hours after admission, before massive hemorrhage ensues. Negative studies do not rule out the diagnosis, and positive findings for other sources (ie, gastroduodenal ulceration, hiatus hernia) that do not demonstrate active bleeding confuse the issue and delay operative intervention.[2]

Diagnostic maneuvers should be accomplished within a few hours after admission and only in patients who are hemodynamically stable.[2] Preoperative studies are of value primarily in patients who are poor operative risks to identify a source of bleeding that is not an aortoenteric fistula and that may be successfully managed without surgery.

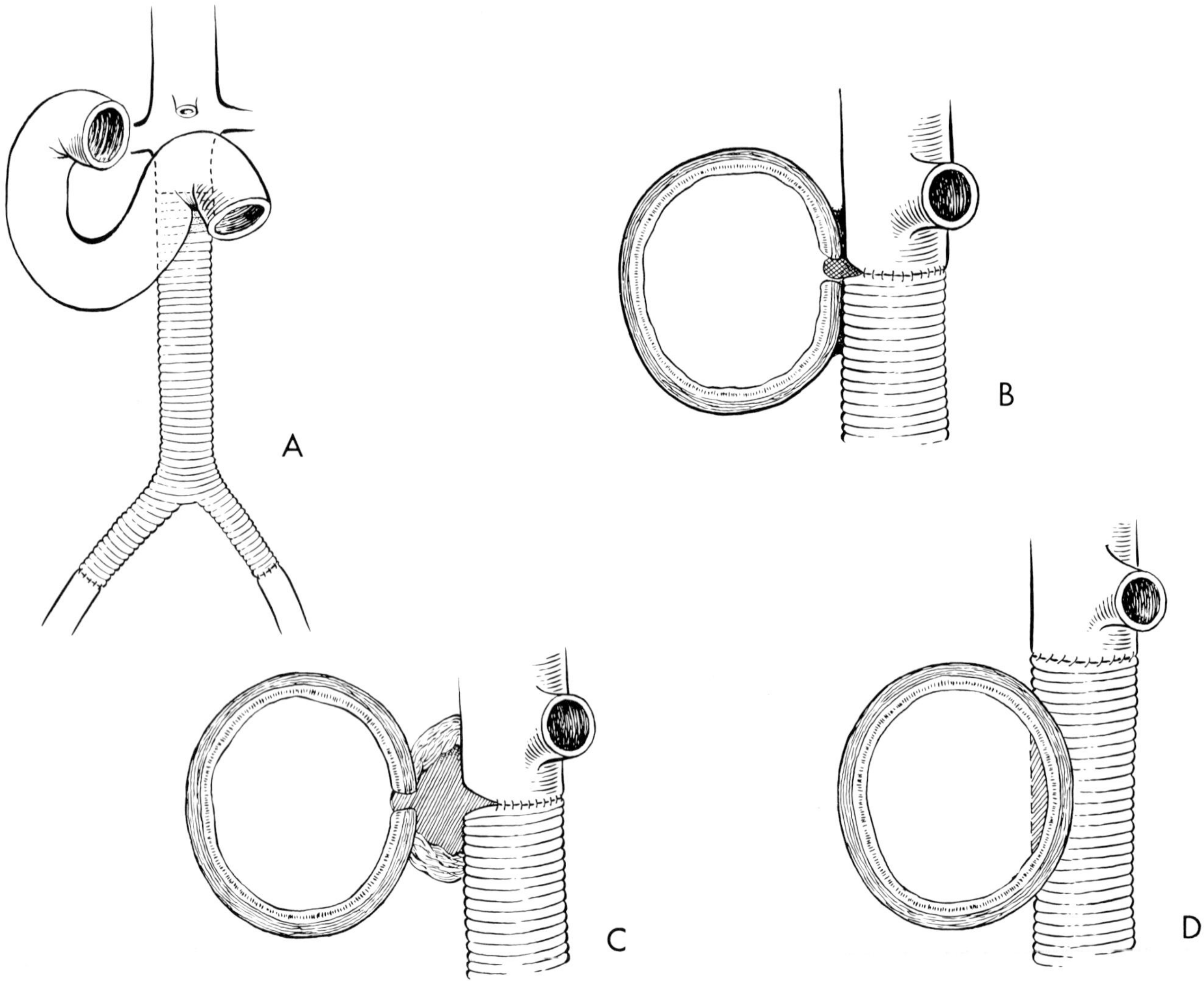

Fig. 1. Anatomy and pathogenesis of secondary aortoenteric fistulas.
(A) The duodenojejunal flexure lies directly over the upper graft and the proximal aortic suture line.
(B) Direct adhesion of the bowel to the proximal aortic suture line. The fistula is temporarily plugged with a thrombus.
(C) Anastomotic aneurysm with intestinal erosion.
(D) Paraprosthetic intestinal fistula.

PREOPERATIVE MANAGEMENT

Preparation for laparotomy should be carried out during the performance of diagnostic investigations. Gastroscopy should be performed in a fully prepared operating room, so that immediate laparotomy can take place in the event that endoscopic maneuvers induce massive hemorrhage from the fistula.

Two large-bore intravenous lines should be inserted as soon as the diagnosis of the aortointestinal fistula is considered. An arterial line should be inserted and an EKG monitor attached early in the preoperative evaluation and management of these patients. If time, facilities, and personnel are available, a Swan-Ganz catheter should be placed to monitor cardiac function and volume replacement. Blood cultures are obtained and broad-spectrum antibiotics started immediately thereafter.

Blood pressure must be checked in both arms to rule out subclavian obstruction, since axillofemoral bypass is the most common method for subsequent lower-extremity revascularization.

In the operating room, the operating team should be scrubbed and gowned during anesthesia induction and preparation of the operative field in order to minimize delay in the event of further massive hemorrhage.

OPERATIVE STRATEGY AND TECHNIQUE

Control of the aorta and closure of the fistula are the first steps in any patient who is actively hemorrhaging or in whom major recurring hemorrhage is imminent. A midline incision should be used since this provides direct, unencumbered access to the fistula and does not invade the territory of a subsequent axillofemoral bypass (Figs. 2, 3A). If the patient is stable and not actively hemorrhaging, a brief exploration is carried out to ascertain that there are no other significant problems.

The proximal aorta should be secured before extensive exploration or other dissection is performed. The segment of aorta just distal to the renal artery may be briefly assessed to determine whether it is readily accessible. However, if the subrenal area appears to be obscured by scar or a diffuse inflammatory process, proximal control at the supraceliac level should be obtained before the infrarenal area is invaded. In those patients who are actively hemorrhaging, direct tamponade with the surgeon's hand or with an aortic compressor at the diaphragm should be carried out as soon as the abdomen is open. Blood volume is rapidly expanded before dissection is carried out to obtain more precise aortic control.

Supraceliac aortic exposure is readily obtained by incision of the gastrohepatic omentum and retraction of the left lobe of the liver. Using the aortic pulse as a guide, the crural fibers of the aortic hiatus are divided and the anterolateral aspects of the aorta are exposed to permit temporary placement of a vascular clamp. The clamp is held in place with its jaws open if the patient is stable and if no significant hemorrhage is encountered during infrarenal aortic dissection (Fig. 3B).

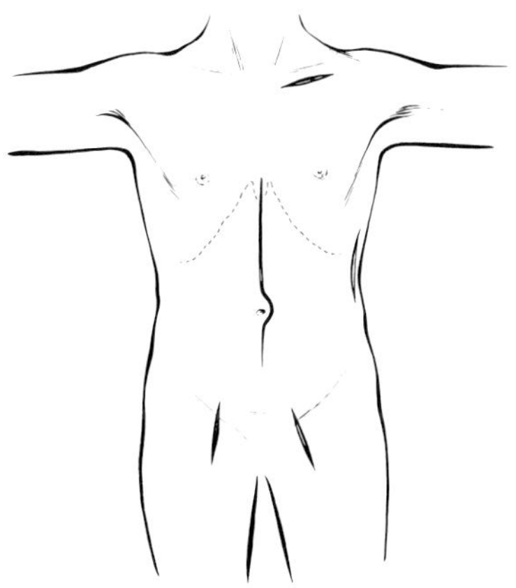

Fig. 2. Proposed incisions for excision of infected prosthesis and subsequent insertion of axillobifemoral grafts. Note that the abdominal incision stops well above the pubis to permit subsequent tunneling for a femoro–femoral graft through fresh, uncontaminated tissue.

Identification of the bleeding site

After aortic control has been achieved, all loops of the small intestine overlying an aortic graft or aneurysm should be gently freed from their adhesions to retroperitoneal tissues. It is especially important to mobilize the duodenojejunal flexure and the third and fourth portions of the duodenum from the retroperitoneum and any underlying graft material, since external inspection and palpation are not adequate to evaluate the posterior aspects of these segments of the bowel. A search for other sources of gastrointestinal bleeding should be carried out *only* after all other potential sites for aortointestinal fistulization have been ruled out. If upper gastrointestinal endoscopy was entirely normal prior to surgery, gastroduodenostomy is unnecessary unless no other bleeding source can be identified.

Frequently, the fistula between the vascular anastomosis and intestine is small, so that simple finger tamponade of the aortic defect is sufficient to control hemorrhage after the fistula has been taken down[4] (Fig. 3B). Prior to this maneuver, however, the supraceliac or infrarenal aorta should be adequately exposed in case immediate clamp application becomes necessary.

Heparinization

Immediately before the aorta is clamped, 5000 units of heparin are instilled directly into the graft or given intravenously to prevent distal arterial thrombosis (Fig. 3C).

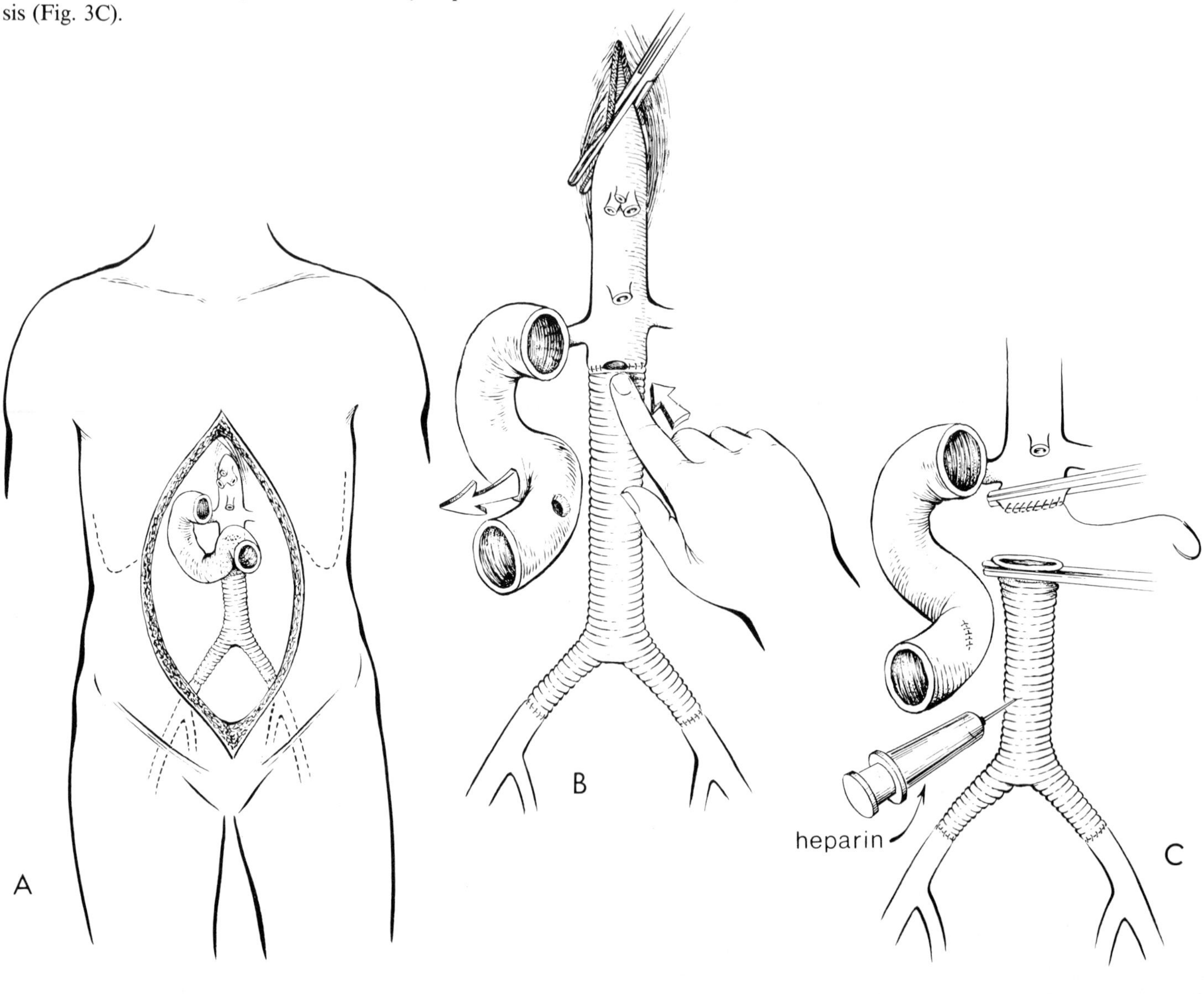

Bowel repair

The bowel defect is usually small and is easily repaired by a transverse two-layer closure in most instances (Fig. 3C). However, when an extensive area of bowel wall has been destroyed by erosion from a paraprosthetic fistula, the involved segment should be resected and continuity restored by end-to-end anastomosis. Extensive destruction of the third and fourth positions of the duodenum makes anastomosis in this area very difficult. Under these circumstances, it may be wise to resect the involved bowel, close the third portion of the duodenum, and anastomose the jejunum to the side of the second portion of the duodenum. Thus, healthy segments of bowel are brought together remote from the septic portion of the operative field (Fig. 4B).

Graft resection

Debridement and direct suture of the aortic defect, usually at the proximal anastomosis, have been successfully reported.[5] Unfortunately, this maneuver is frequently accompanied by recurrent perigraft infection and refistulization or massive retroperitoneal hemorrhage.[2,5] Therefore, it is recommended that all prosthetic material be removed from the retroperitoneal space in addition to careful debridement of necrotic perigraft necrotic tissue. Pieces of graft and excised tissue should be submitted for aerobic and anaerobic cultures.

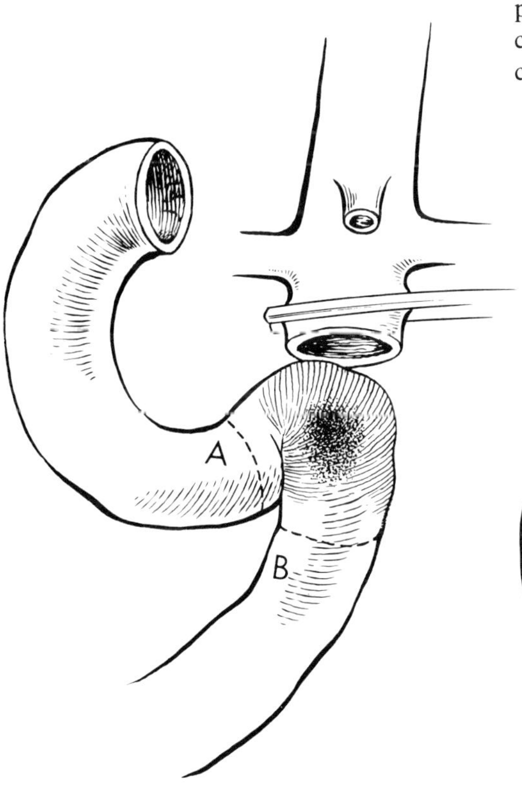

Fig. 3. (A) Midline transabdominal exposure of the aortointestinal fistula.
(B) The aortic hiatus of the diaphragm has been incised to permit application of a supraceliac clamp. The fistula is exposed by dissecting the duodenojejunal flexure from the underlying graft. The aortic defect is usually at the proximal suture line and small enough to permit fingertip control.
(C)The bowel defect is closed with simple sutures. The proximal anastomosis has been dismantled, and the aortic stump is closed with monofilament suture. Heparin may be injected into the graft directly or intravenously to prevent distal thrombosis.

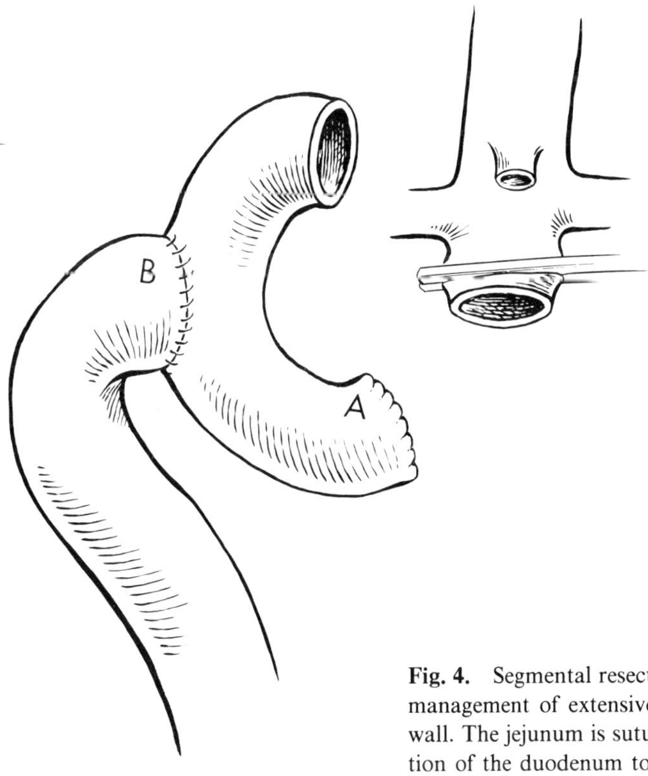

Fig. 4. Segmental resection of the intestine for management of extensive erosion of the bowel wall. The jejunum is sutured to the second portion of the duodenum to avoid anastomoses to the retroperitoneal duodenum in an infected field.

Aortic stump closure

One of the most feared consequences of graft excision is disruption of the aortic stump in the early postoperative period or delayed development of a stump aneurysm with secondary retroperitoneal hemorrhage or intestinal fistula formation.[6] Closure of the aortic stump is difficult when only a short segment of aorta is available below the renal arteries, when infection extends proximally into the aortic tissues, or when healthy periaortic tissue is not available for reinforcement.

Infected aorta adjacent to the proximal suture line is resected as much as possible, and the stump is closed with a row of interrupted mattress sutures and a second running over-and-over stitch of 2–0 monofilament polypropylene. A layer of uninfected tissue is placed around the stump to separate it from the graft bed and adjacent viscera. A pedicle of omentum has been conventionally recommended for this purpose, and we have successfully used it on a few occasions (Fig. 5D).[1,6] Unfortunately, this tissue contributes little to the immediate strength of the stump suture line. A flap of anterior spinous ligament may be employed for this purpose (Fig. 5A–C);[7] however, it is difficult to obtain and is frequently inadequate to provide good stump coverage. Recently, Buchbinder et al[6] demonstrated experimentally that a pedicle flap fashioned from an isolated segment of jejunum from which the mucosa has been stripped will promote solid healing of a transected aortic stump in an infected field. However, human application of this technique has not been reported.[6]

The aortic defect remaining after removal of an end-to-side graft is usually more readily managed. The necrotic and infected rim of tissue at the anastomosis is trimmed and the aortic opening is closed with a double layer of running 3–0 prolene. Although it is ideal to maintain flow through the aorta, in our experience it is rarely possible to restore a patent aortic lumen.

The entire graft can be removed through the abdomen when the prosthesis is interposed in the aortoiliac area. The iliac arteries are readily closed with a double layer of running 3–0 prolene monofilament suture. However, excision of an aortofemoral prosthesis requires counterincisions in the groins so that no graft material is left behind. Femoral arteriotomies may be closed by direct suture or with vein patches to maintain continuity between the profunda and superficial femoral branches (Fig. 7G).

Upon completion of the intraabdominal portion of the procedure, the entire operative field should be liberally irrigated with antibiotic saline solution. Suction drains are placed in the retroperitoneum and brought out through the lower quadrant or flank on the side of the abdomen opposite the anticipated axillofemoral bypass graft (Fig. 7H).

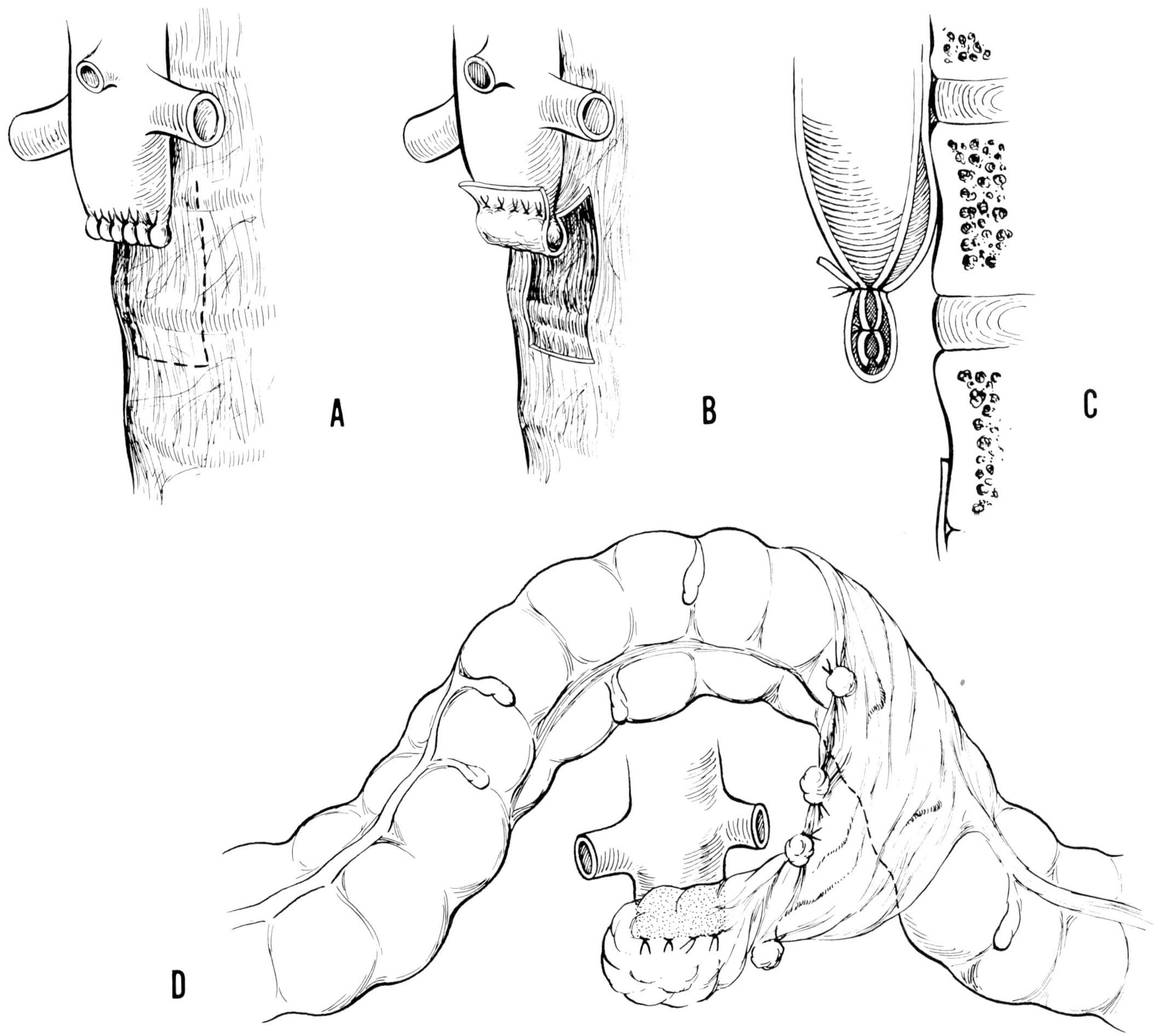

Fig. 5. (A,B,C) Development of a flap of anterior spinous ligament to reinforce the aortic closure (modified from Fry and Lindenauer[7]). (D) A pedicle of omentum may be used to surround the aortic stump with well-vascularized healthy tissue and to separate the stump from adjacent loops of bowel.

Lower-extremity revascularization

Viability of the extremities is primarily dependent upon patency of the involved vascular prosthesis or aortic flow through the lumen of an aneurysm. Abrupt excision of these channels during repair of the fistula precludes timely recruitment of alternate pathways unless prior atherosclerotic obstruction or graft thrombosis has promoted the development of adequate collaterals. The distal colon as well as the extremities may be in jeopardy, and the clinical appearance of the extremities immediately after the removal of the graft is not a reliable sign of eventual viability. On the other hand, patients who have had a major amputation or in whom the aortic graft limb is chronically occluded may have adequate collaterals if these channels are not injured during resection of the contaminated prosthesis.[2]

The vast majority of patients will require revascularization of the lower extremities after resection of an aortic graft or aneurysm.[2,5] This procedure should not be carried out until the abdominal and groin wounds have been closed and sealed with adhesive plastic drapes to prevent contamination of the extra-anatomic bypass. Instruments are changed, the patient is reprepped, and the operative team is freshly gowned and gloved.

Axillofemoral bypass with a femoro–femoral extension is the simplest method for restoring circulation to the lower extremities when the previous aortic graft was entirely confined to the abdominal cavity (Fig. 6). The axillofemoral graft must be placed on the side of the body away from any drains or enterostomy sites. It is prudent to avoid extending the midline abdominal incision all the way to the pubis at the time of infected graft excision, so that a few centimeters of uninvolved subcutaneous tissue will be available above the pubis for passage of the femoro–femoral extension (Fig. 2).

Considerable ingenuity is required to circumvent contaminated areas when the previous graft had extended to the femoral arteries (Fig. 7A–F). The axillofemoral limb may be brought through fresh tissue lateral to the old groin wound by incising the inguinal ligament laterally to produce a trough just medial and deep to the anterior superior iliac spine.[8] The graft is then tracked distally, lateral to the sartorius and rectus femoris, to the midportion of the thigh. The distal superficial femoral or the midprofunda can then be identified in the depths of the intramuscular plane for distal anastomosis of the graft to one or the other of these vessels at a point remote from the infected groin incision (Fig. 7A). The opposite extremity may be revascularized in similar fashion. However, it is usually possible to place a crossover femoro–femoral graft through uncontaminated tissues, depending on the sites of previous incisions and available distal runoff vessels. The femoro–femoral extension may be tunneled from the midportion of the axillofemoral limb through normal tissues below the midline abdominal incision and above the groin incisions to enter the opposite thigh laterally (Fig. 7B–C). Alternatively, a tunnel may be developed along the inner thigh medial to the previous groin incision, extending across to the opposite side just below the pubic symphysis (Fig. 7F). A third possibility utilizes autogenous saphenous vein, which is relatively resistant to infection, to connect the femoral arteries by reopening the old contaminated femoral wounds (Fig. 7E). This crossover graft should not be inserted until all wounds for the axillodistal femoral graft have been closed. These variations are designed to avoid contamination of the extra-anatomic bypass graft, which, at least in part, must be a foreign body conduit.

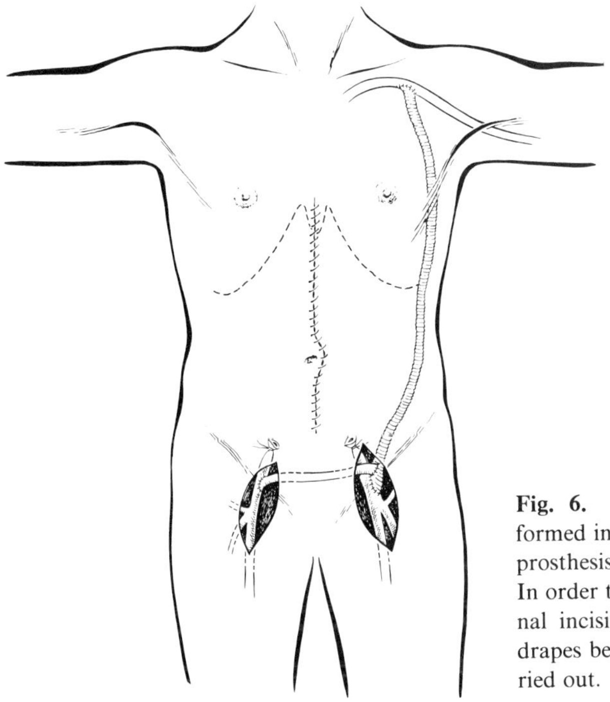

Fig. 6. Axillobifemoral bypass can be performed in the standard fashion when the aortic prosthesis is confined entirely to the abdomen. In order to prevent contamination, the abdominal incision is closed and sealed with plastic drapes before the extra-anatomic bypass is carried out.

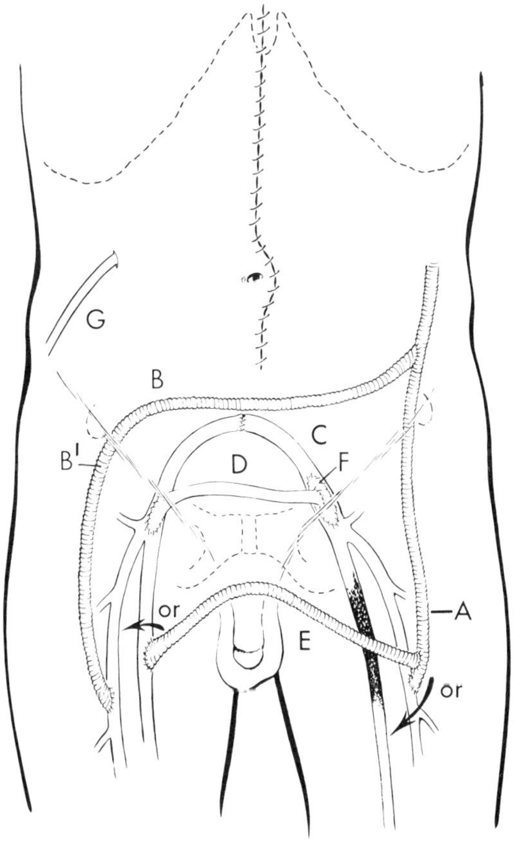

Fig. 7. Variations of the axillobifemoral technique to avoid contamination from the groin wounds required to excise an infected aortofemoral graft.
(A) Lateral placement of the axillofemoral limb just medial and deep to the anterior superior iliac spine with anastomosis to the midprofunda or distal femoral-popliteal segment.
(B) High takeoff of the femoro–femoral limb tunneled between the distal end of the abdominal incision and the pubis but sufficiently proximal to the old femoral incisions to remain in fresh uncontaminated tissue.
(B') The descending limb is placed laterally.
(C) Iliac arteries may be anastomosed to each other to provide transpelvic crossover.
(D) Autogenous saphenous vein femoro–femoral bypass through contaminated groin wounds. This graft is not inserted until the wounds for the lateral axillofemoral graft have been closed.
(E) Femoro–femoral graft tunneled through clean tissue medial and distal to the groin wounds and crossing over to the opposite thigh below the pubic prominence.
(F) Vein-patch closure of common femoral defect after excision of an aortofemoral graft limb.
(G) The retroperitoneal suction drain exits on the opposite side from the axillofemoral conduit.

Management of the primary aortointestinal fistula

Contamination from a primary fistula is usually meager and involves only the sinus tract between the aneurysm and the duodenum. Aortic control can usually be achieved by standard infrarenal application of an aortic clamp. The duodenum can be readily separated from the dome of the aneurysm and the bowel defect closed as described previously. The aneurysm is then incised, and a cuff of aneurysm wall around the fistula is resected. The laminated thrombus and the intima lining the aneurysm should be excised leaving only the muscular adventitial wall of the sac. The aneurysm bed is liberally irrigated with antibiotic saline solution and aortic continuity is restored by insertion of an aortoiliac prosthesis in the standard fashion. The graft itself should be surrounded by a pedicle of omentum to separate it from adjacent viscera and to insure coverage by well-vascularized, healthy tissue. This approach has been recommended by Daugherty and associates,[9] who noted that 13 of 14 patients treated in this fashion for primary fistulas recovered completely with only one recurrence at 2 years. However, if the aneurysm wall is extensively involved in a septic process or if the fistula was initiated by a mycotic aneurysm, resection and extra-anatomic bypass will be required.

REFERENCES

1. Bernhard VM, Kleinman LH: Aorto-enteric fistulas, Bergan JJ, Yao JST (eds): In Surgery of the Aorta and its Body Branches. New York, Grune & Stratton Inc, 1979
2. Kleinman LH, Towne JB, Bernhard VM: A diagnostic and therapeutic approach to aorto-enteric fistulas: A clinical experience with 20 patients. Surgery 86:868, 1979
3. O'Mara C, Imbembo AL: Paraprosthetic enteric fistula. Surgery 81:556, 1977
4. Eastcott HHG: Vascular reconstruction in England, Dardik H (ed): In Graft Materials in Vascular Surgery. Miami, Fl, Symposia Specialists Inc, 1978
5. Ehrenfeld WK, Lord RSA, Stoney RJ, et al: Subcutaneous arterial bypass grafts in the management of fistulae between the bowel and plastic arterial prostheses. Ann Surg 168:29, 1968
6. Buchbinder D, Leather R, Shah D, Karmody, A: Pathological interactions between prosthetic aortic grafts and the gastrointestinal tract. Clinical problems and a new experimental approach. Am J Surg 140:192, 1980
7. Fry WJ, Lindenauer SM: Infection complicating the use of plastic arterial implants. Arch Surg 94:600, 1967
8. Leather RP, Karmody AM: A lateral route for extra-anatomical bypass of the femoral artery. Surgery 81:307, 1977
9. Daugherty M, Shearer GR, Ernst CG: Primary aortoduodenal fistula: Extra-anatomic vascular reconstruction not required for successful management. Surgery 86:399, 1979

Reoperation for Failed Femoropopliteal or Femorotibial Grafts

William R. Flinn, James S.T. Yao, John J. Bergan

In arterial reconstructive surgery, femoropopliteal and femoral-distal bypassing are probably the most performed revascularization procedures. For a variety of reasons including progression of the atherosclerotic process, reocclusion of femoropopliteal or distal bypass grafts is common. In general, graft failure may occur at three different times: (1) during the immediate postoperative period, (2) within 30 days after operation, or (3) late in the follow-up period. Early graft failure is most likely due to technical or thrombotic problems. Later graft failure is often due to progression of the atherosclerotic process with progressive occlusion of distal vessels, intimal hyperplasia at the anastomotic site, and/or stenosis of the autogenous vein secondary to clamp trauma, fibrosis, or valve defects.[1–5] Recently, atheromatous embolism has assumed clinical significance in acute occlusion of arteries.[6] Therefore, the possibility of graft occlusion due to such arteriogenic emboli from proximal atheromatous disease should also be considered.[7] Finally, graft occlusion may be caused by progression of the occlusive process in the proximal, aortoiliac segment.

Occlusion of a bypass graft is often accompanied by severe ischemia. Therefore, the majority of patients require revascularization procedures to relieve their symptoms.[8–10] For claudicants, the mild recurrent symptoms are similar to those found preoperatively, and the decision to proceed with further surgery requires thought by both patient and surgeon.

Reoperation presents a technical challenge because of the previous surgical exposure of various arteries. This is particularly true when a prosthetic graft has been used, the dense adhesions of which make dissection difficult. Decision as to the proper procedure requires careful preoperative evaluation of the groin wound and consideration of the type of graft material used in the previous procedure. Arteriography is mandatory to define the inflow and the distal runoff. Noninvasive testing using Doppler ultrasound flow detection technique offers supplementary information.[11]

Unless there are gross, irreversible ischemic changes of the calf muscle or foot, all patients with occlusion of the previous graft who present with severe ischemia should be considered for reoperation. Failure to visualize arteries below the popliteal trifurcation is not an indication for amputation, as such failure is often due to timing of the exposure, especially when a translumbar aortogram is performed.[12,13] When no arterial filling is seen on routine study, an intraoperative prebypass arteriogram should be done as described in the chapter "Sequential Bypass Grafting" by Flinn et al. Reoperation is terminated if no bypassable distal arteries at the ankle level are seen on the intraoperative arteriogram. Undetectable flow in these arteries on the preoperative Doppler examination reinforces this decision.

SURGICAL PROCEDURE

In reoperation for immediate graft failure, the previous wound can be entered without difficulty. In early or late graft failure, exposure of the artery at a different site requires special consideration.

Exposure of the Common Femoral Artery

The previous surgical scar is excised, and the skin incision is normally extended cephalad for 1 to 3 cm in order to approach the common femoral artery just below the inguinal ligament. Dissection in this fashion avoids the scar tissue that surrounds the previously exposed common femoral artery. Thus, inadvertent injury to the femoral vein is avoided. Once the common femoral artery is identified, the previous anastomotic site can be approached by sharp division of scar tissue. Depending on the ease of the dissection as well as on the available length of the common femoral artery for anastomosis, exposure of the hood of the previous bypass may not be necessary. In immediate failure, the hood of the graft can be exposed without difficulty. In patients with possible narrowing of the profunda femoris artery from previous femoropopliteal bypass, exposure of the profunda femoris is mandatory.

Use of the external iliac artery as the inflow artery must be considered in patients with multiple groin incisions, groin hematoma, or wound problems. The bypass can then be routed through the obturator foramen, sparing the groin and thus eliminating possible graft infection or difficult dissection of the groin arteries.

Depending on the previous site of anastomosis and the arteriographic findings, the distal anastomosis of the femoral graft is placed either in the midcalf or at ankle level. Exposure of the anterior tibial, peroneal, or posterior tibial artery at these two levels is as follows.

Exposure of the Anterior Tibial Artery

A vertical incision is made over the anterior compartment about 2 fingerbreadths from the tibial crest (Fig. 1). After the fascia is excised, the groove between the extensor digitorum longus and anterior tibial muscle is split bluntly. After placement of a self-retaining retractor between these two muscles, the neurovascular bundle sheath is opened. The artery is often seen between two anterior tibial veins. Care must be taken to free the artery from the veins as well as from the deep branch of the peroneal nerve. Multiple branches of the anterior tibial artery must be carefully preserved. Avulsion of these branches may cause oozing of blood, obscuring the surgical field. Approximately 3 to 4 cm of the artery are exposed to allow adequate length for anastomosis. The artery is then encircled by silastic tapes for proximal and distal control.

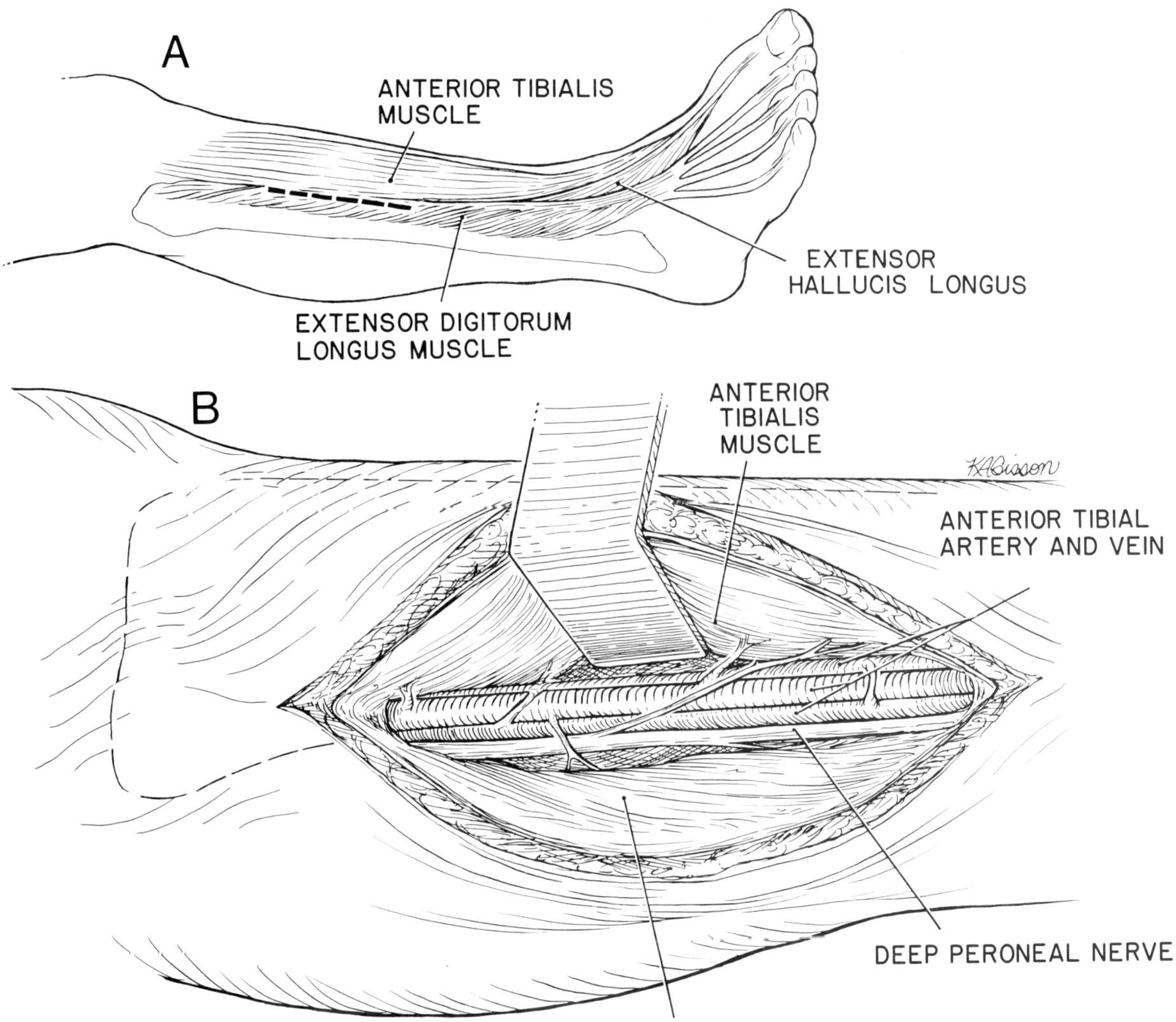

Fig. 1. Exposure of the anterior tibial artery: A skin incision is made about 2 fingerbreadths from the tibial bone over the anterior compartment. The anterior tibial artery is readily identified by the muscle-splitting technique.

Exposure of the Popliteal Artery and Tibioperoneal Trunk

A skin incision is made 10 to 12 cm in length along the medial aspect of the calf about 1 fingerbreadth from the tibia (Fig. 2). The skin incision is carried to the lower part of the joint line. After the fascia is divided, the popliteal space is readily entered. The gastrocnemius muscle is then retracted downward. A self-retaining retractor (Garrett type) is placed inside the space. The semimembranosus and semitendinosus (gracilis) tendons may be divided to facilitate the exposure of the popliteal artery. In this position, the artery normally lies slightly behind the popliteal vein. The vein is retracted gently, and the sheath of the popliteal artery is entered by sharp dissection using scissors (Fig. 2). Once the popliteal artery is encircled with silastic tape, the artery is pulled toward the wound to facilitate the exposure. Dissection is then carried out distally. The anterior tibial artery is often crossed by a large tributary of the popliteal vein (anterior tibial vein), which may be ligated and transected to allow adequate control of the anterior tibial artery. The tibioperoneal trunk can be exposed by further dissection distally (Fig. 3).

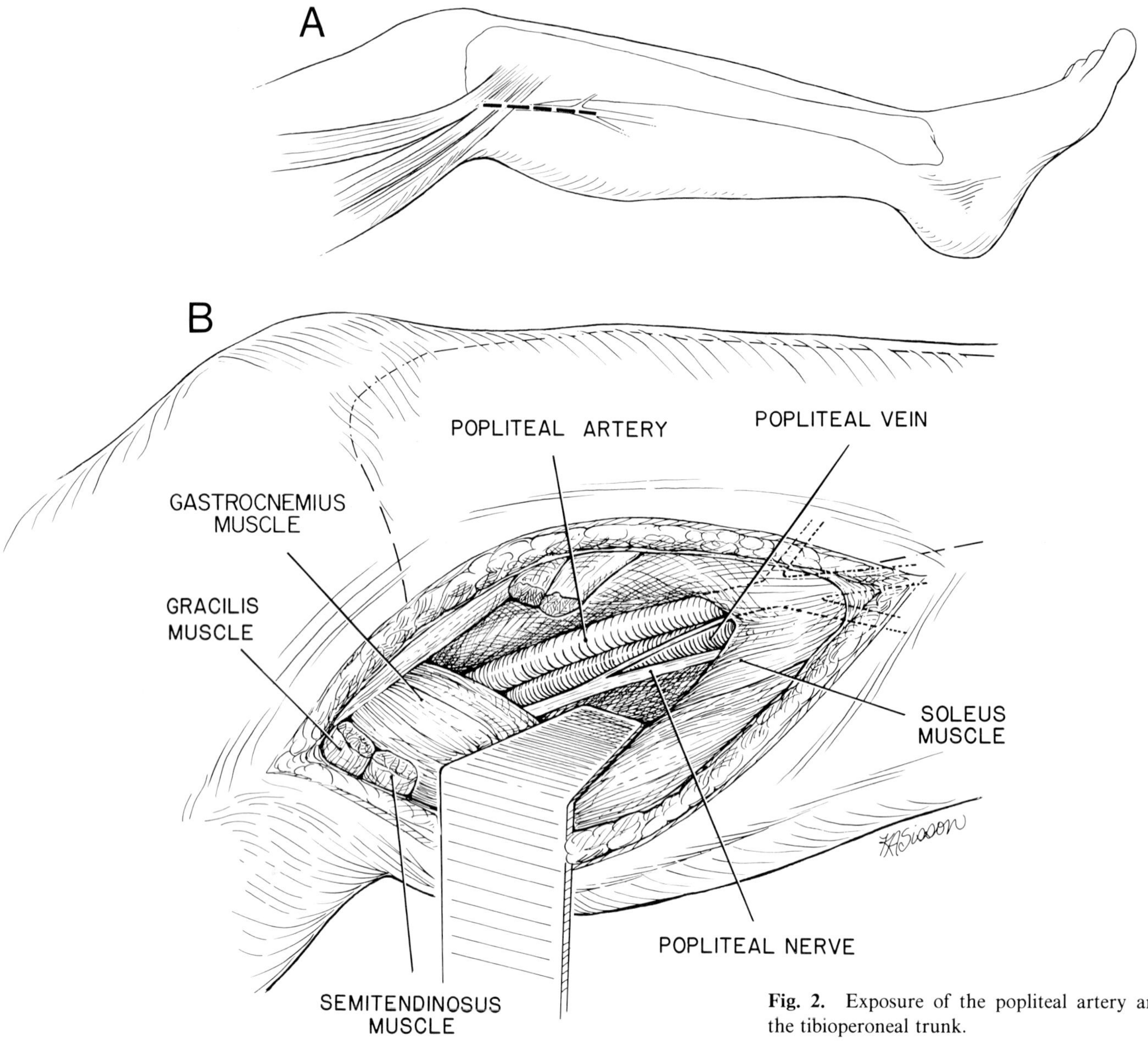

Fig. 2. Exposure of the popliteal artery and the tibioperoneal trunk.

Exposure of the Peroneal or Posterior Tibial Artery

Both arteries can be approached by extending the medial calf incision as depicted in Figure 3. In our experience, there is no need to remove the fibula to expose the peroneal artery. The soleal muscle is detached from the tibia; such a maneuver allows adequate exposure of both the posterior tibial and the peroneal artery.

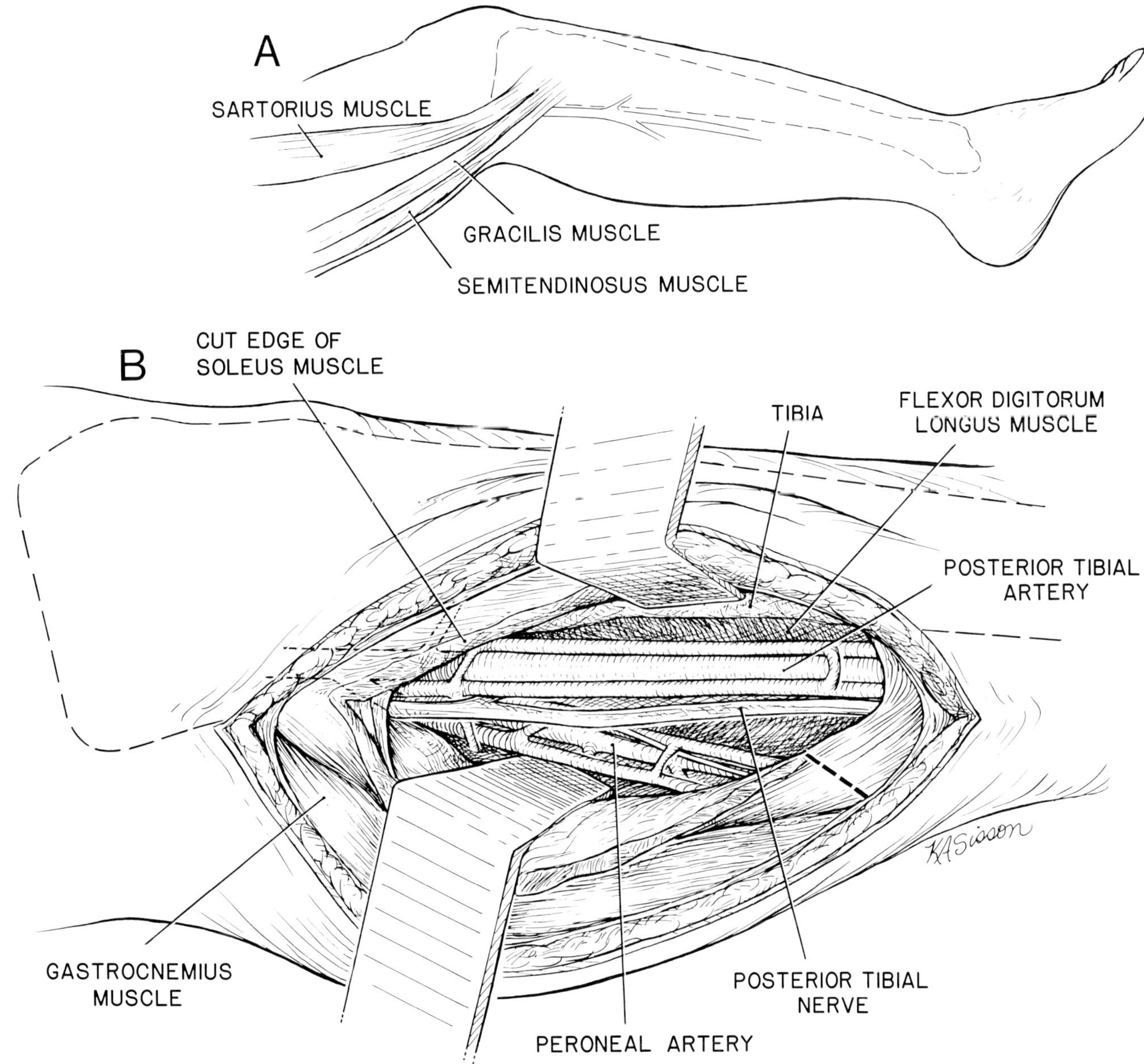

Fig. 3. Both the peroneal and the posterior tibial arteries can be exposed by extending the incision as depicted here. The soleus muscle is detached from the tibial bone to facilitate the exposure of these two arteries.

Exposure of the Posterior Tibial Artery at Ankle Level

The posterior tibial artery is exposed at the ankle level by an incision placed posterior to the malleolus. The posterior tibial artery is often seen between the flexor digitorum longus and the flexor hallucis longus muscles (Fig. 4).

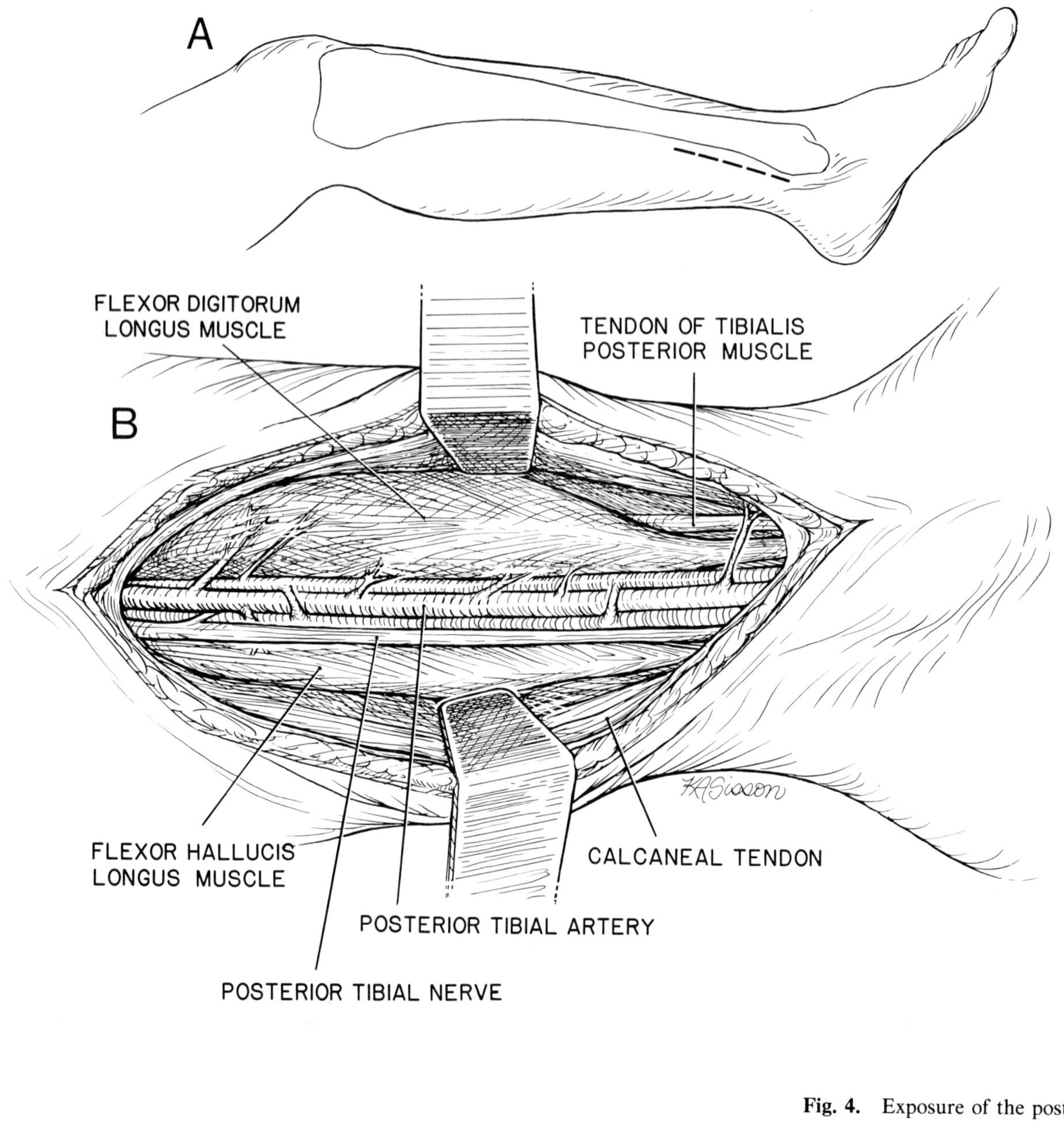

Fig. 4. Exposure of the posterior tibial artery at the ankle level.

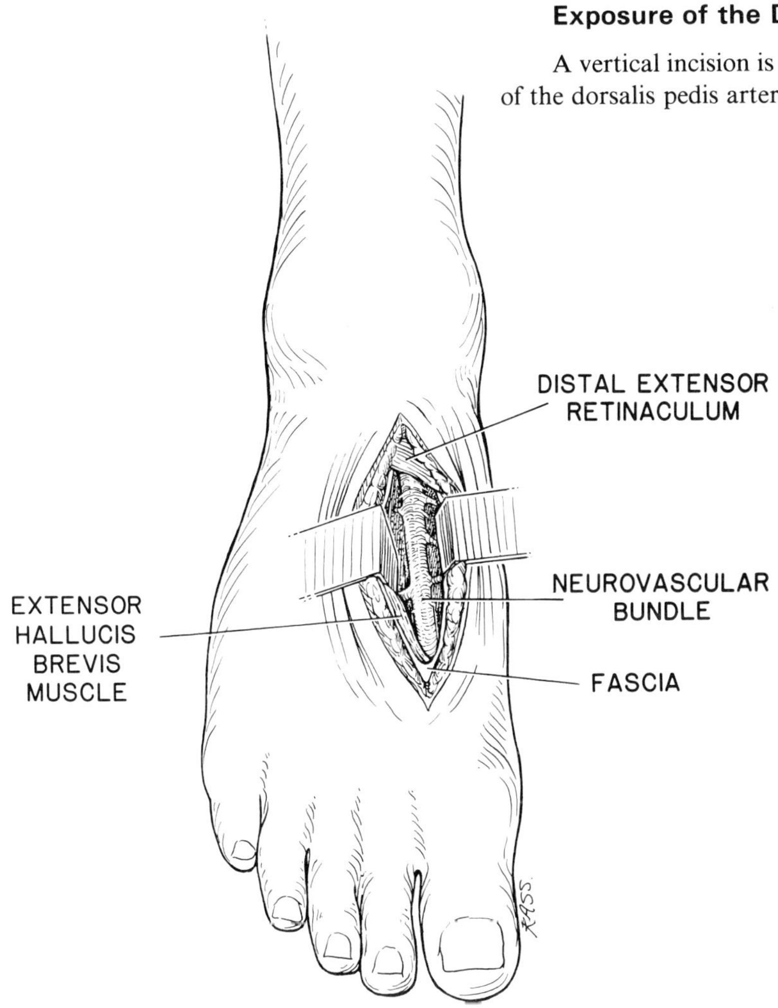

Fig. 5 Exposure of the dorsalis pedis artery. (Reprinted with permission from Flanigan DP: in Nyhus LM, Baker RJ (eds): Mastery of Surgery. Boston, Little, Brown & Co. [in press])

Exposure of the Dorsalis Pedis Artery

A vertical incision is made on the dorsum of the foot over the usual location of the dorsalis pedis artery (Fig. 5).

REOPERATION PROCEDURES

Immediate Failure

Most graft failures during the immediate postoperative period are due to technical fault or to thrombosis from severely atherosclerotic arteries distal to the anastomosis. Frequently, atheromatous embolism from a proximal artery (aorta, iliac, or common femoral) may be the cause of graft occlusion. Exploration of immediate graft failures often begins with the distal anastomosis, which can be exposed simply by reopening the distal wound. After proximal and distal control and heparinization, the hood of the distal anastomosis is opened by a longitudinal incision. This incision allows full inspection of the anastomotic site for atheromatous debris or technical fault such as an intimal flap. After this, thrombectomy of the distal vascular bed is done with a No. 3 or No. 2 Fogarty catheter, depending on the size of the artery. For thrombectomy of the proximal artery and the graft itself, a No. 4 Fogarty catheter is used. After restoration of flow, the longitudinal incision is closed with 7–0 polypropylene suture. An intraoperative arteriogram is then performed to ensure integrity of the anastomosis as well as patency of the distal vessels. Reanastomosis in a new location is often distal to the previous site and is performed when an intimal flap exists or when the original graft was placed on an atherosclerotic plaque not previously recognized.

Immediate graft failure is commonly encountered with a polytetrafluoroethylene (PTFE) graft.[14,15] An aggressive surgical approach is necessary to maintain graft patency (see chapter "Femoral-Distal Artery Bypasses" by Veith and Gupta). Thrombectomy of the PTFE graft is often successful if thrombosis is detected early, ie, within 6 hours after completion of the procedure. If the thrombus is older than 24 hours, the entire PTFE graft may need to be replaced because of adherence of the thrombus to the wall of the graft which prevents effective removal by the Fogarty catheter. In this circumstance, the groin must be reopened and prepared for reanastomosis. Proximal anastomosis of the new PTFE graft can be performed in the following fashion: First, the thrombosed PTFE graft is transected right at the hood and an end-to-end anastomosis done between the new and old grafts (Fig. 6). Second, the hood of the proximal graft can be opened longitudinally for inspection of the luminal surface, with the new graft resutured to the opening in end-to-side manner and the thrombosed graft left in place (Fig. 7). The new graft can be sutured onto the transected end of the thrombosed graft and pulled through the old tunnel, thus avoiding reopening of the thigh incision.

If no apparent cause of immediate graft failure is found, embolization from a proximal artery must be kept in mind. Re-examination of the arteriogram at the aortoiliac level may help plan a further procedure. On occasion, an aortofemoral graft is necessary to eliminate the problem.[7]

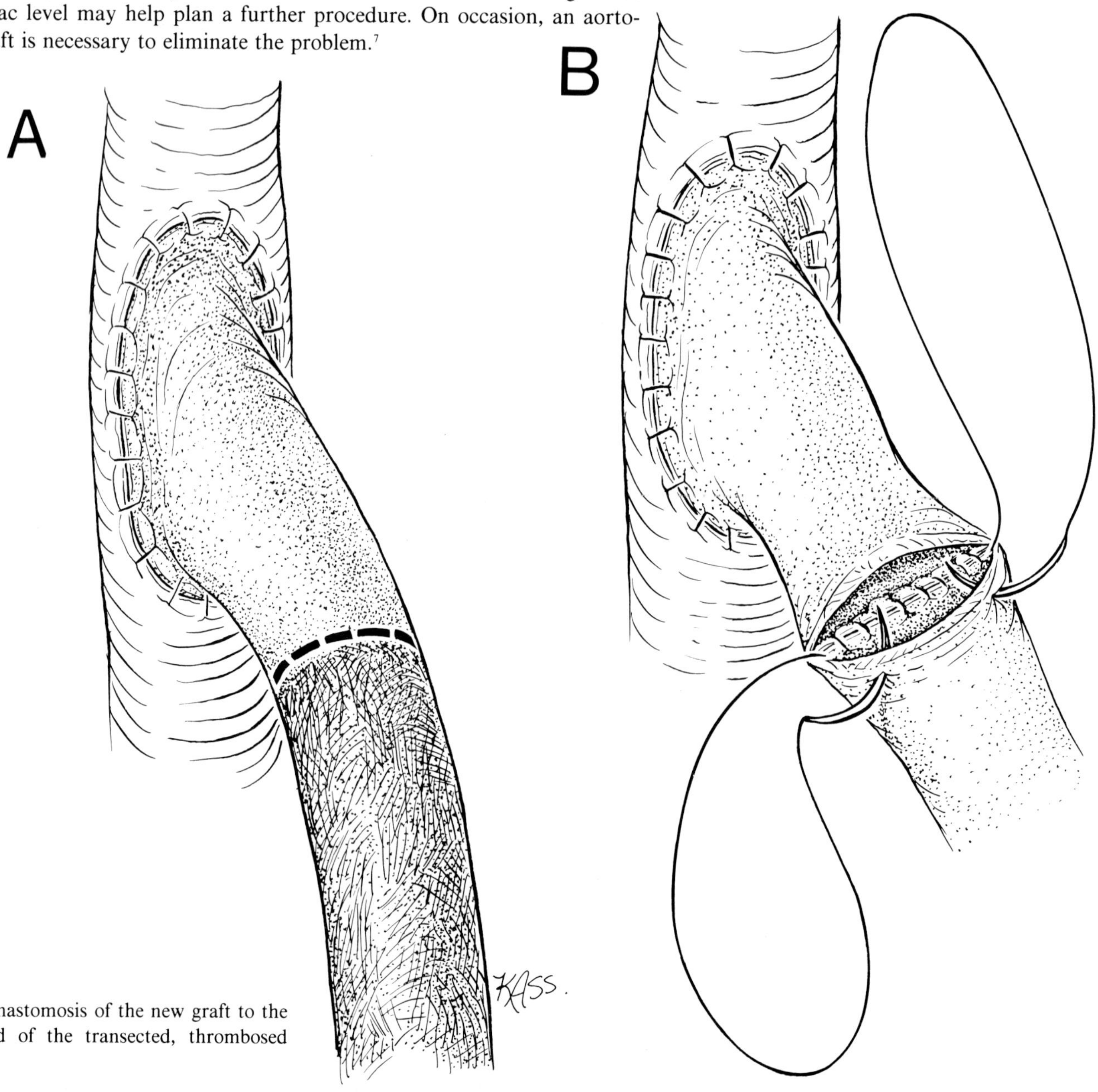

Fig. 6. Reanastomosis of the new graft to the proximal end of the transected, thrombosed PTFE graft.

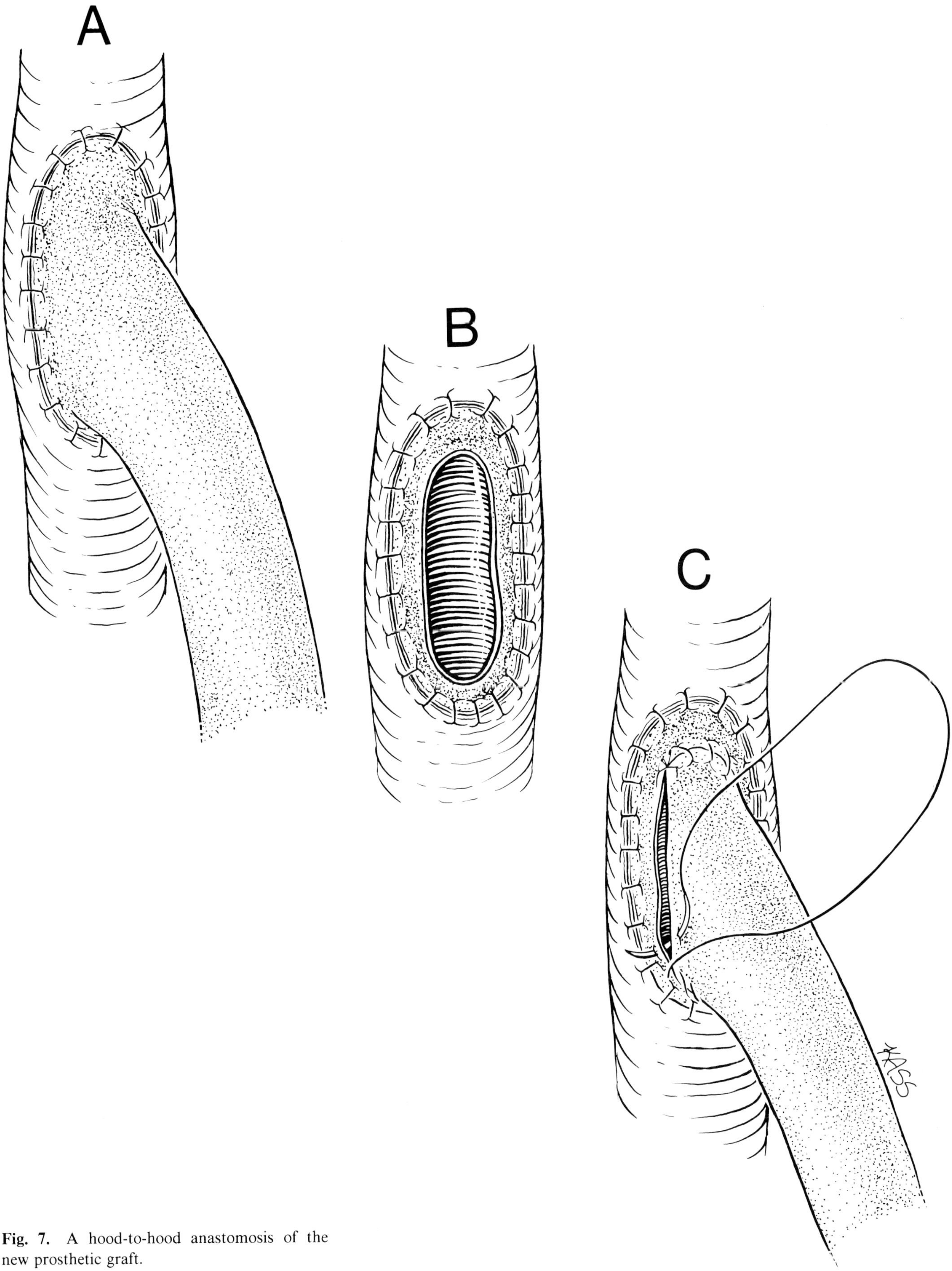

Fig. 7. A hood-to-hood anastomosis of the new prosthetic graft.

Delayed or Late Graft Failure

Delayed (30 days) or late graft failure must be dealt with by placement of a new graft. Depending on the availability of autogenous vein and the disease status of the contralateral limb, a prosthetic (PTFE) graft is often used if autogenous vein is not available. Reanastomosis of the proximal end of the graft to the common femoral artery depends on the condition of the groin, as described previously. Preferably, the arteriotomy is made in a more proximal area free of the atherosclerotic process. In the presence of a previously implanted aortofemoral Dacron graft and a failed femoropopliteal bypass, the limb of the Dacron graft is exposed by a longitudinal incision over the capsule of the Dacron limb to expose the graft (Fig. 8A). This maneuver avoids unnecessary dissection around the adherent tissue surrounding the graft and greatly facilitates the exposure of the Dacron graft without unwanted venous bleeding. Anastomosis of the proximal end of the graft is then performed by removal of an elliptical portion of the Dacron graft (Fig. 8B), with suturing done in the usual manner.

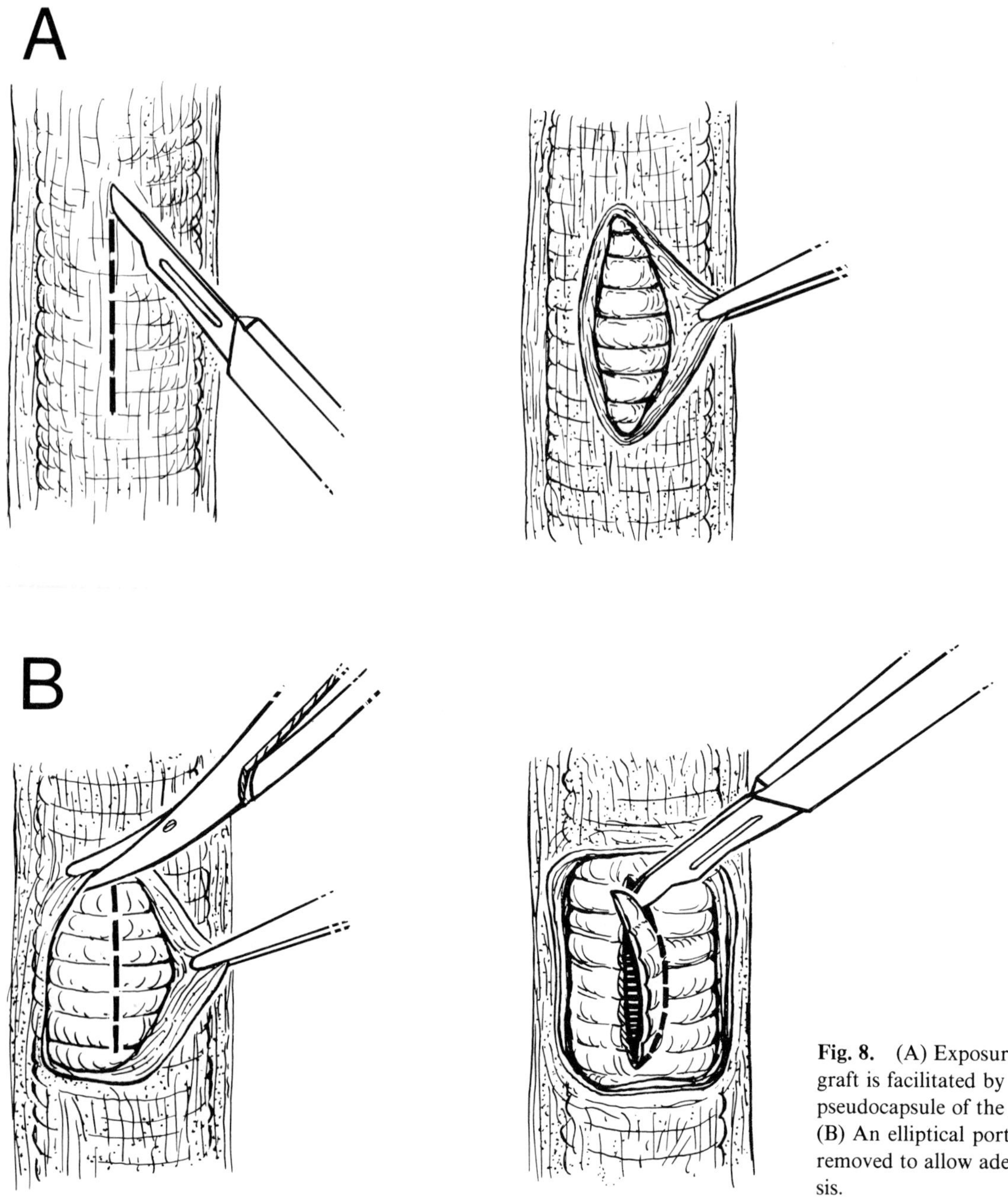

Fig. 8. (A) Exposure of the implanted Dacron graft is facilitated by an incision made over the pseudocapsule of the graft.
(B) An elliptical portion of the Dacron graft is removed to allow adequate room for anastomosis.

For distal anastomosis, the choice of the site depends on the new arteriographic findings (prebypass arteriogram) and noninvasive flow detection. A careful review of the previous arteriogram, especially the intraoperative arteriogram, will help in planning the distal anastomosis. Often, a new site for the distal anastomosis, either at the previous anastomosed artery or at another tibial or peroneal artery, is needed for restoration of perfusion. If the previous operated artery is used, anastomosis is often done in the more distal part of the artery. In the presence of occlusion of the femoropopliteal artery above the knee, anastomosis is often performed at the infrapopliteal level or infrageniculate arteries. Likewise, a failed femorotibial bypass may necessitate a more distal anastomosis at the ankle level to restore flow to the extremity.

Problems associated with autogenous vein grafts are unique, including spoon-bowl deformity,[16] progression of the proximal atherosclerotic process, intimal hyperplasia, or stenosis due to fibrous or venous valve deformity.[17–19] Many of these grafts are patent by arteriography, but with such defects they cause recurrent symptoms. All these graft defects can be dealt with by local angioplasty or interposition graft. For inflow problems, a formal aortofemoral graft may be needed to restore flow through the graft.

Reoperation presents a challenge to vascular surgeons. A planned approach is necessary to achieve good results.

REFERENCES

1. Reichle FA, Rankin KP, Tyson RR, Finestone AJ, Shuman C: Long-term results of 474 arterial reconstructions for severely ischemic limbs: A fourteen year follow-up. Surgery 85:93–100, 1979
2. DeWeese JA, Rob CG: Autogenous venous grafts ten years later. Surgery 82:775–784, 1977
3. Mozersky DJ, Sumner DS, Strandness DE Jr: Disease progression after femoropopliteal surgical procedures. Surg Gynecol Obstet 135:700–704, 1972
4. Szilagyi DE, Hageman JH, Smith RF, Elliott JP, Brown F, Dietz P: Autogenous vein grafting in femoropopliteal atherosclerosis: The limits of its effectiveness. Surgery 86:836–851, 1979
5. Buda JA, Weber CJ, McAllister FF, Voorhees AB Jr: Factors influencing patency of femoropopliteal artery bypass grafts. Am J Surg 132:8–12, 1976
6. Brenowitz JB, Edwards WS: The management of atheromatous emboli in the lower extremities. Surg Gynecol Obstet 143:941–945, 1976
7. Flinn WR, Yao JST, Bergan JJ: Atheromatous embolization as a cause of femorotibial graft failure (ms in preparation)
8. Painton JF, Avellone JC, Plecha FR: Effectiveness of reoperation after late failure of femoropopliteal reconstruction. Am J Surg 135:235–237, 1978
9. Sproul G, Pinto JM, Trummer MJ, Stevens DM: Reoperation for early complications of arterial surgery. Arch Surg 104:814–816, 1972
10. Tyson RR, Grosh JD, Reichle FA: Redo surgery for graft failure. Am J Surg 136:165–170, 1978
11. Yao JST, Nicolaides AN: The use of Doppler ultrasound in reconstructive surgery, in Nicolaides AN, Yao JST (eds): Advances in Investigation of Peripheral Vascular Disease. New York and London, Churchill Livingstone (in press)
12. Knox WG, Finby N, Moscarella AA: Limitations of arteriography in determining operability for femoropopliteal occlusive disease. Ann Surg 161:509–515, 1965
13. Nicholas GG, Latshaw RF: Femoropopliteal bypass grafting: Predictive value of preoperative angiography. Am J Surg 138:672–674, 1979
14. Echave V, Koornick AR, Haimov M, Jacobson JH II: Intimal hyperplasia as a complication of the use of the polytetrafluoroethylene graft for femoral-popliteal bypass. Surgery 86:791–798, 1979
15. Veith FJ, Moss CM, Daly V, Fell SC, Haimovici H: New approaches to limb salvage by extended extra-anatomic bypasses and prosthetic reconstruction to foot arteries. Surgery 84:764–773, 1978
16. Root JA, Giustra PE: "Spoon bowl" deformity of proximal femoral bypass vein graft. Arch Surg 112:166–169, 1977
17. Karayannacos P, Hostetler JR, Bond MG, Kakos GS, Williams RA, Kilman JW, Vasko JS: Late failure in vein grafts. Ann Surg 187:183–188, 1978
18. Fuchs JCA, Mitchener JS III, Hagen P: Postoperative changes in autologous vein grafts. Ann Surg 188:1–15, 1978
19. Bosher LP, Deck JD, Thubrikar M, Nolan SP: Role of the venous valve in late segmental occlusion of vein grafts. J Surg Res 26:437–446, 1979

Reoperation For the Infected Aortic Graft

Roger F. Smith

An infected aortic graft remains one of the most feared and devastating complications in vascular surgery. Fortunately it is a relatively rare occurrence but will still be encountered in 1 to 2 percent of patients undergoing prosthetic aortic reconstructions.[1,2] In our own reported experience[3] there was a 1.3 percent incidence of abdominal aortic graft infection. Currently with the use of prophylactic antibiotics, the infection rate has been reduced to less than 1 percent. The aortofemoral group of cases comprised the largest number of patients with this complication, because of the frequency of an associated groin-healing problem. The serious consequences of these infections are well illustrated by the fact that there was a 50 percent mortality rate, and of those patients surviving, 17 percent required a major amputation. Only one third of the patients eventually recovered without significant disability.

There is no place in the management of prosthetic graft infection for procrastination or a nonoperative approach. The only acceptable form of treatment is aggressive surgical intervention, which is a demanding and challenging endeavor that requires an individualized approach but at the same time follows the well-established surgical principles of appropriate antibiotic therapy, complete removal of the infected prosthesis, and vascular reconstruction when needed through noninfected tissues.

It is not the primary purpose of this discussion to deal with the etiology, diagnosis, or clinical presentation of infected aortic grafts. However, since these are important aspects of this subject, it should be noted that in our experience all but one case of infection limited to the aortoiliac segment developed as a result of a visceroparaprosthetic fistula. These cases characteristically tend to occur as late complications and present as either fever of unknown origin or as a metastatic abscess.[4] The treatment of this type of graft complication has been described elsewhere in this symposium and will therefore not be dealt with in detail here. Suffice it to state that the surgical principles of management are again straightforward and consist of (1) closure of the visceral perforation, (2) removal of the prosthesis, and (3) construction of a remote bypass when required. Because the groins are usually uninvolved in these cases, the technical considerations are often less demanding than when dealing with an infected aortofemoral prosthetic reconstruction.

The most common manifestation of an aortic graft infection is that associated with aortofemoral grafting and secondary to a groin complication such as an infected false aneurysm or a deep-wound infection. We have observed only one instance of late secondary hematogenous spread from a severe staphylococcus skin infection that resulted in a late graft infection. It is this major group of aortic graft infections that comprises the bulk of our clinical experience and on which I wish to focus attention.

GENERAL CONSIDERATIONS

Antibiotics

Antibiotic administration should be based upon specific bacteriologic culture information whenever possible. This may be obtained from peripheral venous or distal arterial blood sampling and by direct wound culture. On occasion, needle aspiration from either a groin swelling or the para-aortic retroperitoneal space by a translumbar puncture will be helpful. Preoperative administration of the appropriate antibiotic in the indicated dosage is essential and should be continued until the infected prosthesis has been removed and the infectious process controlled. The systemic route of administration is preferred but can be supplemented by local topical irrigations both intraoperatively and postoperatively.

Timing and Staging of Operations

The surgical approach to an aortic graft infection must usually consist of two separate operations: one to provide adequate distal circulation, and another to remove the infected prosthesis. The timing of these operative interventions and the order in which they are performed will vary according to certain clinical considerations. If the extent of the infectious process is known and if it is adequately controlled by antibiotics and, if necessary, by drainage, it is best to proceed directly with a remote bypass, prior to removing the infected prosthesis in a second operation. On the other hand, it is mandatory that the contaminated-prothesis operation be performed as the first step when: (1) the diagnosis is uncertain (rare with aortofemoral graft infection), (2) the septic process cannot be adequately controlled, or (3) there has been a hemorrhagic complication, such as anastomotic disruption. Under these latter circumstances, after the arteries have been ligated and the prosthesis removed a determination must immediately be made regarding the adequacy of the collateral circulation to the extremities. Doppler ankle/brachial indices may be helpful when clinical doubt exists. If revascularization is deemed necessary, a second reconstructive operation can be promptly performed under the same anesthetic with the patient systemically heparinized and with a completely new operative setup. In some cases it may be possible and even desirable to closely observe the patient's limbs before deciding to proceed with a remote bypass.

Extent of Infection

The anatomical extent of the infection involving an aortofemoral graft will in most instances determine the operative approach. There are three basic patterns of the infectious process that are usually encountered: (1) infection limited to the groin wound (Fig. 1A), (2) infection involving the entire aortic prosthesis and both groins (Fig. 3A), and (3) rarely, infection limited to one limb of the aortic prosthesis and to the groin without involvement of the contralateral iliac limb or groin (Fig. 4A).

Fig. 1. First operative stage for aortofemoral graft infection limited to the groin.
(A) Extent of infectious process.
(B) Suprainguinal approach to noninfected portion of proximal iliac limb with clean transsection and separation.
(C) Ilio-superficial-femoral obturator bypass.

In planning an operative approach to any of these clinical situations, the surgeon must first make a judgement, to the best of his or her ability, regarding the extent of the pathologic process and the adequacy of the collateral circulation. Sinogram injections, noninvasive blood flow studies, and angiography may be of considerable help in arriving at this determination. In each case an individualized plan of treatment must then be developed, which requires careful thought and, at times, considerable ingenuity.

For purposes of illustrating the various surgical techniques that are employed in these three types of infectious involvement, I have assumed that the diagnosis is known, the extent of infection is well established, and that a distal arterial reconstruction is required.

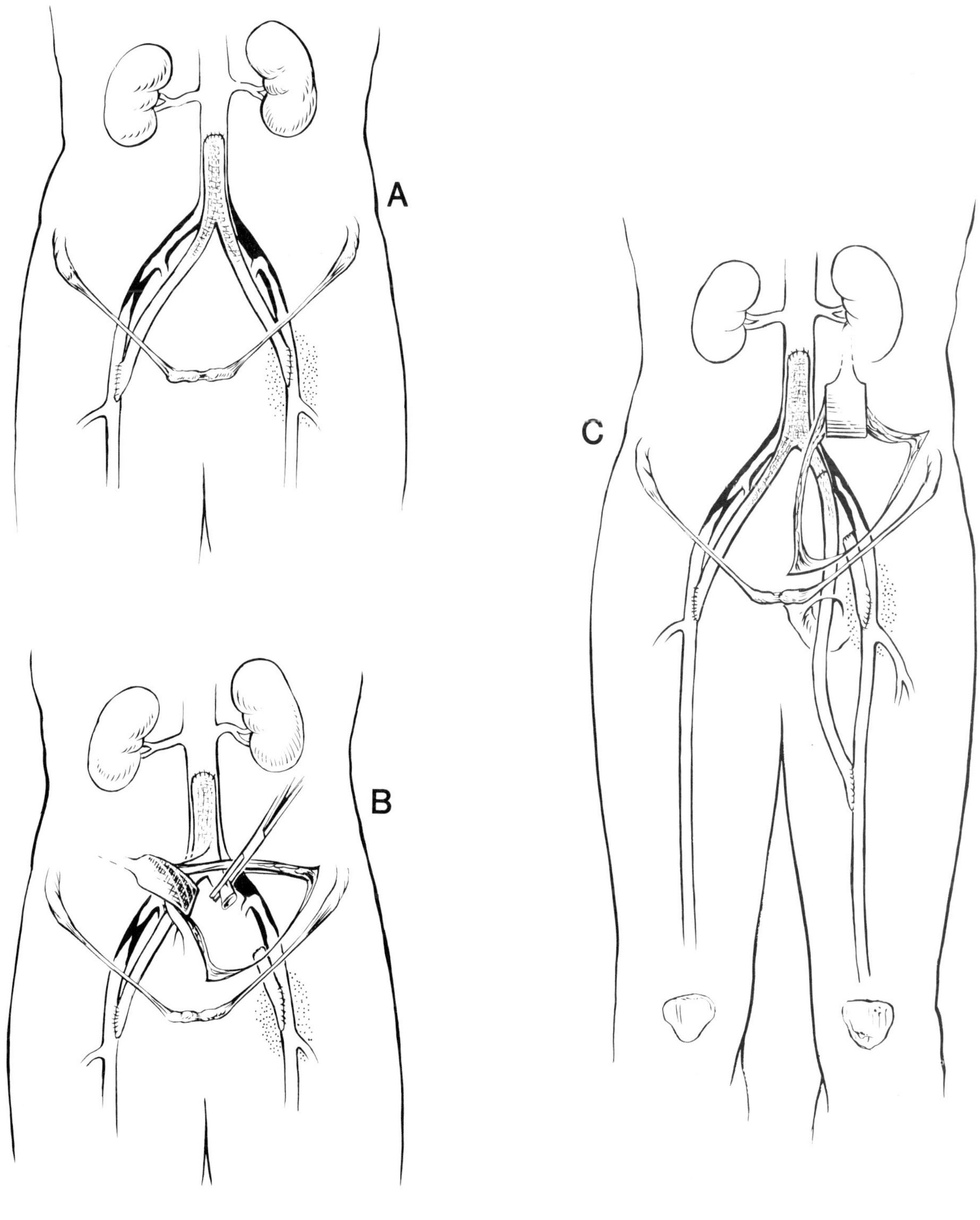

SURGICAL TECHNIQUE

Aortic Graft Infection Limited to the Groin

Providing there is no evidence of hemorrhage, the first step in the treatment of graft infection limited to the groin is the control of the infection by systemic antibiotics and the provision of drainage if there is an associated abscess. Packing the wound with antiseptic gauze or using topical antibiotics may be of benefit. If the infectious process is brought under control and if it is determined that only a limited portion of the prosthesis is involved and the anastomotic suture line is not affected, conservative management may be considered. Needless to say, this method of treatment is rarely applicable. The patient remains in the hospital for local wound care, which is continued until the infection is well controlled and healthy granulation tissue appears. At this point it may be possible to proceed with secondary closure of the wound, rather than continuing prolonged local treatment. If technically possible, it is desirable to transpose viable muscle tissue (eg, sartorius muscle) over the exposed prosthesis to obtain good graft coverage and thereby increase the chances of successful healing.

It should again be emphasized that this conservative form of management is not recommended if the deep-wound infection is virulent, if there has been any sign of hemorrhage, or if the anastomotic suture line is exposed.

The customary two-phase surgical approach to the infected groin wound with prosthetic involvement is illustrated in Figures 1 and 2. After the initial antibiotic therapy and local wound care have been instituted, a clean retroperitoneal operation is planned as the first phase. In this phase the noninfected portion of the graft is isolated from the infected area, and adequate circulation is provided to the limb. The patient is carefully prepped and extensively draped with adhesive plastic sheets in order to completely isolate the infected groin wound. General anesthesia is administered, and a suprainguinal transverse incision is made and extended retroperitoneally to expose the uninvolved segment of the iliac limb of the prosthesis. The patient is heparinized (5000 to 10,000 units controlled by activated clotting time), and the prosthetic limb is divided between vascular clamps (Fig. 1B). A short segment of the graft is excised and the distal end oversewn with a nonabsorbable vascular suture. Surrounding tissues are then used to cover and isolate the distal segment of the graft from the clean operative wound. In those patients who do not require vascular reconstruction, the proximal limb of the prosthesis may also be ligated and the incision closed. Usually however, distal reconstruction is accomplished by performing an obturator bypass between the prosthesis and the midportion of the superficial femoral artery, taking great pains to avoid any contamination from the infected groin wound (Fig. 1C). For the latter purpose, an anterior medial thigh incision is made well below the groin, the superficial femoral artery is dissected free, and a site is selected for anastomosis. The obturator foramen is identified and the heavy obturator membrane incised, taking care not to injure the obturator vessels. A tunnel is initiated both proximally and distally with finger dilatation. An end-to-end anastomosis is then made to the proximal limb of the prosthesis, using braided Dacron vascular suture. The wounds are connected by the use of a flexible tunneler inserted through the obturator foramen. The new segment of prosthesis is then drawn through the lumen of the instrument to lie in the proper position for an end-to-side anastomosis with the prepared superficial femoral artery. All vascular clamps are removed and the wounds are closed. As the second phase of the procedure, under the same anesthesia but with completely new draping and instruments, the infected segment of graft may now be removed. Under some circumstances it may be desirable to wait until the clean wounds have sealed and the patient has established a well-functioning obturator bypass before proceeding to the removal of the infected graft.

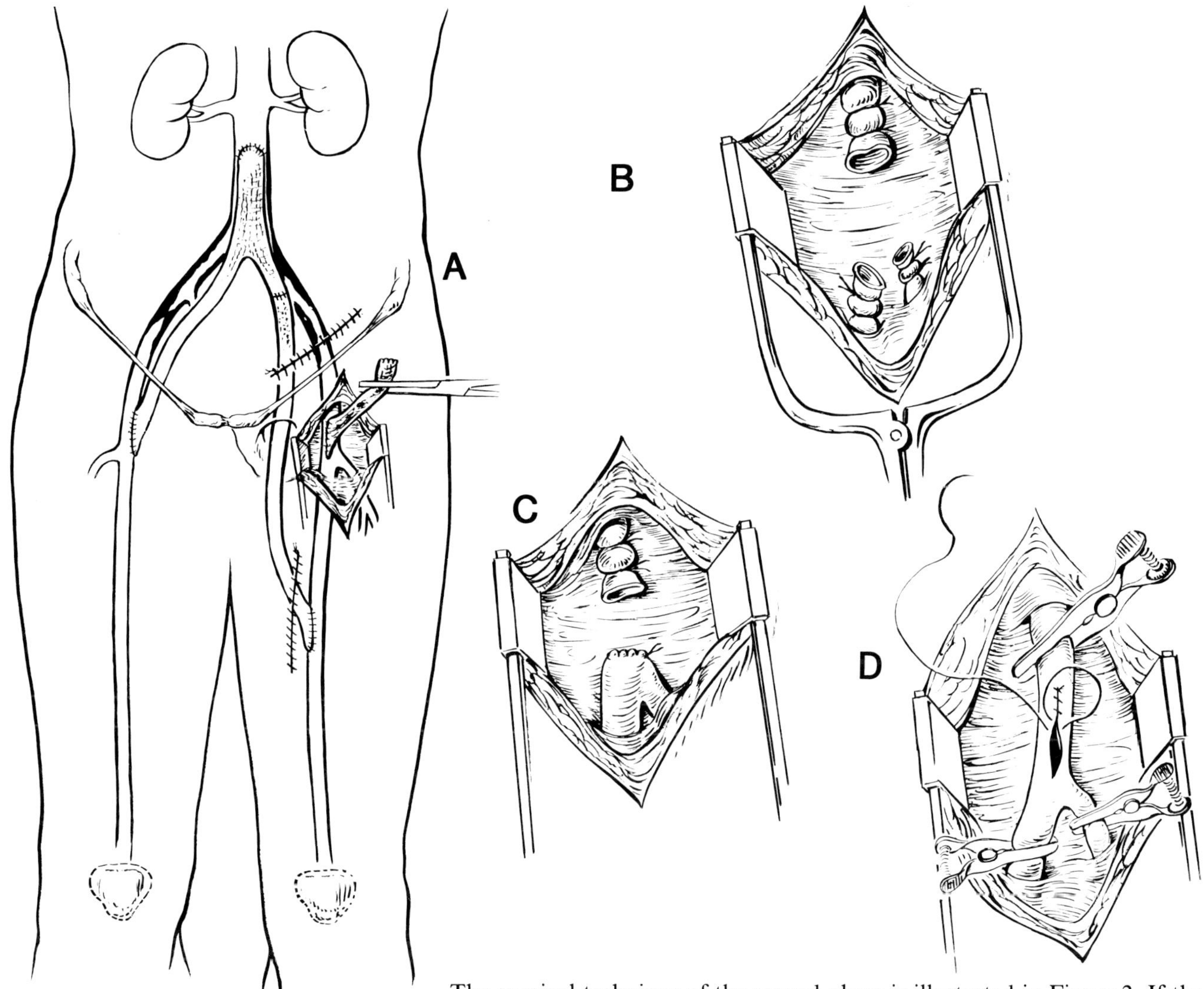

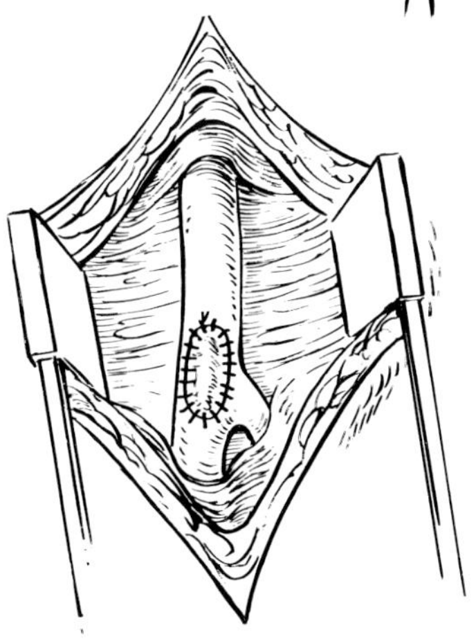

Fig. 2. Second operative stage for aortofemoral graft infection limited to the groin.
(A) Excision of infected graft segment.
(B) Ligation of common, superficial, and deep femoral arteries.
(C) Ligation of common femoral artery with functional preservation of bifurcation.
(D) Arterioplasty with monofilament vascular suture.
(E) Autogenous vein-patch arterioplasty.

The surgical technique of the second phase is illustrated in Figure 2. If the removal of the infected graft is carried out as a delayed procedure, it is performed 1 to 2 weeks after the first phase. Care is again taken with the surgical draping. The infected groin wound may be extended or excised, depending upon the need for adequate exposure. The previously isolated prosthetic limb is dissected, gently freed proximally, and delivered from beneath the inguinal ligament (Fig. 2A). The final step is the complete excision of the prosthesis, which requires vascular control of the common, superficial, and deep femoral vessels under heparinization. The remaining arterial defect may be closed in a variety of ways. The safest and most definitive method is to ligate all three branches (Fig. 2B); this method is preferred when the infectious process has destroyed the common femoral artery or when preservation of its function is deemed unnecessary. In some cases where the proximal end of the artery requires ligation, it will still be possible to preserve communication between the superficial and deep femoral arteries by carefully oversewing the common femoral bifurcation with polypropylene monofilament suture (Fig. 2C). If the wall of the artery has been fairly well preserved and common femoral arterial flow is considered essential, closure may be accomplished by means of a continuous monofilament suture (Fig. 2D). Assurance of the patency of the common femoral artery may require the use of a vein patch (Fig. 2E). The patch technique should not be used routinely, since its employment in the presence of infection increases the risk of secondary hemorrhage. A small soft drain is placed under the inguinal ligament in the bed of the removed infected graft, and the wound is left open, loosely packed with antiseptic gauze. Prompt healing by second intention occurs when the infected foreign material has been eliminated.

Infection Involving Entire Aortofemoral Graft

The most life-threatening and difficult graft infection to treat is that represented in Figure 3A, in which the entire aortofemoral prosthesis has been extensively involved. In this circumstance, the first step in surgical treatment is to perform bilateral axillofemoral bypasses under proper antibiotic management (Fig. 3B). The distal anastomosis is ideally made to the midportion of a patent superficial femoral artery. When the superficial femoral artery is occluded, the distal anastomosis may be done in a patent popliteal segment above the knee. It has been our policy not to perform an axillopopliteal bypass with the distal anastomosis below the knee because of the poor patency performance of such vascular reconstructions. An available alternative under these circumstances might be to use a well-developed deep femoral artery if it can be exposed distally without contamination from the infected groin wound. There are some patients, however, who do not have any satisfactory outflow below the groin, and an adequate, safe, remote bypass therefore may be technically impossible. Should the collateral circulation prove to be insufficient, amputation will be necessary to save the patient's life. Figure 3B illustrates the two patterns of distal reconstruction with the superficial femoral artery patent (right limb) and with a segmental occlusion (left limb).

The axillofemoral bypass is performed under general anesthesia with the patient extensively draped. A transverse infraclavicular incision is made by splitting the pectoralis major muscle and exposing the axillary artery medial to the pectoralis minor muscle. The latter muscle may be divided if necessary for improved exposure. The distal incision is placed well below the infected area of the groin and connected to the proximal incision by a subcutaneous tunnel utilizing small stepwise incisions and an appropriate tunneling device. Care is taken to keep the course of the new graft lateral to the anterior superior iliac spine and away from the infected groin. It has been helpful on occasion to "notch" the iliac crest in order to avoid impingement on the graft. The distal anastomoses are usually made end-to-side. If the superficial femoral artery is patent with good proximal inflow, this vessel must be ligated (as shown in the right limb of Figure 3B) just proximal to the anastomosis in order to establish the necessary pressure differential between the two ends of the graft.

Antibiotics are continued postoperatively until the infected graft has been removed and the infection completely controlled. This is important in order to prevent bacterial seeding of the new prosthesis.

When the patient has recovered from the first operation, the next step is to remove the infected aortic graft (Fig. 3C). The retroperitoneal aortic graft is exposed through a midline abdominal incision by retracting the small intestine and placing it in a protective bowel bag. The proximal infrarenal aorta is dissected and prepared for clamping as is the distal aorta below the aortic graft anastomosis. Systemic heparinization is used if preservation of the patency of the abdominal aorta is planned. Vascular clamps are applied above and below the aortic anastomosis, and the prosthesis is clamped and detached. The aortotomy incision is then closed (following a limited endarterectomy if needed) with 3–0 monofilament polypropylene continuous suture (Fig. 3C). When this has been accomplished the groin wounds are opened, the distal limbs of the prosthesis are detached, and the common femoral artery is closed or ligated, as illustrated in Figure 2. The next step is to remove the infected prosthesis, which is easily accomplished as there usually is no incorporation of the graft because of the extensive infection.

When there has been a previous end-to-end aortic anastomosis, the aortic stump must be securely closed, as shown in Figure 3D. At times this will require that the aortic occluding clamp be placed above the renal arteries to obtain satisfactory aortic stump tissue. In some instances the clamp may even have to be placed at the level of the diaphragm. The aortic stump is closed with monofilament sutures in two layers. The first row is comprised of interrupted mattress stitches, and the second row is a reinforcing double running suture.

Fig. 3. Aortofemoral graft infection involving entire prosthesis:
(A) Extent of infection.
(B) Bilateral axillofemoral bypasses: right, patent superficial femoral artery; left, occluded superficial femoral artery.
(C) Excision of prosthesis with primary closure of aortotomy.
(D) Suprarenal aortic clamping with closure of infrarenal stump.
(E) Retroperitoneal closure with omental pedicle graft.

With either type of aortic closure, the last step of the operation is to prepare a viable pedicle of omentum and bring it through the transverse mesocolon to lie in the retroperitoneal bed of the removed infected prosthesis. The pedicled omental graft is also tacked to isolate the closed aortic stump from the duodenum and the infected graft bed, as shown in Figure 3E. Topical antibiotic irrigation is carried out, and soft drains are placed from below in the tunnels of the removed iliac limbs to exit in the groin incisions to establish the most efficient dependent drainage. The abdominal closure is reinforced with retention sutures, and the groin wounds are left open, as previously described.

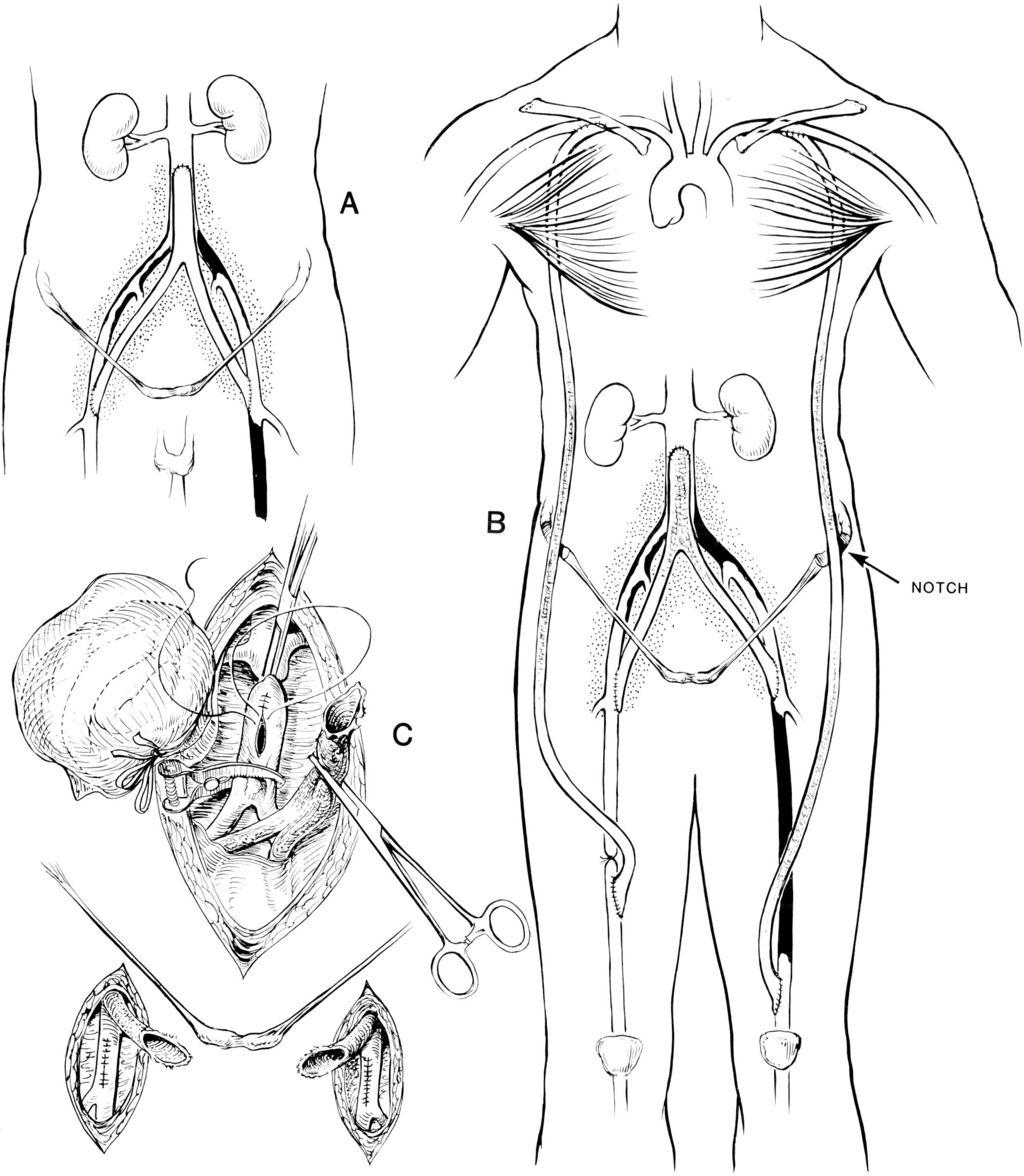

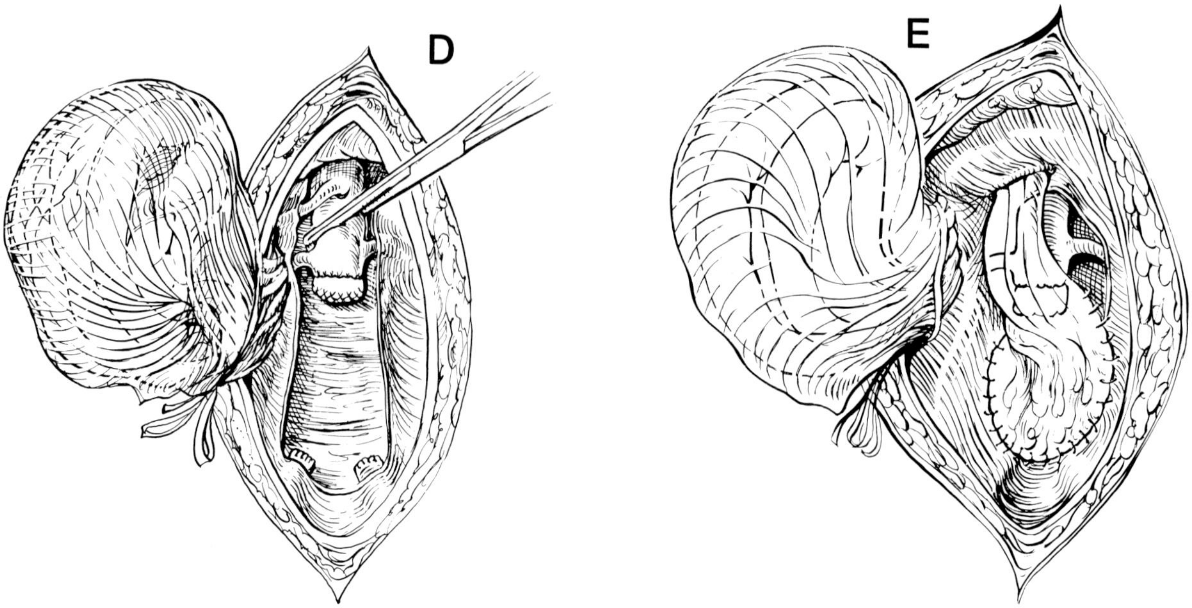

Infection Limited to Aortic Shaft and One Limb Including the Groin

A relatively rare situation is depicted in Figure 4A, in which the infectious process involves the aortic prosthesis and only one limb of the graft, sparing the contralateral groin. However, under these circumstances it may be feasible to perform an axillobifemoral bypass, as would be done for an infected aortoiliac prosthesis (Fig. 4B). The initial approach is through a suprainguinal retroperitoneal incision to the noninfected distal iliac limb, which is divided as shown in Figure 1B following systemic heparinization. The incision is then closed, and the same steps are followed as in a unilateral axillofemoral bypass, with the exception that a cross-femoral limb is attached (freshly sutured or preformed) and brought across suprapubically to a clean groin incision in such a manner as to avoid the infected groin. After dissecting the common femoral bifurcation and freeing the detached limb from beneath the inguinal ligament, it is trimmed and an end-to-end anastomosis is made to the residual stump of the graft (Fig. 4B, insert). This step greatly simplifes the amount of dissection usually required in a secondary operation. Assuming the previous anastomosis is satisfactory, no further angioplasty is necessary. All of the clean wounds are then closed. At a subsequent combined abdominal–groin operation, as illustrated in Figure 4C, the remaining infected aortofemoral prosthesis is excised as detailed in Figure 3. Drainage is provided via the open infected groin wound.

At times, modifications of the surgical approaches described above will be required, depending upon each patient's individual circumstances, particularly the extent and virulence of the infection and the adequacy of collateral circulation. In some cases of limited aortoiliac occlusive disease or richly developed collateral circulation, it may very well be possible to proceed directly with the graft excision as the only operation required. Several months later if the clinical situation warrants, another attempt at aortofemoral grafting might be considered. Some success has been achieved with use of the distal descending thoracic aorta for the proximal site of anastomosis under these circumstances.

Whatever approach is chosen, the principles of management remain the same: namely, determination of the extent of infection and an attempt to control it with drainage and antibiotic therapy; provision of adequate circulation to the affected limbs when the graft is sacrificed; complete excision of the infected foreign material with debridement of nonviable tissues; and institution of adequate drainage and antibiotic therapy until the wounds are healed. It is hoped that, in the future, this form of prompt and aggressive surgical treatment may save more lives and limbs.

Fig. 4. Aortofemoral graft infection limited to shaft, one iliac limb, and groin:
(A) Extent of infection.
(B) Axillobifemoral bypass with clean graft-to-graft anastomosis.
(C) Excision of infected prosthesis.

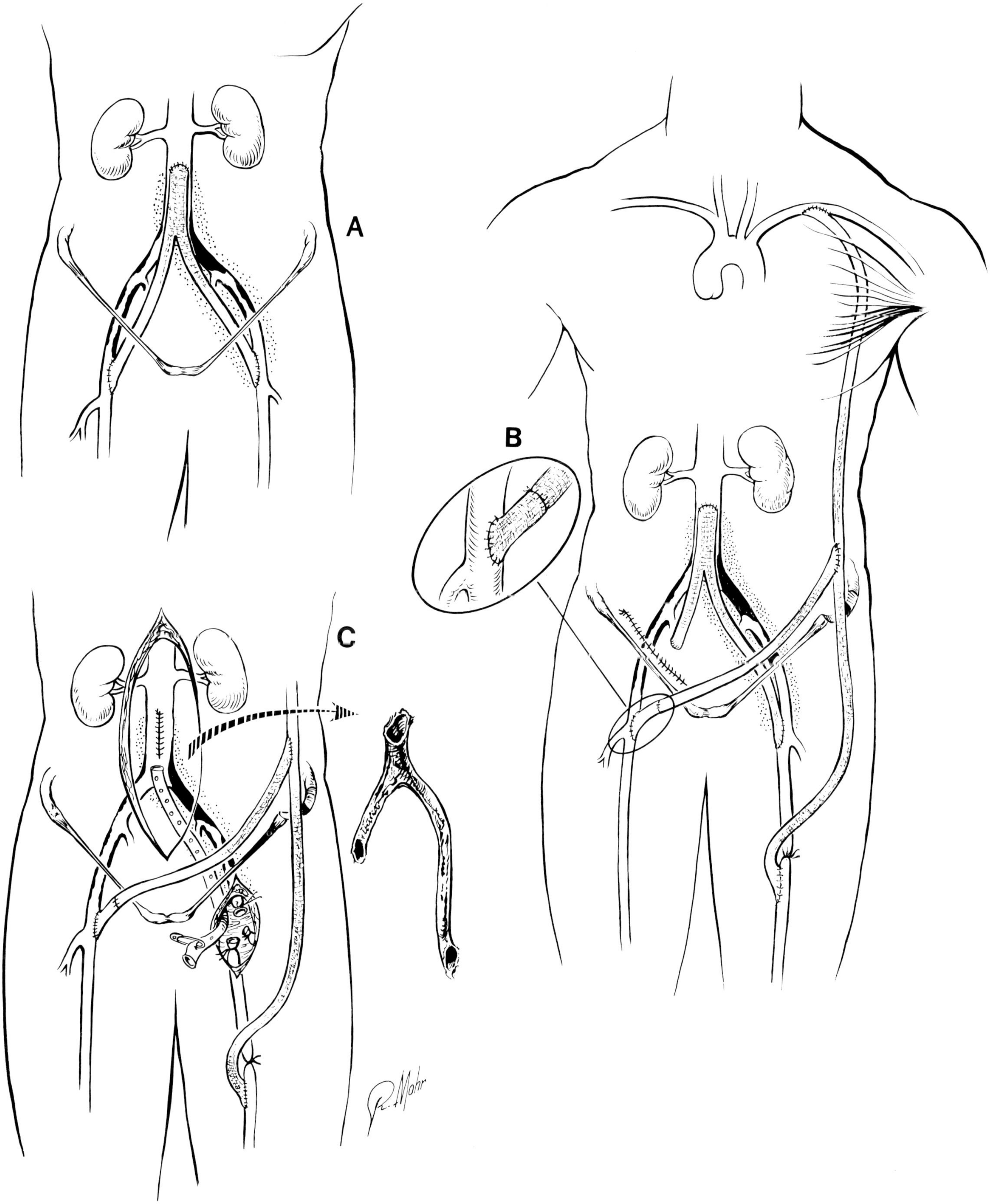
A
B
C

REFERENCES

1. Wilson SE, Wagenen, Passaro E Jr: Arterial infection. Curr Probl Surg 15:1–89, 1978
2. Moore WS: Infection in prosthetic vascular grafts, in Rutherford RB (ed): Vascular Surgery. Philadelphia, WB Saunders Co, 1977, pp 385–396
3. Szilagyi DE, Smith RF, Elliott JP Vrandecic MP: Infection in arterial reconstruction with synthetic grafts. Ann Surg 176:321–333, 1972
4. Elliott JP, Smith RF Szilagyi DE: Aortoenteric and paraprosthetic-enteric fistulas. Arch Surg 108:479–490, 1974

Obturator Bypass in Reoperations for Graft Complications

Ralph G. DePalma

Obturator bypass was originally used to manage sepsis and false aneurysm complicating femoral grafts.[1–5] It is also useful in other situations when the femoral artery in the groin is rendered unavailable because of, for example, extensive shotgun wounds, mycotic aneurysms, neoplasms, irradiation with skin loss, or aneurysms of the external iliac or common femoral artery.[4] Its use for these indications has been detailed in a recent publication summarizing experience with obturator bypass.[5] The present chapter outlines the technique of obturator bypass for sepsis complicating grafts in the femoral triangle.

PREOPERATIVE MEASURES

Once the diagnosis of graft sepsis or false aneurysm is established, operation should be planned as an urgent procedure. Once cultures have been obtained, prompt treatment with broad-spectrum antibiotics is mandatory. The author's current preference remains penicillin (2 million units) and chloramphenicol (0.5 grams) intravenously every 6 hours. In anticipation of an intra-abdominal vascular procedure, a formal bowel preparation is also begun preoperatively. To plan an adequate reconstruction, transaxillary or lumbar arteriography is performed to view proximal and distal arterial anatomy. In this situation, it is not advisable to use a retrofemoral arteriographic approach, since this might further compromise the uninvolved graft limb. Computerized axial tomographic (CAT) scanning is also of great value in selecting a proximal anastomotic site for the obturator graft origin, which is away from any potential septic collection. Thus, in many instances of localized groin sepsis, it is not always necessary to remove the entire graft. If one can accurately localize the infection to the femoral or distal pelvic portion of one limb of the graft, obturator bypass can be safely performed without radical graft excision.

REVASCULARIZATION TECHNIQUE

Either general or epidural anesthesia is preferred. The patient is placed in supine position and a Foley catheter inserted to decompress the bladder. Slight elevation of the affected side with flexion, abduction, and external rotation of the hip aids exposure. At this point the surgeon must inspect the infected groin and mechanically cleanse it of adherent tape and debris. The groin area is then screened using an impervious drape covered with a sterile, sewn-down towel conforming to the area of potential contamination in the femoral triangle. Following this, a standard wide skin preparation is done by another assistant and the patient is draped to accomplish exposure sufficient for proximal aortic and distal popliteal anastomoses.

The proximal anastomosis of the obturator graft may originate in the abdominal aorta, the proximal portion of a bifemoral graft limb, or the iliac arteries. Either intraperitoneal or extraperitoneal exposure can be used. It is essential that the approach chosen assures optimal control for the proximal anastomosis as well as avoiding any proximal septic extension.

Figure 1 shows the details of an extraperitoneal transverse approach. Note the draping of the femoral contaminated area, the salient principle in carrying out this operation. After exposure of the proximal anastomotic site, the obturator canal is located using the obturator nerve as a landmark (Fig. 2). In men, an incision just at the lateral vesicle cul de sac will expose the obturator foramen; in women, the parietal peritoneum can be opened at its junction with the anterior leaflet of the broad ligament. The author prefers blunt dissection to locate the obturator canal and nerve. In addition, it is not always necessary to dilate the canal itself to pass the graft. Depending upon the availability of uninvolved distal planes in the thigh, the tough obturator membrane itself can be perforated more posteriorly or laterally.

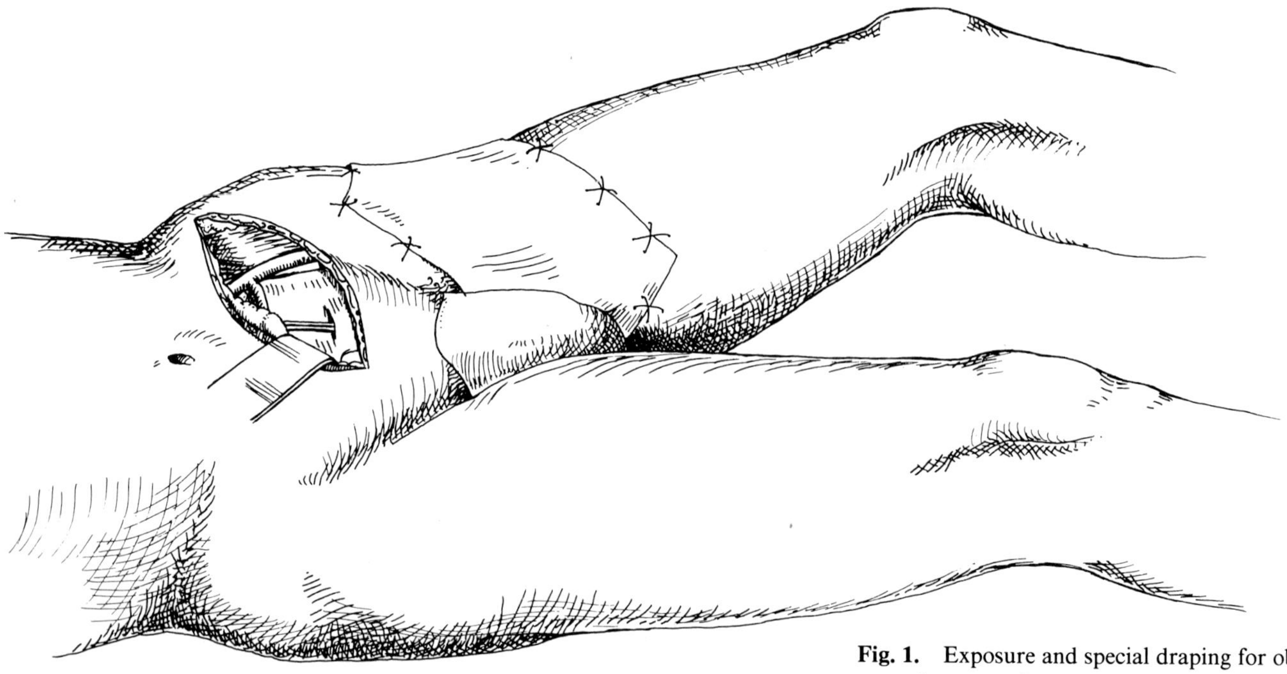

Fig. 1. Exposure and special draping for obturator bypass using transverse retroperitoneal approach. Note extensive exposure and protection of septic femoral triangle by sewn down drape over an impervious drape. (From Nyhus L, Baker R (eds): Mastery of Surgery. Boston, Little Brown and Co. (in press)

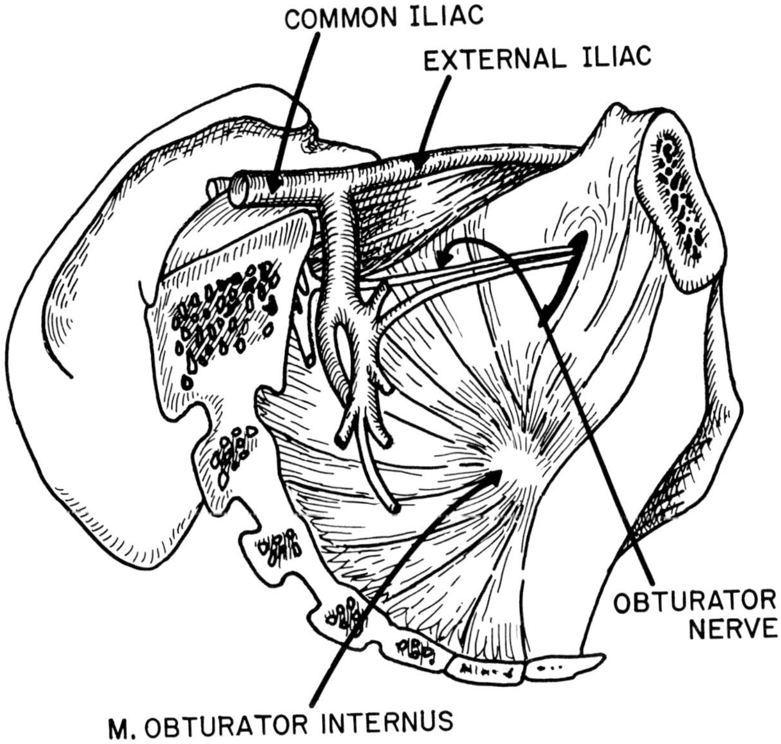

Fig. 2. Schematic view of male pelvis illustrating obturator foramen. Note course of obturator nerve as a guide to the foramen. (From Nyhus L, Baker R (eds): Mastery of Surgery. Boston, Little Brown and Co. (in press)

The essential step at this stage of the operation is identification and protection of the obturator neurovascular bundle and associated collateral vessels. A passage of sufficient size to accomodate a new graft without kinking or constriction is created. Figure 3 shows the author's preferred method of perforating the obturator membrane using a blunt uterine forceps. During this maneuver, the surgeon protects the neurovascular bundle with the index finger in the pelvis as the clamp is passed proximally from the thigh. The hand within the pelvis also serves as a guide to the proper plane. This step is especially important when extensive collaterals exist about the obturator canal, as in cases of arteriovenous fistula. The distal anastomosis is usually carried out in the middle or distal reaches of the superficial femoral artery. Occasionally the graft may pass to the popliteal artery itself, though this is not desirable. As in any vascular procedure, arteriography is critical in determining the site of distal anastomosis and the adequacy of runoff.

The obturator nerve also serves as a guide to the proper dissection plane in the thigh. It courses upon the adductor brevis muscle; the new graft plane will pass between the adductor longus anteriorly and the adductor medius posteriorly. To enter this plane, the distal portion of the gracilis muscle is reflected medially. On some occasions, the thigh dissection plane must be located more posteriorly, that is, posterior to the adductor magnus and anterior to the hamstrings. The tunneling clamp will then pierce the adductor magnus before it enters the obturator foramen. Using this passage, it is also possible to use the distal profunda femoris artery as an alternative outflow anastomotic site.

A variety of reconstructive options are available to deal with septic grafts. Figures 4 and 5 show the use of proximal and distal anastomoses as originally applied by us in 1968[4] for septic aortic and femoral popliteal grafts. More commonly, however, the surgeon will now encounter infection of one limb of a bilateral aortofemoral graft.

Since 1977, a new twist, as it were, was added by my colleagues[6] in the form of cross-obturator bypass grafts, which traverse the space of Retzius. Figure 6 shows a cross-obturator bypass for a localized left pelvic limb infection involving a bilateral aortofemoral graft. Note that it was not necessary to remove the entire aortofemoral graft. Figure 7 shows a cross-obturator reconstruction to salvage a septic left axillofemoral–femoral bypass.

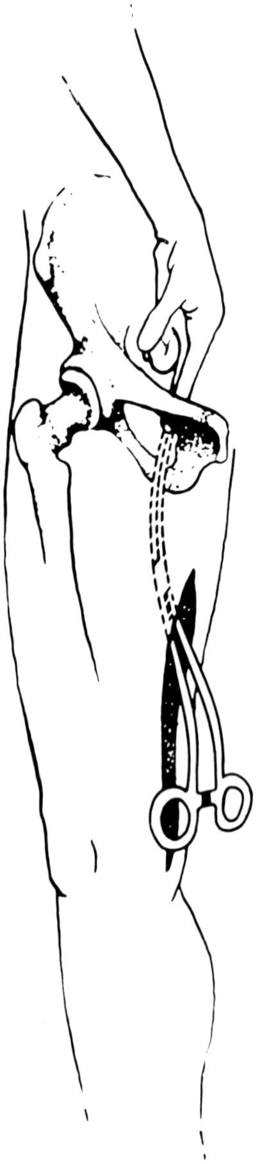

Fig. 3. Method used for creation of tunnel and entry through obturator membrane. Note use of long, blunt, uterine forceps and position of fingers during this maneuver. (From DePalma RG, Hubay CA: Arterial bypass via the obturator foramen. An alternative in complicated vascular problems. Am J Surg 115:323–328, 1968.)

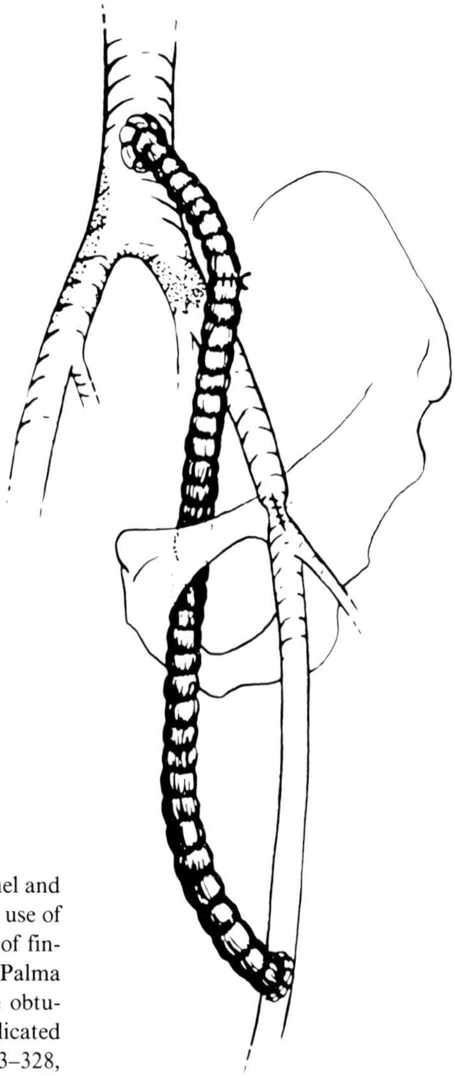

Fig. 4. Schematic of obturator bypass for a proximal aortic graft. Note anastomosis to the uninvolved graft segment. (From DePalma RG, Hubay CA: Arterial bypass via the obturator foramen. An alternative in complicated vascular problems. Am J Surg 115:323–328, 1968.)

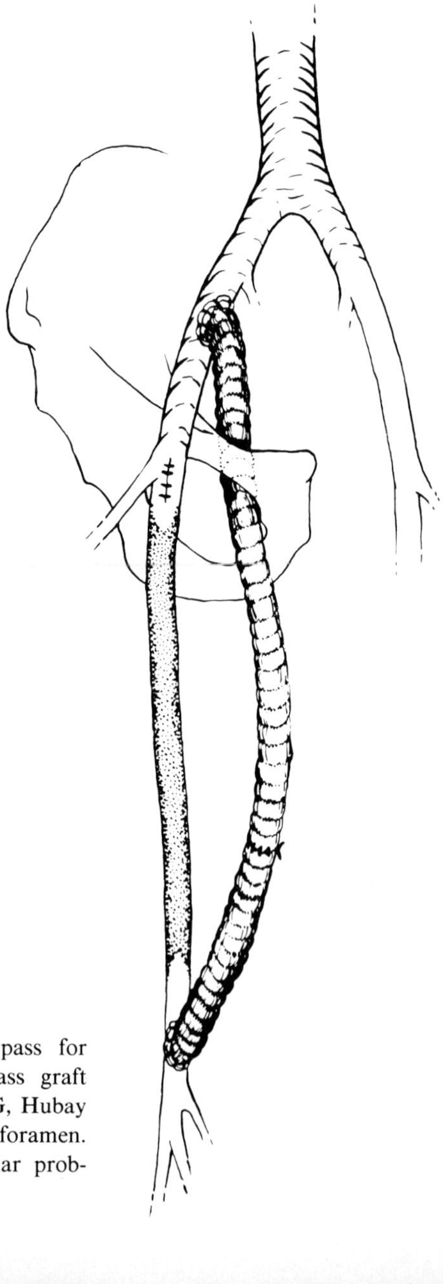

Fig. 5. Schematic of obturator bypass for treatment of a femoropopliteal bypass graft with groin sepsis. (From DePalma RG, Hubay CA: Arterial bypass via the obturator foramen. An alternative in complicated vascular problems. Am J Surg 115:323–328, 1968.)

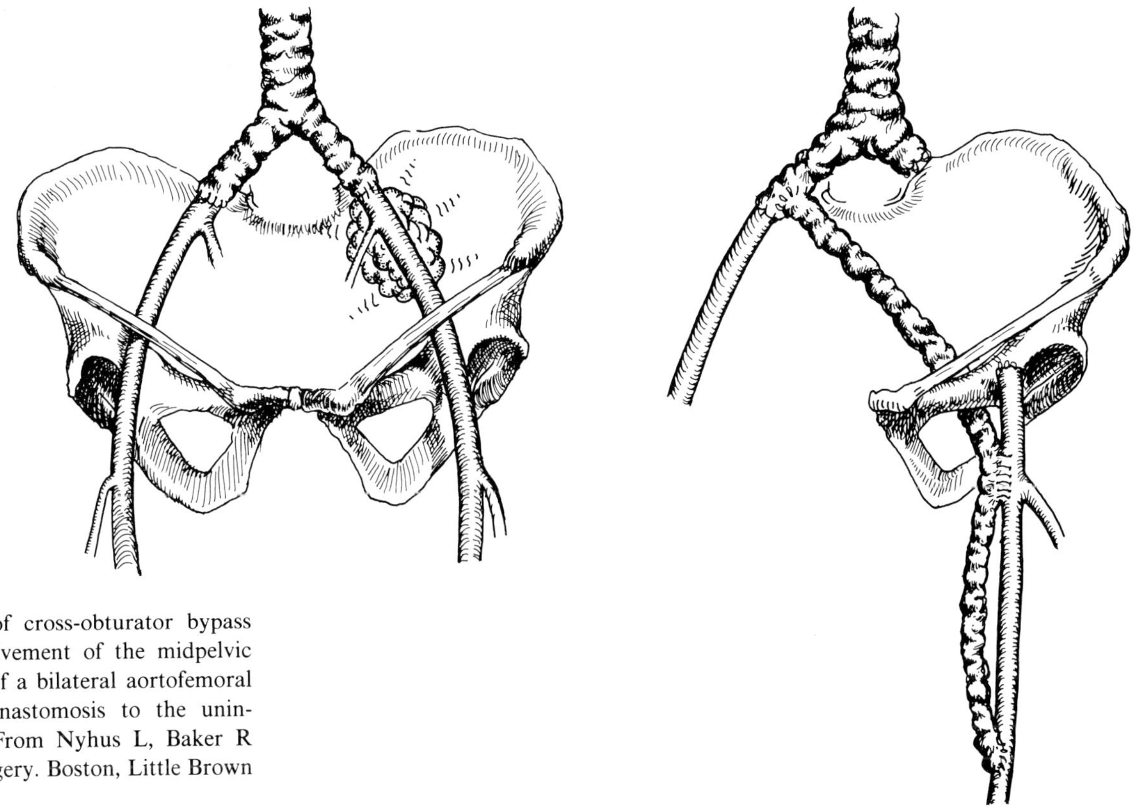

Fig. 6. Schematic of cross-obturator bypass graft for septic involvement of the midpelvic portion of left limb of a bilateral aortofemoral bypass. Note side anastomosis to the uninvolved right limb. (From Nyhus L, Baker R (eds): Mastery of Surgery. Boston, Little Brown and Co. (in press)

MANAGEMENT OF GROIN WOUND

When revascularization has been completed and all access wounds have been closed, the operative field is revised to approach the septic groin. The aim of this stage is to excise the affected graft from below the inguinal ligament. The involved femoral artery can often be exceedingly friable; blood loss remains a serious threat at this stage should the septic graft be separated prematurely from the femoral artery. An adequate amount of blood must be available. In addition, due to scarring it is sometimes difficult to obtain circumferential control of the groin vessels. Control can be achieved in some cases by proximal external iliac artery ligation in continuity. A heavy-caliber nonabsorbable tie such as No. 1 silk can be safely used for this purpose. On occasion, ties or sutures are inadequate for very friable arteries; large metal hemoclips are also useful to achieve control of such arteries. The use of metal hemoclips within the abdomen should be avoided, as these seriously cloud subsequent CAT scans. After excision of the graft, a formal suture in the defect of the wall of the femoral artery is placed with standard arterial suture material. The author prefers polypropylene for this purpose. The operation is completed by achieving soft-tissue coverage to avoid further exposure of the femoral artery in the groin. The wound is closed insofar as possible using a variety of methods to achieve adequate drainage without actually exposing the femoral artery. The skin can be partially or completely closed depending upon its condition. On occasion, it is advisable to divide the origin of the sartorius muscle and rotate the muscle to insure arterial protection.

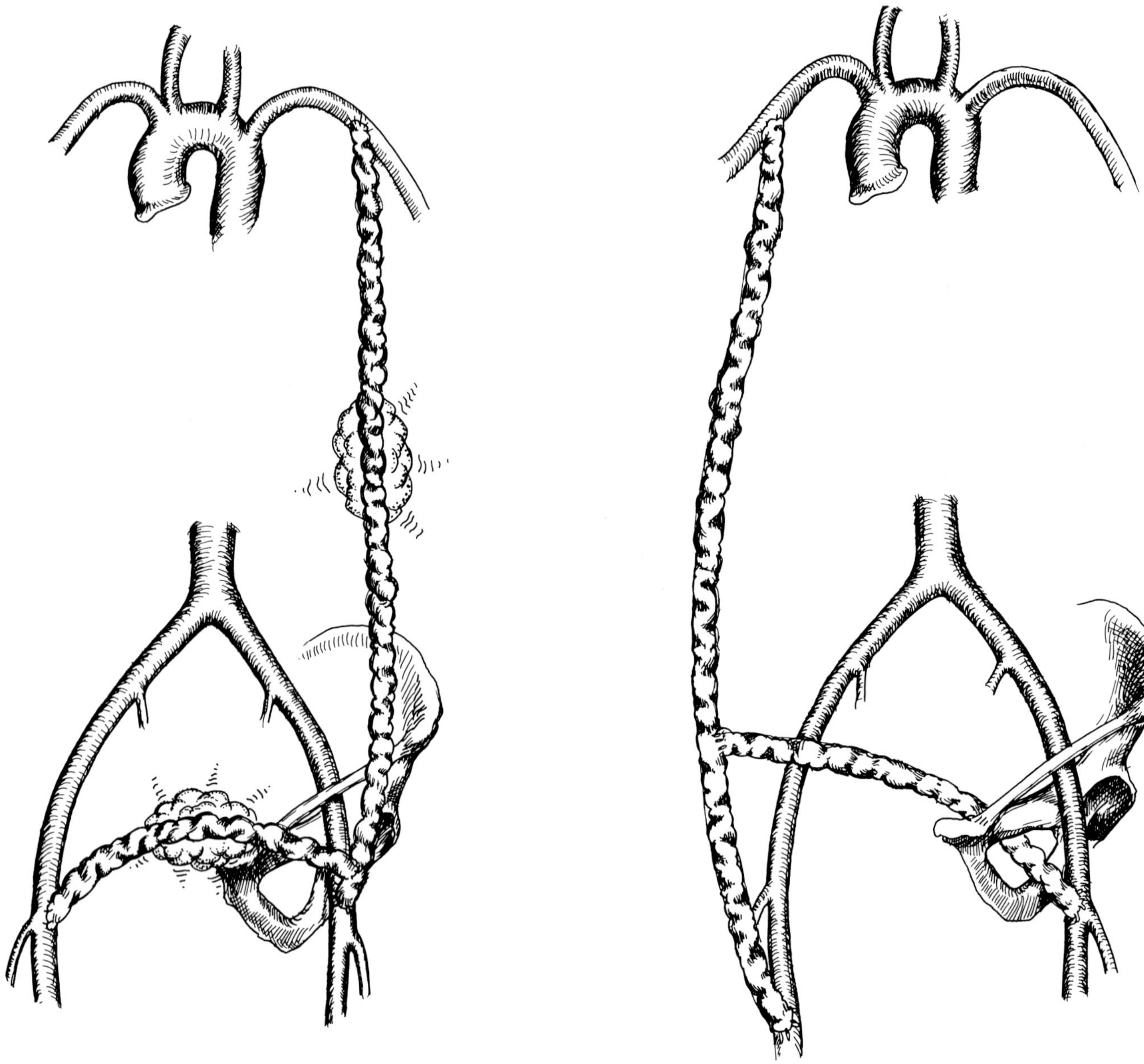

Fig. 7. Schematic of cross-obturator bypass to correct two areas of sepsis involving a left axillo-femoro–femoral bypass. Note new bypass anastomosed to a newly placed right axillo-superficial femoral artery graft. (From Nyhus L, Baker R (eds): Mastery of Surgery. Boston, Little Brown and Co. (in press)

POSTOPERATIVE CARE AND RESULTS

Postoperative care in these cases involves careful continued observation for sepsis. The author feels it wise to continue intravenous antibiotics for a total of 7 to 10 days postoperatively. With broad spectrum antibiotic therapy, recurrent sepsis has not occurred in a personal series of 7 cases. There have been 54 reported cases of obturator bypass in the literature recently reviewed.[6] Postoperative arterographic observations[5,7] demonstrate that these grafts will pass through the obturator membrane without kinking and follow a mechanically sound course when the hip flexes. Extended patency has been reported in two cases, one for 5 years and one for 9 years.[8] Thus, obturator bypass is a particularly attractive alternative for localized aortofemoral graft limb infection in the groin. It is also useful as a secondary procedure for limb salvage in sepsis involving other types of extra-anatomic bypass grafts.

REFERENCES

1. Shaw RS, Baue AE: Management of sepsis complicating arterial reconstructive surgery. Surgery 53:75, 1963
2. Mahoney WD, Whelan TJ: Use of obturator foramen in iliofemoral artery grafting: Case reports. Ann Surg 163:215, 1966
3. Macpherson AIS: Iliofemoral arterial bypass through the obturator foramen. Br J Surg 54:946, 1967
4. DePalma RG, Hubay CA: Arterial bypass via the obturator foramen: An alternative in complicated vascular problems. Am J Surg 115:323, 1968
5. Mentha Ch, Launois B, Delaere J: Les pontages arteriels ilio-femoraux par le trou obturateur. J Chir (Paris) 90:131, 1965
6. DePalma RG, Niemczura RT, Wolkoff JS: Arterial bypass via the obturator foramen, in Nyhus LM, Baker RJ (eds): Mastery of Surgery. Little Brown and Co, Boston, Mass (in press)
7. Gruss JD: Le pontage-obturateur. Indication, Technique, Resultats. Chirurgie 97:220, 1971
8. Tilson MD, Sweeney T, Gusberg RJ, Stansel HC: Obturator canal bypass grafts for septic lesions of the femoral artery. Arch Surg 114:1031, 1979

Use of the Profunda Femoris Artery for Secondary Revascularization

Terry A. King, Robert S. Rhodes, Ralph G. DePalma

Late failure of grafts placed in the common femoral artery is a difficult problem. For example, Kanaly et al[1] reported a 45 percent amputation rate in patients requiring secondary operations after aortic reconstruction. The availability of relatively undiseased previously undissected profunda femoris artery can avert some of the problems associated with local endarterectomy and reanastomosis of a graft in the common femoral artery.

We have therefore recommended the use of the profunda femoris as an inflow or outflow conduit for secondary revascularization of critically ischemic lower limbs.[2] This reduces the difficulties caused by intense scarring, distorted local anatomy, and progressive atherosclerosis during secondary procedures. This chapter describes the anatomy of the deep femoral artery and provides technical information to facilitate exposure of the profunda femoris system, thus avoiding dissection in a "concrete groin."

Angiographic data were collected from 20 femoral and translumbar arteriograms to provide baseline information about the size and branching of the profunda femoris. Diameters and distances of origin of the branch vessels were measured and then corrected for magnification. The distances to the major branches of the profunda femoris system were measured from the midpoint of a line between the anterior superior iliac spine (ASIS) and the pubic tubercle to the midpoint of vessel origin. Vessel diameters were measured just distal to each bifurcation. The accuracy of the angiographic data was confirmed by in situ measurements in six cadavers. Figure 1 shows the average diameters of the vessels of the profunda femoris system and the origins of its important collateral branches.

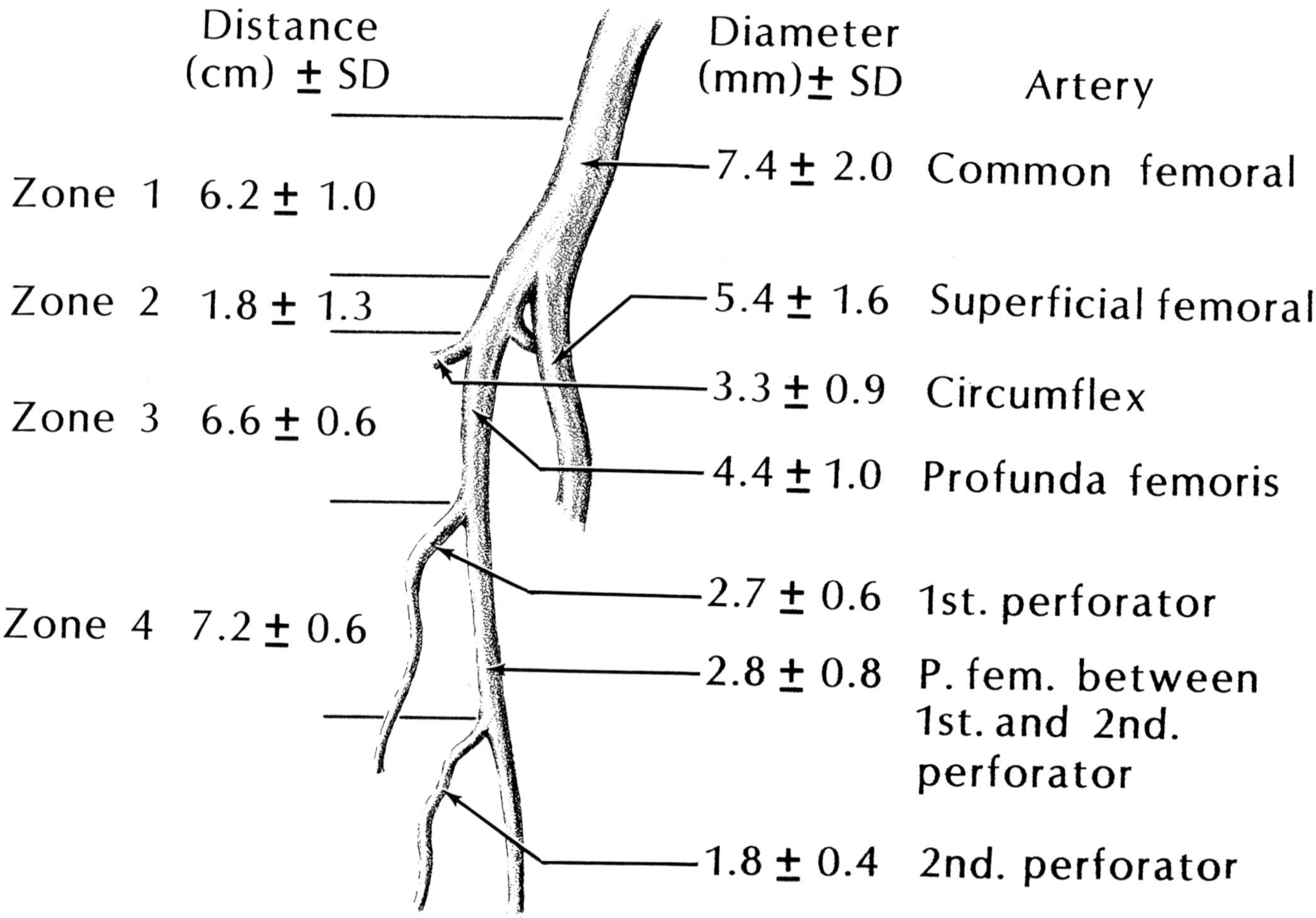

Fig. 1. Average diameters of the profunda femoris artery and its branches as measured from the midpoint of a line between the anterior superior iliac spine and the pubic tubercle.

To expose the artery for secondary revascularization, the medial aspect of the sartorius muscle is identified topographically by a line drawn from the ASIS to the posterior aspect of the medial femoral condyle. An incision is then made along this line the appropriate distance from the midpoint of the line between the ASIS and the pubic tubercle (Fig. 2). The sartorius muscle, superficial femoral artery, and femoral vein are retracted (Fig. 3), and the origin of the profunda artery is identified if possible. Careful dissection is then used to separate the bundles of the vastus medialis and adductor longus muscles. The profunda artery and its branches can be found near the insertion of these muscles on the femur, resting on the adductor brevis. Using this approach the artery can be easily exposed and mobilized, skin incisions are kept to a minimum, and dissection through a scarred groin is avoided. Final exposure and arteriotomy are shown in Figure 4. Figures 5 and 6 show application of profunda bypass for late occlusion of proximal or distal grafts.

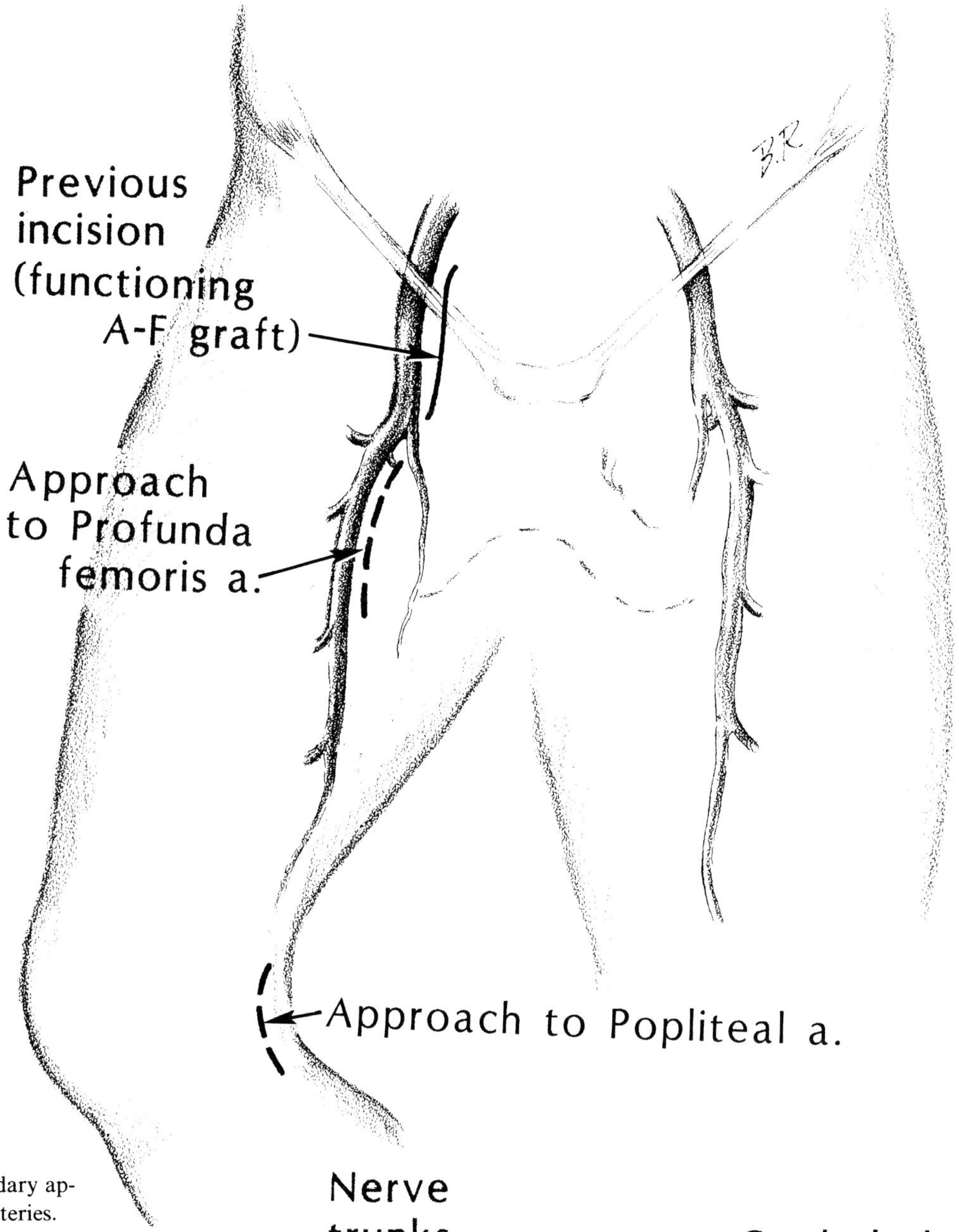

Fig. 2. Location of incisions for secondary approach to the profunda and popliteal arteries.

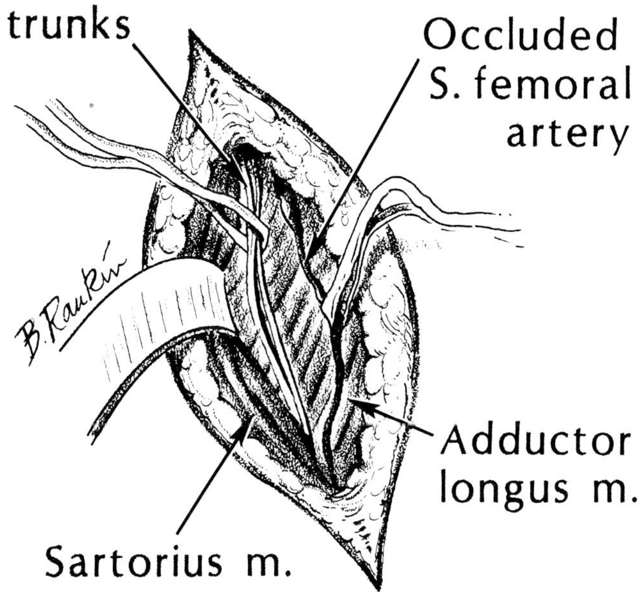

Fig. 3. Initial exposure and approach to the profunda femoris artery.

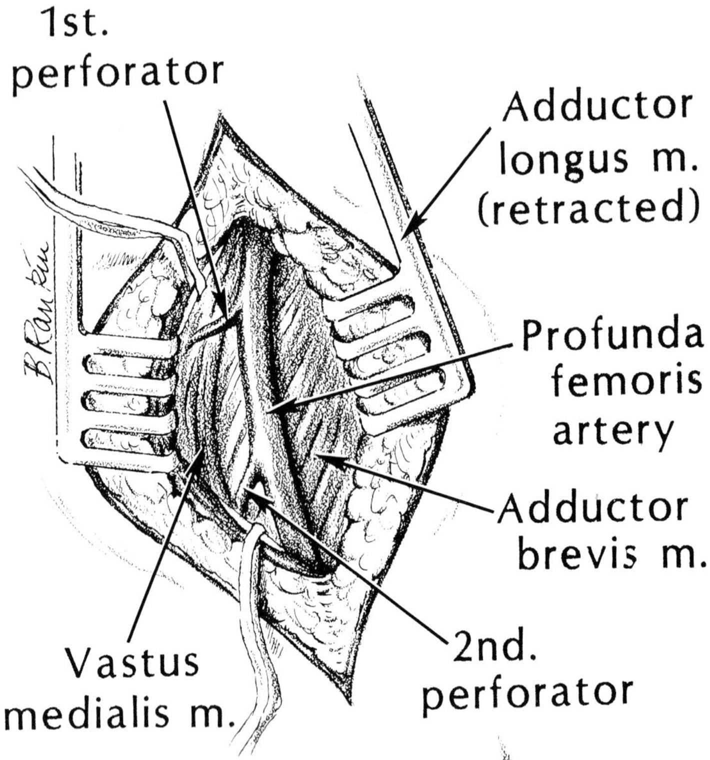

Fig. 4. Exposure of the profunda femoris with arteriotomy at the origin of the second perforator.

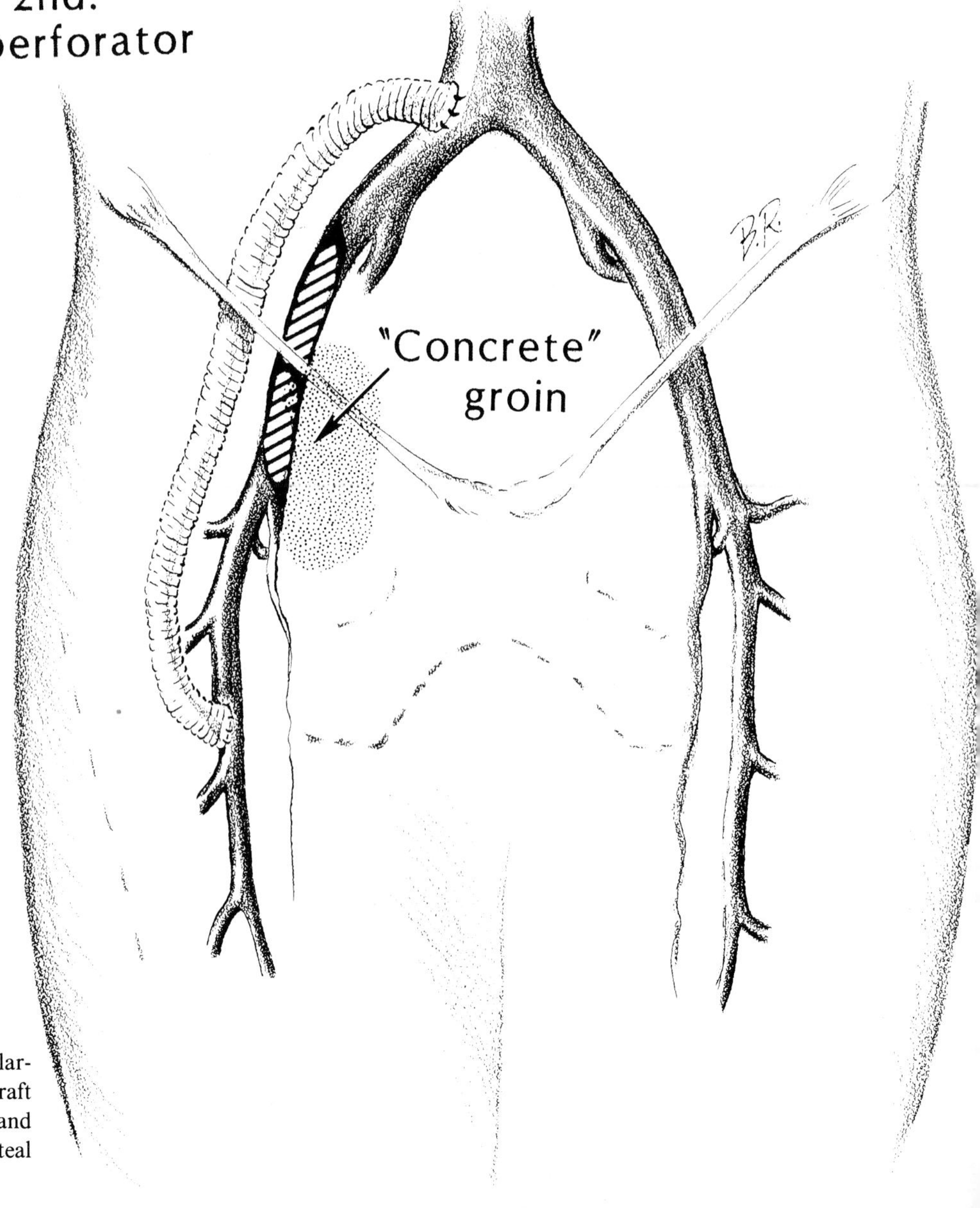

Fig. 5. Schematic of ilea profunda revascularization for failure of a femoropopliteal graft that resulted in proximal iliac thrombosis and clamp trauma. The previous femoropopliteal graft is not shown.

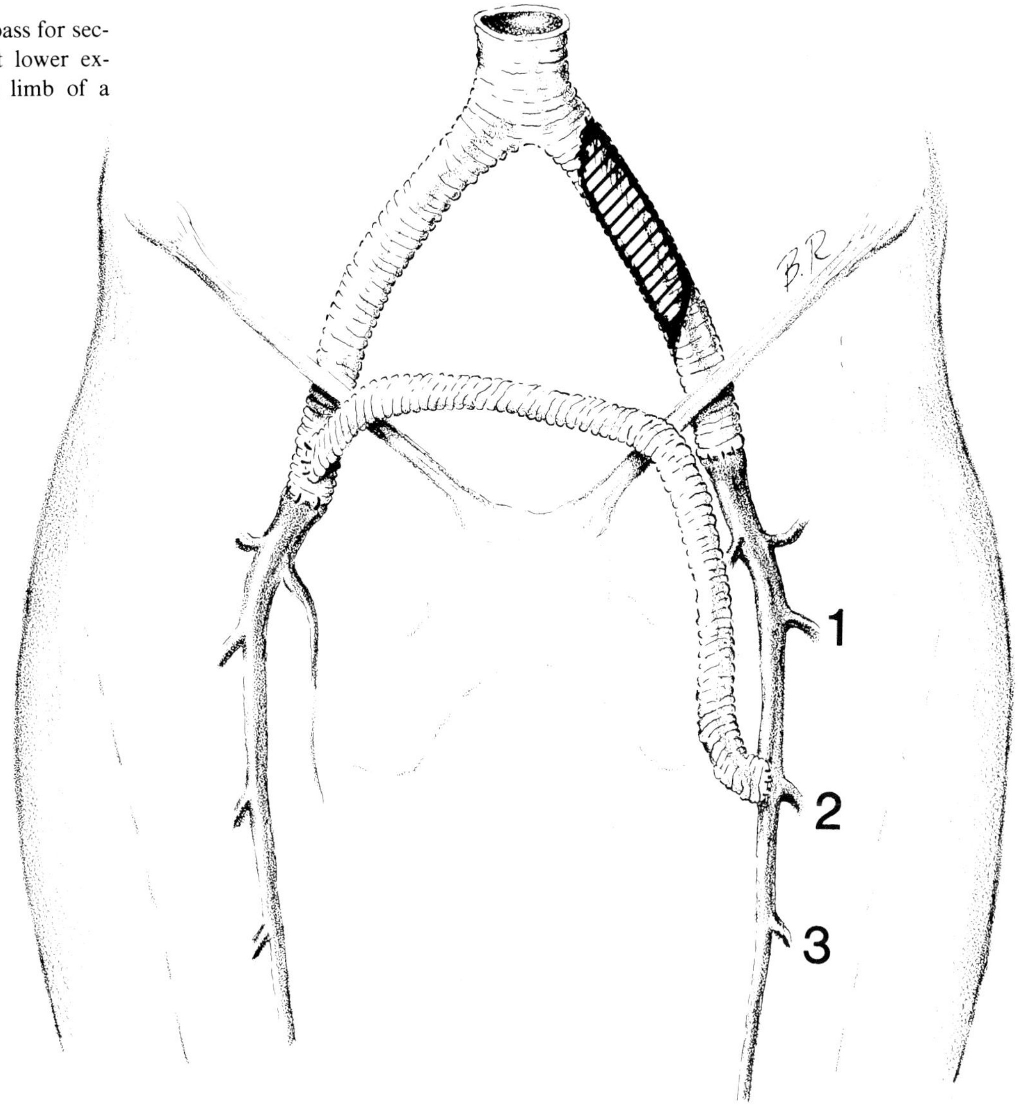

Fig. 6. Cross femoral profunda bypass for secondary revascularization of the left lower extremity following occlusion of left limb of a previous aortofemoral bypass.

We have used this approach in 17 patients: 7 required proximal secondary reconstructions, 8 required distal reconstructions, and 2 needed both proximal and distal reconstructions. Loupe magnification, gentle vascular occlusion, and fine polypropylene sutures have been found to be important technical factors in dealing with the small and more delicate deep femoral artery. Vein grafts should be used whenever possible; reinforced polytetraflouroethylene (PTFE) has been used when a vein was not available. All procedures resulted in increased Doppler ankle-to-arm pressure ratios and immediate limb salvage.

At present, we have been following these patients from 6 to 36 months. There have been two late failures, both of which involved secondary revascularizations using reinforced PTFE grafts originating in the zone of the second perforator and extending below the knee. In both of these instances, thrombosis and amputation resulted 8 months and 12 months, respectively, after the secondary limb salvage procedure. Neither sympathetectomy nor attempts at thrombectomy appeared of benefit in this situation.

Profunda bypass, either proximal or distal, appears to be an excellent option for secondary lower-extremity revascularization. If below-knee reconstruction is needed, a vein graft may yield better long-term results.

REFERENCES

1. Kanaly PJ, Dilling EW, Robinson HB, Eldins RC: Discussion and management of late failures in reconstructive procedures involving the abdominal aorta. Am J Surg 136: 709, 1978
2. DePalma RG, Malgieri JJ, Rhodes RS, Clowes AW: Profunda femoris bypass for secondary revascularization. Surg Gynecol Obstet (in press)

EXTRA-ANATOMICAL BYPASS

Axillary-Bifemoral Bypass Graft

Robert B. Rutherford

This operation is normally performed under general endotracheal anesthesia, but because it involves only relatively superficial dissection and subcutaneous tunneling, deep levels of anesthesia and profound relaxation are not required. Also because this operation is usually performed as an alternative to an aorto-bifemoral bypass, the patient is likely to be a poor risk and have signifcant cardiopulmonary disease. Therefore either light general or balanced anesthesia supplemented with local lidocaine is usually employed.

The patient is placed in the supine position with the "donor" arm abducted no more than 90 degrees. Ordinarily the donor axillary artery is on the same side as the lower extremity with the most severe ischemic symptoms, but this may be varied if vascular laboratory studies show better systolic pressures and plethysmographic tracings on the contralateral side. If there is any question about occlusive disease proximal to the prospective "donor" axillary artery, arteriography is mandatory. Because of the large surface area left exposed, the patient should either be placed on a warming blanket or the temperature of the room should be above normal, as for operations on infants. Until completion of the upper dissection and anastamosis, the table should be flexed approximately 15 degrees and rotated toward the contralateral side until the plane of the upper incision is horizontal and accessible to both surgeon and first assistant. The contralateral upper extremity ordinarily serves for both blood pressure monitoring and intravenous infusions. The radial artery is cannulated to provide continuous blood pressure monitoring and intermittent blood gas analysis. This not only has obvious advantages in patients with severe cardiopulmonary disease but is preferable to a syphgmomanometer cuff because, when intermittently inflated, the latter can cause irregular intravenous infusion rates and result in extravascation of irritating or necrotizing drugs. After the arterial and venous cannulas are securely in place, the arm is positioned at the side and protected with a curved metal shield, because, if it is abducted like the donor extremity, it will get in the way of the first assistant.

An area of skin is prepared with antiseptic solution to include the base of the neck, the ipsilateral clavicle and adjacent shoulder, the thorax, both lower quadrants, and the upper thighs. On the donor side, the area prepared and draped should extend to the posterior axillary line. The genitalia are excluded from the operative field with a folded towel. The entire operative field should be covered with an adhesive plastic drape to avoid contact between the prosthesis and the skin. The position of the patient, the extent of the operative field, the location of the incisions, the subcutaneous course of the grafts, and the subcutaneous tunneling maneuvers are shown in Figure 1.

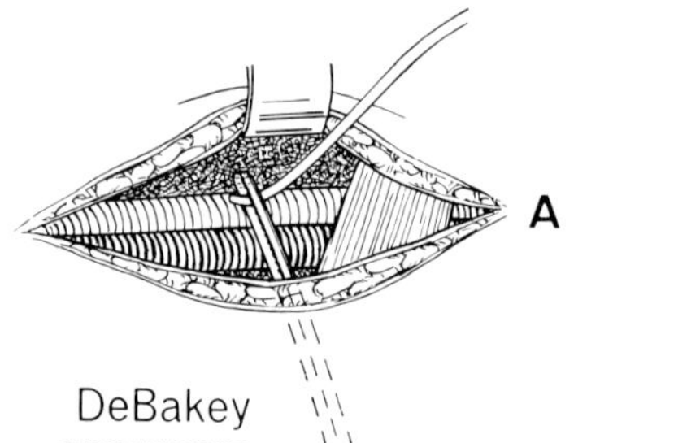

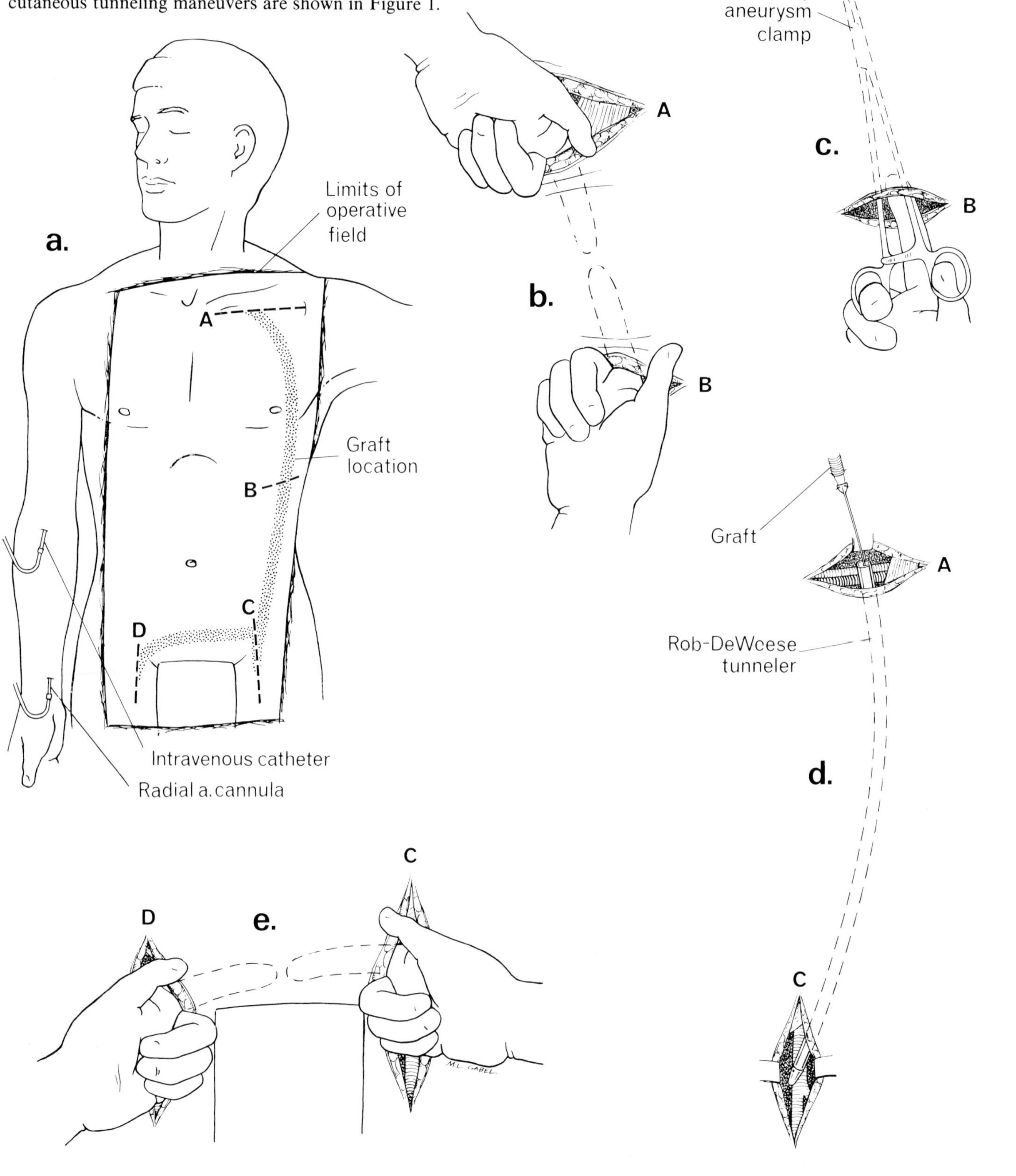

The upper incision (A) is made over the axillary artery, from a point 1 cm lateral to the inferior aspect of the medial attachment to the clavicle, at least three-fourths of the distance to the edge of the deltoid muscle and in line with the medial termination of the deltipectoral groove (Fig. 2a). The incision slants slightly upward with the patient's arm abducted but will be almost transverse and horizontal when the arm is in its normal, adducted position. After opening the skin, subcutaneous tissue, and pectoral fascia, the natural separation between the fibers of the pectoralis major muscle, which run in the same direction as the incision, is exploited. Often this will carry one down between the two heads of the pectoralis major muscle, but just as commonly the opening will be made superior to this. In either event, only minimal bleeding will be encountered. When the fibers of the pectoralis major muscle are separated throughout the length of the wound, the clavipectoral (or costocoracoid) fascia and the adipose tissue overlying it are exposed. The inferior edge of the first part of the clavicle will be encountered medially and, as the incision is deepened, the pectoralis minor muscle will be exposed in the lateral third of the wound, in continuity with the clavipectoral fascia (Fig. 2b). In many individuals it is possible to preserve and retract the pectoralis minor muscle, although many surgeons (including the author) prefer to divide it at its insertion to gain better exposure and assure that it will not compromise the position of the graft. This decision can be deferred until later if exposure is not a problem. Dissection is carried downward through the overlying adipose tissue towards the palpable pulse of the axillary artery. In the course of this dissection, axillary artery branches or axillary vein tributaries may be encountered (Fig. 2b). The latter may need to be divided, but the former can be followed down to the axillary artery since they are branches of the thorocoacromial trunk. The axillary artery lies slightly superior but deep to the axillary vein and inferior to the brachial plexus. One of the nerves supplying the pectoralis muscles may cross over it laterally. It is important to initially approach the axillary artery in the medial half of the incision where it is more accessible. As soon as this artery is visualized and freed-up enough to pass a right angle clamp around it, a moist unbilical tape should be passed around this artery and upward traction exerted. This greatly facilitates its mobilization from the vein inferiorly and the brachial plexus superiorly. (Fig. 2c). Usually the thorocoacromial trunk must be ligated at its origin to allow an adequate length of axillary artery to be dissected free. In addition, the axillary artery should be mobilized close to the chest wall where it emerges from underneath the clavicle. This allows one to place the anastomosis as medially as possible in order to avoid the shearing forces otherwise produced by movement of the upper extremity.

Having mobilized the axillary artery and encircled it medially and laterally with double-looped broad silastic rubber tapes, the upper subcutaneous tunnel is prepared down to an approximately 6-cm counterincision (B) placed obliquely over the sixth or seventh intercostal space in the midaxillary line (Fig. 2a). It is important that the position of the graft not be located anteriorly to the midaxillary line, because it may kink when the patient is seated in the usual partially flexed position.[1] In addition, a more anterior position may cause the graft to ride over a prominent costal margin. Breakdown of the fabric and aneurysm formation have been reported in this location.[2] The tunneling should initially be performed with the tips of the index fingers inserted through each incision (Fig. 1b). The upper part of the tunnel should pass anteriorly to the axillary vein and, if it has not been divided, in front of the pectoralis minor muscle.[3] Inferiorly it should follow the loose areolar tissue right on the chest wall, as deep as possible to the skin, subcutaneous tissue, and fascia. Once the opposing index fingers have made free contact with each other and gained an additional fingerbreadth or two of lateral freedom, a long curved (e.g., DeBakey aneurysm) clamp is passed through this tunnel, an umbilical tape withdrawn through it, and its ends are clamped (Fig. 1c). This allows the tunnel to be easily found later. (In smaller, shorter patients, a tunnel all the way from the axillary to the ipsilateral groin incision can be developed using a Rob-DeWeese tunneler, as shown in Fig. 1D.

Fig. 1. Position of patient, extent of operative field, location of incisions, subcutaneous course of grafts, and subcutaneous tunneling maneuvers for axillary bifemoral bypass.
(a) The extent of the prepared operative field, showing the eventual location of the incisions and grafts.
(b) Tunnel is made with tips of opposing index fingers inserted through each incision.
(c) After opposing fingertips have made contact and gained an additional fingerbreadth or two of lateral freedom, a long curved clamp is passed through the tunnel. An umbilical tape is withdrawn through the tunnel, and its ends are clamped.
(d) In smaller, shorter patients, a tunnel can be made from the axillary to the ipsilateral groin incision using a Rob-DeWeese tunneler.
(e) The final tunnel is made suprapubically by inserting the index fingers medially up over the inguinal ligaments to meet in the midline.

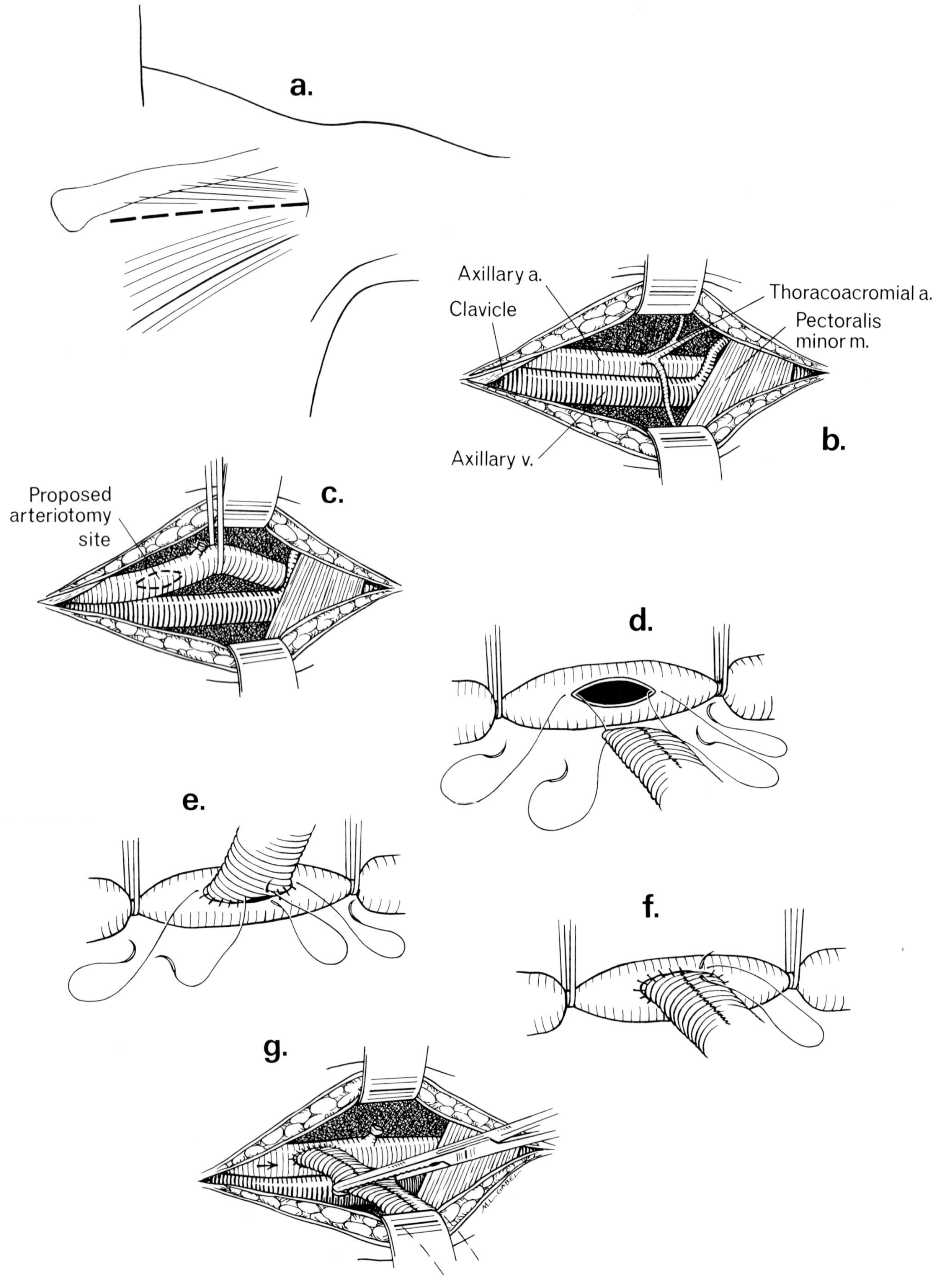
a.
Axillary a.
Clavicle
Thoracoacromial a.
Pectoralis minor m.
Axillary v.
b.
Proposed arteriotomy site
c.
d.
e.
f.
g.

Next, attention is turned to the groin incisions. Standard vertical incisions for exposure of the femoral artery bifurcation are made bilaterally, but on the donor side this incision is extended higher than usual so that not only the inguinal ligament but at least 3 to 4 cm of the external oblique aponeurosis are exposed (Fig. 3a). Care is taken in these incisions to avoid injury to the saphenous vein medially, since it may be required for later operations, and to fibers of the femoral nerve laterally, particularly those that may cross over close to the superficial femoral artery in the lower part of the incision. In the upper part of the incision, an attempt is made to avoid open transection of lymphatic channels. For this purpose, a combination of cautery and suture ligation is employed, and the main cluster of lymph nodes is skirted laterally. The common femoral artery and its superficial and profunda branches are dissected free and each is encircled with double-looped silastic tapes for later hemostatic control. Smaller branches are controlled with double loops of 0 silk. If there is significant superficial femoral artery occlusive disease, the profunda femoris artery is exposed down to its first perforator branch. During this dissection, one must avoid injurying the corresponding tributary of the profunda femoris vein, which crosses over the upper profunda femoris artery. It is often necessary to ligate and divide this vein in order to obtain sufficient exposure to perform a concomitant profundaplasty.

Having completely mobilized the femoral arteries bilaterally, the subcutaneous tunneling is completed by first linking the femoral incisions on donor side (C) with a counter incision in the midaxillary line above the lower ribs (B). The proper plane is easily developed if one stays just above the external oblique aponeurosis. Again, an umbilical tape is left in the tunnel to facilitate later passage of the graft from incision to incision. The final tunnel is made suprapubically by inserting the two index fingers medially up over the inguinal ligaments to meet in the midline (Fig. 1e). It is necessary to break through some adherent tissue in the midline; otherwise this plane of dissection meets little resistance. In a very obese patient with a protuberant abdomen, it may be advisable to tunnel behind some or all of the lower abdominal musculature. This can be accomplished by dividing the inguinal ligament and carrying the dissection up into the properitoneal plane, then medially until the two fingers meet in the midline behind the rectus abdominus muscles. This must be done gently and carried high enough to avoid bleeding from veins in the space of Retzius. Alternatively, one can tunnel under the external oblique aponeurosis and then pass anteriorly or posteriorly to the rectus muscles. These additional maneuvers are justified only if subcutaneous passage might cause kinking or undue angulation of the graft.

Once all the incisions have been prepared and tunneling is completed, heparin (100 units/kg) is administered intravenously, and all incisions but the axillary are packed with antibiotic soaked sponges. A prosthetic graft the diameter of which matches the recipient vessel, usually 8 mm, is selected. If a double velour knitted Dacron graft is used, it is preclotted prior to administering heparin; if an expanded polytetraflouroethylene (PTFE) prosthesis is used, this is not necessary. The end of the prosthetic graft is trimmed at a 30-degree angle with its apex medially, so that it will angle slightly outward from the point of anastomosis. Using the cut end of the graft for sizing purposes, a longitudinal arteriotomy is made on the inferior and anterior aspect of the axillary artery about 2 cm beyond its emergence from underneath the clavicle (Fig. 2d). Using 4–0 coated braided Dacron suture with swaged-on needles at each end, the corners of the anastomosis are begun with an everting horizontal mattress suture. When these have been tied, the anastomosis is completed by running the suture in a continuous over-and-over fashion from each corner towards the middle (Fig. 2e). By completing the more difficult "corners" first, there is less danger of narrowing the axillary artery at either edge of the anastomosis. The graft can be lifted upward or downward as necessary to facilitate the anastomosis (Fig. 2f).

Fig. 2. (a) The upper incision is made over the axillary artery from a point 1 cm lateral to the inferior aspect of the medial attachment to the clavicle, at least three fourths of the distance to the edge of the deltoid muscle and in line with the medial termination of the deltipectoral groove.
(b) As the incision is deepened, the pectoralis minor muscle is exposed in the lateral third of the wound, in continuity with the clavipectoral fascia.
(c) Passage of a moist umbilical tape around the axillary artery and exertion of upward traction upon the artery greatly facilitates its mobilization from the vein inferiorly and from the brachial plexus superiorly.
(d) A longitudinal arteriotomy is made on the inferior and anterior aspect of the axillary artery about 2 cm beyond its emergence from below the clavicle.
(e) Suture is run in a continuous over-and-over fashion from each corner towards the middle to complete the anastomosis.
(f) The graft can be lifted upward or downward as necessary to facilitate the anastomosis.
(g) The graft is crossclamped about 3 cm from the anastomosis and is tested for hemostasis.

After the anastomosis has been completed, it is tested for hemostasis by releasing the silastic loops and restoring flow through the axillary artery while the graft is crossclamped about 3 cm from the anastomosis (Fig. 2g). Using the linear markers on a Dacron prosthesis or indelible ink marks along the PTFE graft to assure maintenance of correct orientation during passage, the graft is passed between the upper incision and ipsilateral groin incision, if necessary using the counterincision to facilitate this maneuver.

The graft should neither be redundant nor under undue tension. If the table has been jack-knifed to facilitate operating in the upper incision, it should be straightened at this time so that the correct length of the graft can be determined. Too much tension, after the desmoplastic reaction around the graft matures, will result in the axillary artery being pulled down to form a "U"-shaped bend that will create turbulence and in turn encourage platelet deposition and/or intimal hyperplasia at or near the anastomosis.

When there is no superficial femoral occlusive disease, the anastomosis to the femoral artery can be made in the standard end-to-side fashion to an arteriotomy placed in the anterior surface of the common femoral artery just above its bifurcation. However, because this operation is most commonly performed for limb salvage indications in patients with multilevel occlusive disease, there usually *is* significant superficial femoral artery occlusive disease. In this circumstance, the common femoral incision should be carried down into the profunda femoris artery almost to the origin of its first perforator branch (Fig. 3a). In either event, an end-to-side anastomosis is performed between the graft and the arteriotomy after an acutely angled cut (60 degrees) is made across the prosthesis, trimming it to proper length. The first suture is placed as a horizontal everting mattress at the "heel" or proximal angle of the anastomosis. After this is tied, the needle on each end of the suture is run, in continuous, everting, through-and-through fashion, towards the midlateral aspects of the anastomosis (Fig. 3b). At this point additional adjustments are made in the arteriotomy or occasionally the prosthesis, to correct for any discrepancies in length, before the distal tip or "toe" of the anastomosis is begun with another everting mattress suture (Fig. 3c). The ends of this suture are run in continuous fashion back up along either side of the anastomosis to meet the upper suture. Back-bleeding is allowed to fill the graft and evacuate any air before the last sutures are tied. Then the upper clamp is released while the runoff vessels are briefly compressed to divert the initial surge of blood back up into the common femoral artery and avoid the risk of distal embolization or "trash foot."

After achieving adequate hemostasis at the second anastomosis, attention is directed towards the third anastomosis, between the prosthesis in the upper part of this incision and a second segment of the prosthesis, which is to be brought over to the contralateral femoral artery. Some Dacron prostheses are specially constructed with this anastomosis already completed, but in the absence of such luxury, an end-to-side anastomosis is fashioned between an extra length of the prosthesis and an arteriotomy made in its medial aspect as high as possible in this incision (Fig. 3d). Two vascular clamps are placed across the graft above and below the proposed arteriotomy site and then rotated 90 degrees so that the anastomosis can be faciliated by having the opening in the graft facing superiorly (Fig. 3e). An end-to-side anastomosis is performed in similar fashion to the upper anastomosis, but with at least a 30-degree angle. After this is performed and tested for hemostasis, the graft is passed across to the opposite groin incision through the soprapubic tunnel (Fig. 3f). There the final anastomosis is completed in exactly the same fashion described for the second anastomosis in the ipsilateral groin (Fig. 3g).

After a final check for hemostasis, the wounds are irrigated with topical antibiotics and the incisions closed. In the upper incision, the two edges of the pectoralis major muscle are approximated with 2–0 braided Dacron suture. In all incisions, the subcutaneous tissue and deep fascia are separately closed with interrupted 3–0 absorbable sutures, after which the skin is closed with interrupted 4–0 polypropylene sutures.

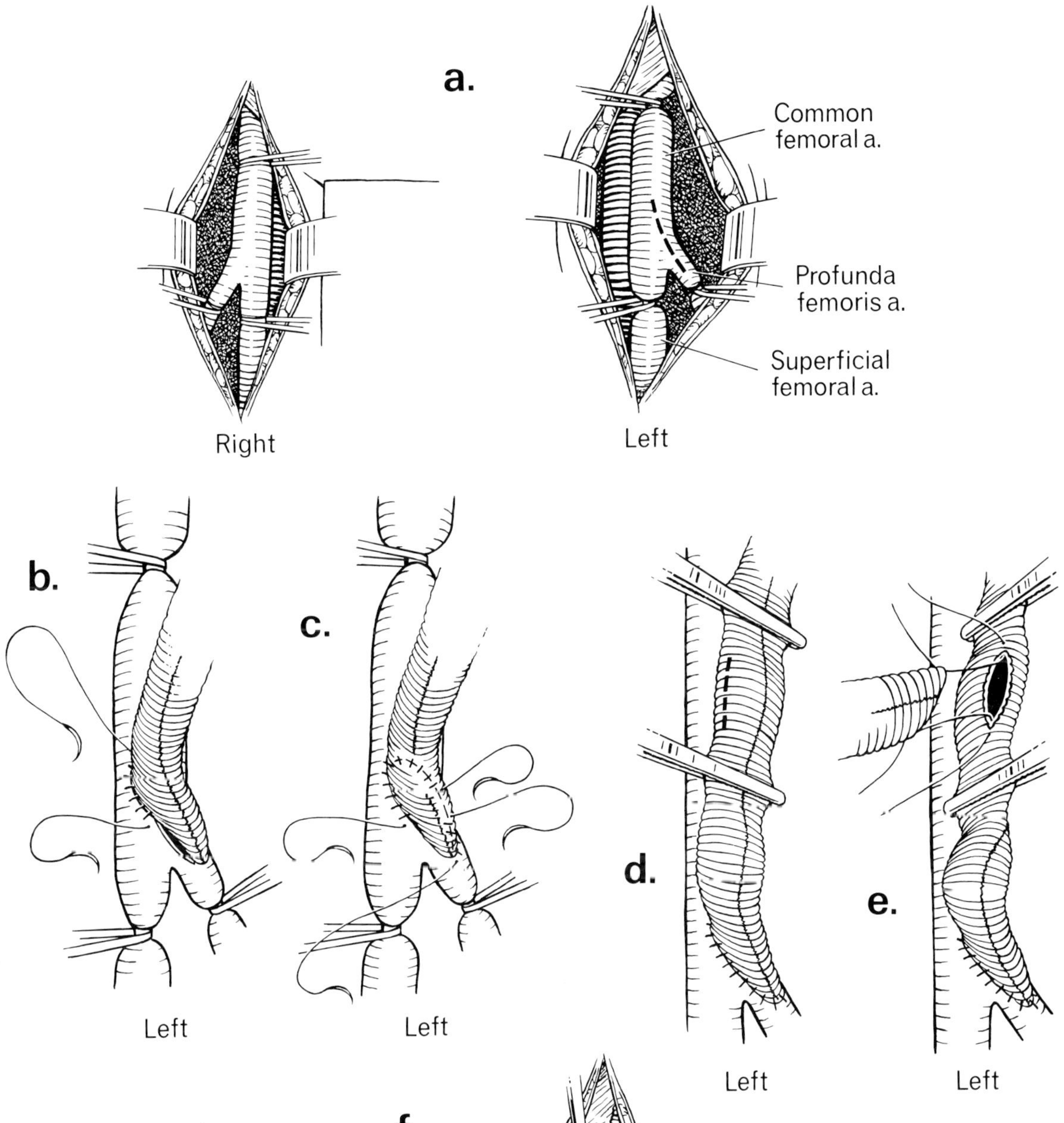

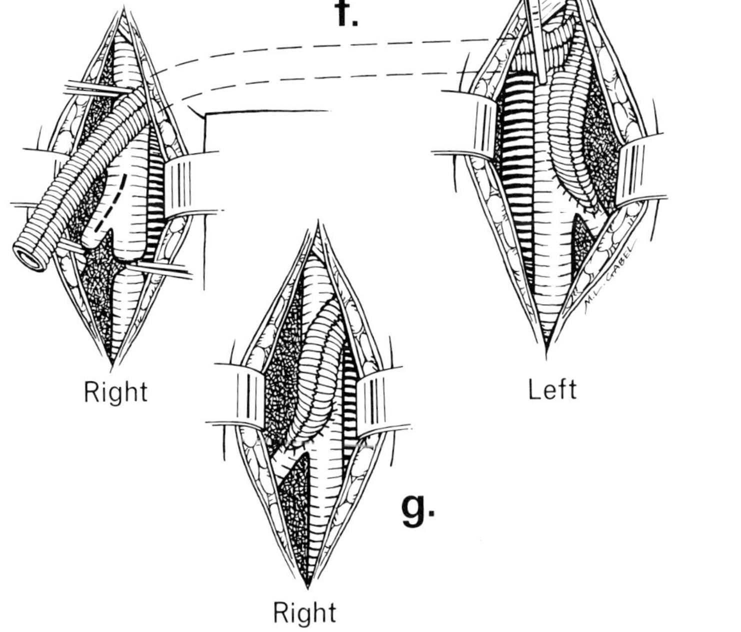

Fig. 3. (a) Exposure of the femoral part of the operation.
(b) After the first suture is placed, the needle on each end of the suture is run towards the midlateral aspects of the anastomisis in continuous, everting, through-and-through fashion.
(c) Adjustments in the arteriotomy or the prosthesis to correct for discrepancies in length before the distal tip or toe of the anastomosis is begun.
(d) An end-to-side anastomisis is fashioned between an extra length of the prosthesis, and an arteriotomy is made in its medial aspect as high as possible in the incision.
(e) Anastomisis with the opening in the graft facing superiorly.
(f) Graft is passed across to the opposite groin incision through the suprapubic tunnel.
(g) Completion of the final anastomosis.

This operation is usually well tolerated, for there is minimal blood loss or hemodynamic disturbance. Nasogastric intubation is rarely necessary; in fact, the patient can usually begin oral feedings the day after surgery. Intravenous antibiotics, which are begun preoperatively, are continued until the third postoperative day or until all indwelling catheters have been removed. However, antibiotic coverage should be reinstituted in the future whenever an invasive procedure that may cause a bacteremia (dental procedure, urethral catheterization, etc) is contemplated. The patient should be given antiplatelet drugs for at least six months postoperatively and at no time be allowed to sleep on the donor side. This can be prevented by attaching a loose wrist gauntlet from the donor wrist to the opposite side of the bed at night. If the patient needs crutches, it is important that the "Canadian" type with forearm grips are used rather than the standard variety. The patient should be taught to feel the pulse in both limbs of the graft on a daily basis to detect graft thrombosis and ensure early presentation should this complication develop.

REFERENCES

1. DeLaurentis DA, Sala LE, Russell E, McCombs PR: A twelve year experience with axillofemoral and femorofemoral bypass operations. Department of Surgery, Pennsylvania Hospital, and University of Pennsylvania School of Medicine, Philadelphia.
2. Orringer MB, Rutherford RB, Skinner DB: An unusual complication of axillary femoral artery bypass. Surgery 72:769, 1972
3. Johnson WC, LoGerfo FW, Vollman RW: Is axillo bilateral femoral graft an effective substiture for aorto bilateral iliac femoral graft? Ann Surg 186:123–128, 1976

ADDITIONAL SOURCES

Blaisdell FW, Hall AD: Axillary femoral artery bypass for lower extremity ischemia. Surgery 54:563–568, 1963

Ernst CB: Axillary femoral bypass graft without aorto femoral pressure differential. Ann Surg 181:424–427, 1974

Eugene J, Goldstone J, Moore WS: Fifteen year experience with subcutaneous bypass grafts for lower extremity ischemia. Ann Surg 186:177–182, 1976

LoGerfo FW, Johnson WC, Corson JD, et al: A comparison of the late patency rates of axillobilateral femoral and axillo unilateral femoral grafts. Surgery 81:33–40, 1977

Mannick JA, Williams LE, Nabseth DC: The late results of axillofemoral grafts. Surgery 68:1038, 1970

Parsonnet V, Alpert J, Biref DK: Femoral femoral and axillofemoral grafts: Compromise of preference. Surgery 67:26–33, 1970

Plecha FR, Pories WJ: Extra-anatomic bypasses for aortoiliac disease in high-risk patients. Surgery 80:480–487, 1976

Crossover Femoro-Femoral Bypass

D. Preston Flanigan

The crossover femoro-femoral bypass, as initially described by Vetto,[1] is a low-risk alternative method of vascular reconstruction when iliac artery occlusive disease is unilateral in nature (Fig. 1A). The nondiseased or minimally diseased contralateral femoral artery serves as the donor vessel.

The patient is positioned supine on the operating table. General or regional anesthesia is usually employed. If necessary, in particularly high-risk patients, the procedure may be carried out under local anesthesia. A Foley catheter is inserted to decompress the bladder, monitor urine output, and avoid contamination of the operative field secondary to urinary incontinence. The patient is antiseptically prepared with providone iodine from the nipple to the knees. A sterile towel is folded, placed over the groin, and sutured in place.

The first step in the operation involves dissection of both femoral arteries. The groin dissections may be carried out either consecutively or simultaneously. The groin incisions are vertical in orientation and are made over the femoral artery from the inguinal ligament (not the groin crease) to a point approximately 8 to 10 cm distally. The location of the inguinal ligament may be estimated by a line from the pubic tubercle to the anterior superior iliac spine (Fig. 1B). The incision is carried sharply through the skin, subcutaneous tissue, and fascial layers, using the scalpel. Continued dissection through the femoral sheath and around the artery is usually more facile with Metzenbaum scissors. The dissection plane should be made between the adventitia of the vessel and the surrounding structures. Dissection wide of this plane may cause injury to the femoral vein medially or the femoral nerve laterally (Fig. 1C). In reoperated groins or when considerable fibrosis and inflammation are present around the artery following arteriography, care should be taken to avoid subadventitial dissection of the artery.

Dissection of the vessels should begin with the proximal common femoral artery near the inguinal ligament. Dissection should begin anterior to the artery, as generally no branches are present in this location. Occasionally, however, the lateral and deep circumflex iliac veins course anterior to the artery to enter the common femoral vein at this location, the normal position of these veins being proximal to the inguinal ligament where they course anterior to the external iliac artery to enter the external iliac vein. These circumflex iliac veins may be sacrificed to facilitate exposure of the femoral artery, if necessary. Lateral and medial dissection of the common femoral artery is usually not impaired by branch vessels; however, like the circumflex iliac veins, arterial branches, which most commonly originate from the external iliac arteries, may originate below the inguinal ligament from the proximal common femoral artery. Medially, these branches are the inferior epigastric and external pudendal arteries; laterally are the superficial and deep circumflex iliac arteries and the superficial epigastric artery (Fig. 1C). Rarely does the common femoral artery have posterior branches. All branches should be preserved. Once the proximal common femoral artery is dissected, it is encircled with a silastic sling for proximal control and the dissection carried distally.

The extent of the distal arterial dissection is variable but should at least encompass the proximal portions of the superficial femoral artery and the profunda femoris artery (Fig. 1D). These vessels should be gently palpated to assess the extent of orificial disease. If preoperative angiographic and intraoperative assessments of the vessels dictate anastomosis to the common femoral artery, no further distal dissection of the vessels is required, and they are controlled at their origins with silastic slings (Fig. 1D). If the anastomosis is to be more distal, dissection of the more distal superficial femoral artery and/or profunda femoris artery will be required. Dissection of the superfical femoral artery is generally unencumbered by branch arteries or crossing veins, but profunda femoris artery dissection is more difficult. The profunda femoris artery usually originates postero-laterally from the common femoral artery, usually as a single trunk but occasionally as two major vessels. The best landmark for the location of the profunda femoris artery is the sudden narrowing of the common femoral artery as it becomes the superficial femoral artery. At a variable distance from the origin of the profunda femoris artery (1 to 3 cm), the lateral circumflex femoral veins cross the anterior surface of the artery to enter the profunda femoris vein (Fig. 1C). These veins are large and can result in significant blood loss if injured. Like the circumflex iliac veins, these veins may also be sacrificed, if necessary, for arterial exposure. Within the first centimeter of the profunda femoris artery, the lateral circumflex femoral artery usually takes its origin. This branch, as well as the more distal perforator branches of the profunda femoris artery, should be preserved. With more distal profunda dissection, care must be exercised in avoiding crossing branches of the femoral nerve. All branches of the femoral arteries are encircled with silastic vessel loops for vascular control. The distal superficial femoral and profunda femoris arteries are likewise controlled.

Knitted or woven Dacron (8- or 10-mm) is the most commonly used graft material, although adequate-size saphenous vein or polytetrafluoroethylene is also acceptable. If Dacron is used, blood is drawn from the common femoral vein to preclot the graft.

Fig. 1. (A) Crossover femoro-femoral bypass. (B) The location of the inguinal ligament may be estimated by a line from the pubic tubercle to the anterior superior iliac spine.
(C) Dissection plane between the adventitia of the vessel and the surrounding structures. Dissection wide of this plane may cause injury to the femoral vein medially or the femoral nerve laterally.
(D) Dissection should encompass the proximal portions of the superficial femoral artery and the profunda femoris artery. These vessels are controlled at their origins with silastic slings.

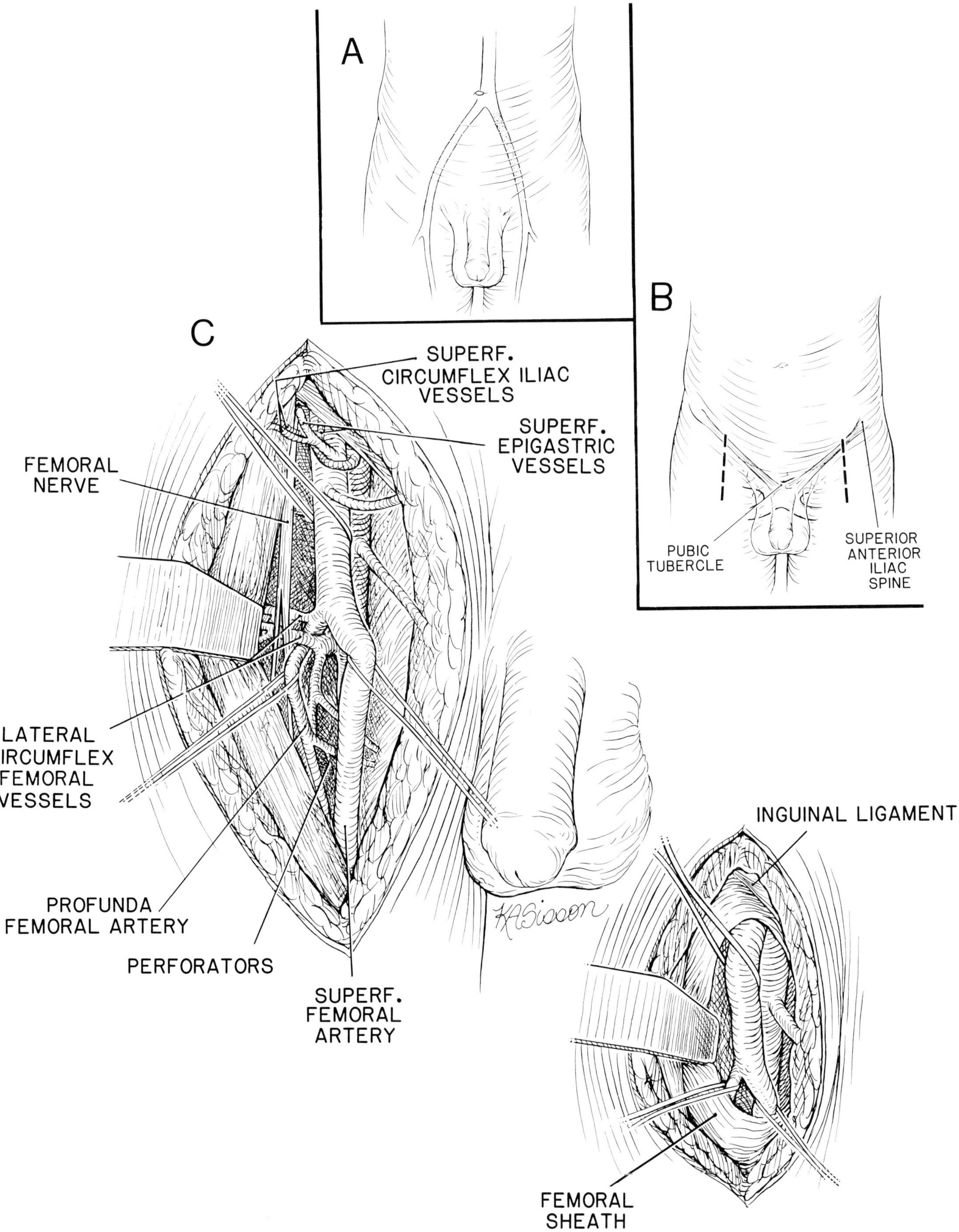
A
B
PUBIC
TUBERCLE
SUPERIOR
ANTERIOR
ILIAC
SPINE
C
SUPERF.
CIRCUMFLEX ILIAC
VESSELS
SUPERF.
EPIGASTRIC
VESSELS
FEMORAL
NERVE
LATERAL
CIRCUMFLEX
FEMORAL
VESSELS
PROFUNDA
FEMORAL ARTERY
PERFORATORS
SUPERF.
FEMORAL
ARTERY
INGUINAL LIGAMENT
FEMORAL
SHEATH

Once the graft has been prepared, a tunnel is created across the lower abdomen just superior to the pubis. The tunnel is made by finger dissection (Fig. 2) and may be placed in the subcutaneous position[1] (Fig. 2A) or in the space of Retzius[2] (Fig. 2B). No difference in patency rate has been noted based on the location of the tunnel.[3] The tunnel should be constructed in such a way that no kinking of the graft will occur at the entrances to the tunnel from the groins. Once the tunnel is constructed, a large curved DeBakey aneurysm clamp is passed through the tunnel and used to pull the graft back through the tunnel. At this time, 5000 units of heparin are given intravenously, and after 3 minutes, atraumatic vascular clamps are applied to the common femoral, superficial femoral, and profunda femoris arteries (Fig. 3A).

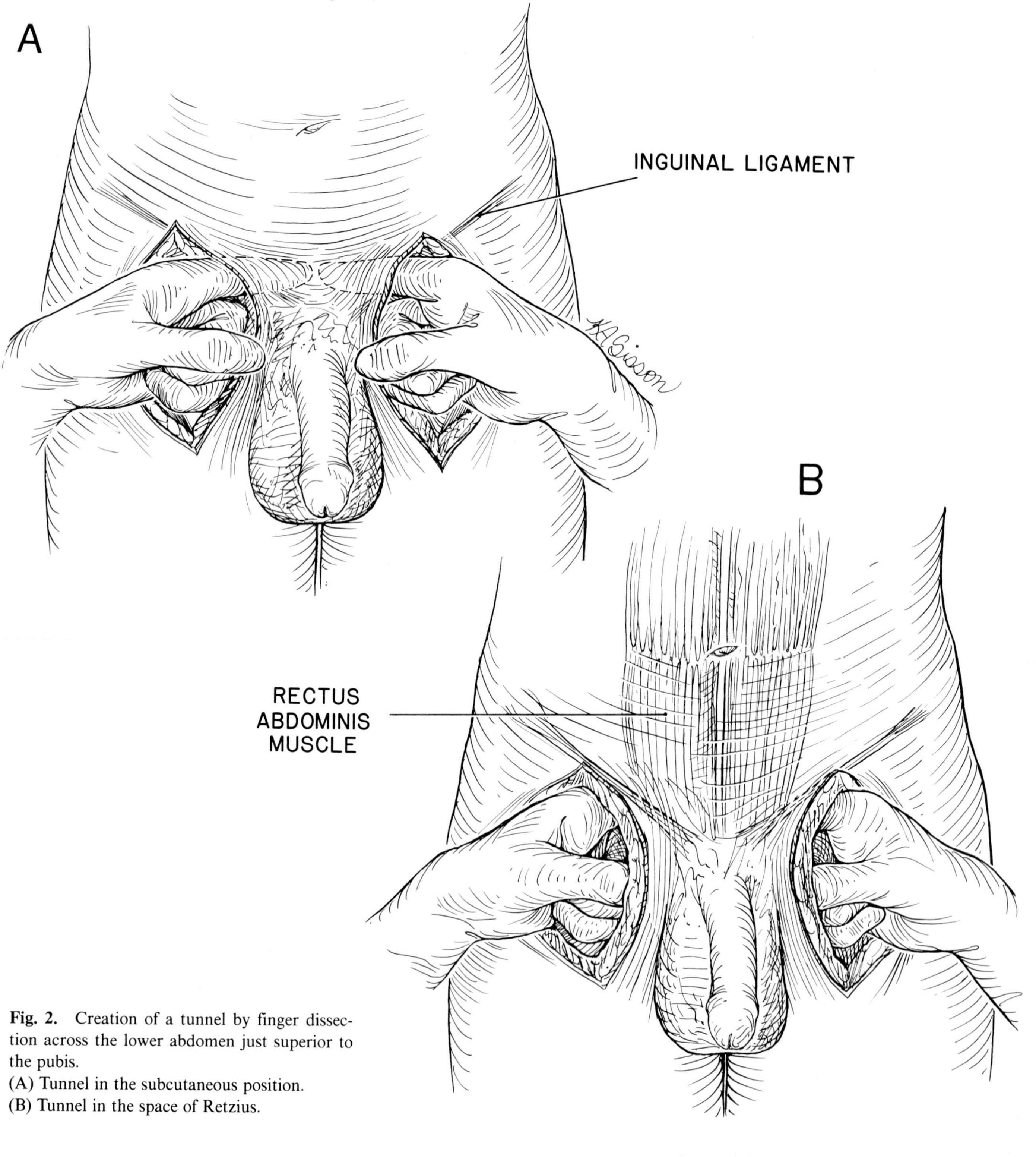

Fig. 2. Creation of a tunnel by finger dissection across the lower abdomen just superior to the pubis.
(A) Tunnel in the subcutaneous position.
(B) Tunnel in the space of Retzius.

The placement of the arteriotomies depends on the distribution of any athrosclerotic occlusive disease in the femoral vessels. If no significant occlusive disease is present, the arteriotomy is made only on the common femoral artery for a distance of 2 to 2.5 cm (Fig. 3B). Commonly, the superficial femoral artery is occluded at its origin and there is also disease in the orifice of the profunda femoris artery. In this situation the arteriotomy should be extended through the profunda stenosis so that the hood of the graft will act as a patch to widen the artery and provide adequate runoff for the graft (Fig. 3C).[4] This maneuver, although important on the recipient limb, may also be employed on the donor vessel to provide increased flow to the donor limb.

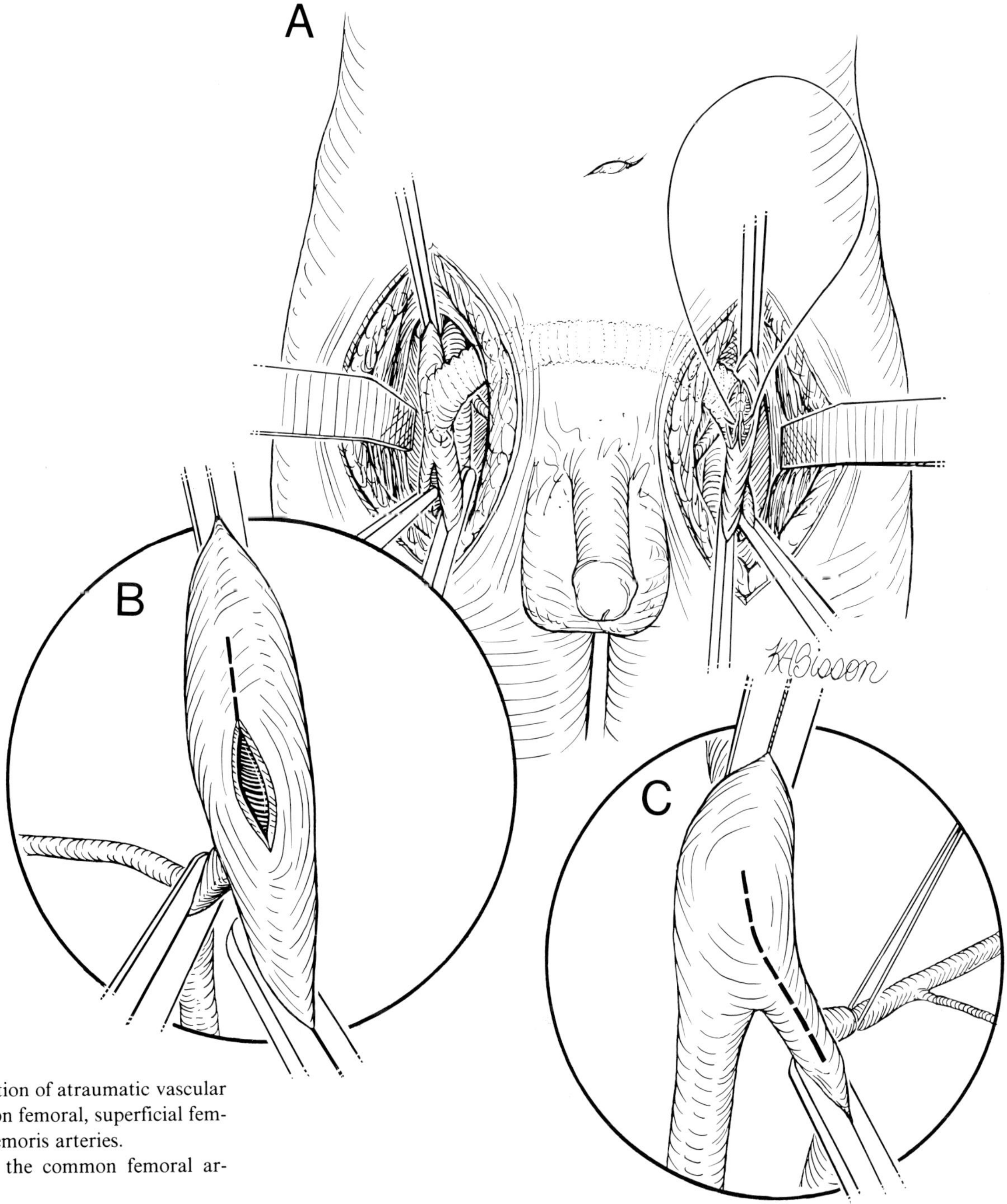

Fig. 3. (A) Application of atraumatic vascular clamps to the common femoral, superficial femoral, and profunda femoris arteries.
(B) Arteriotomy on the common femoral artery.
(C) Arteriotomy is extended through the profunda stenosis so that the hood of the graft will act as a patch to widen the artery and provide adequate runoff for the graft.

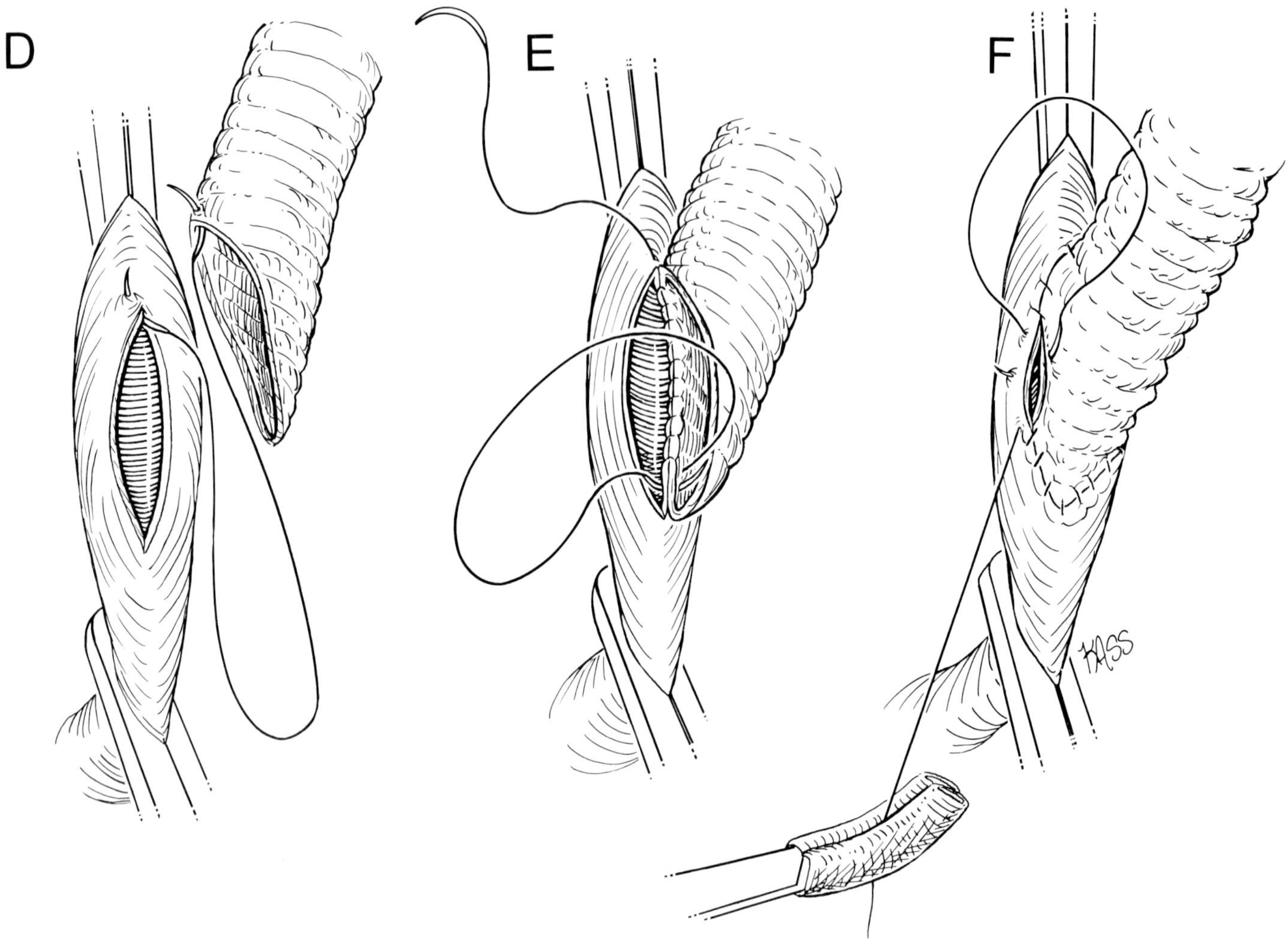

(D) Heel stitches are placed first, from inside to outside the lumen on both the artery and the graft.
(E) Medial rotation of the graft to give wide-open exposure for placement of apical and periapical stitches.
(F) One end of suture is held on tension in rubber-shod clamp while the other end is used to complete the lateral wall of the anastomosis.

The anastomoses may be performed either consecutively or simultaneously and are performed with end of graft attached to side of femoral artery (Fig. 3A). The anastomoses are sutured with 5–0 or 6–0 monofilament polypropylene in a continuous fashion. The anastomoses are begun by placing the heel stitch first, using a double-armed suture such that the stitches are taken from inside to outside the lumen on both the artery and graft (Fig. 3D). Stitches through the artery are always started from the inside, so that the effect is to tack down rather than elevate the intima. The medial side of the anastomosis is performed first. The toe of the graft is not sutured prior to suturing of the medial wall of the anastomosis, as this hinders visibility during placement of the distal medial-wall stitches. By not placing tacking sutures, the graft can be rotated medially, giving wide-open exposure for placement of the all-important apical and periapical stitches (Fig. 3E). Using this same suture, the suture line is carried around the apex to begin suturing the lateral wall of the anastomosis distally to a point approximately one third of the distance from the toe to the heel of the anastomosis. This end of the suture is then held on tension in a rubber-shod clamp as the other end is used to complete the lateral wall of the anastomosis (Fig. 3F).

On the recipient limb, the configuration of the anastomosis is always made such that it points distally in the normal direction of blood flow. On the donor limb, the anastomosis may be oriented either proximally (the so-called "S"-shaped graft as in Figure 4A), or distally (the so-called "C"-shaped graft as in Figure 4B). Before completing the recipient anastomosis, the graft should be flushed by removing the donor limb clamps on the superficial femoral, profunda femoris, and finally the common femoral artery. The graft is then occluded, and the recipient limb profunda femoris artery and superficial femoral artery are unclamped and flushed as well. Following flushing, the recipient anastomosis is then completed. After completion of this anastomosis, all clamps are removed.

Fig. 4. (A) "S"-shaped graft.
(B) "C"-shaped graft.
(C) Fascial layer is closed with interrupted 2–0 synthetic absorbable suture.
(D) Subcutaneous closure is accomplished with interrupted 3–0 synthetic absorbable suture.

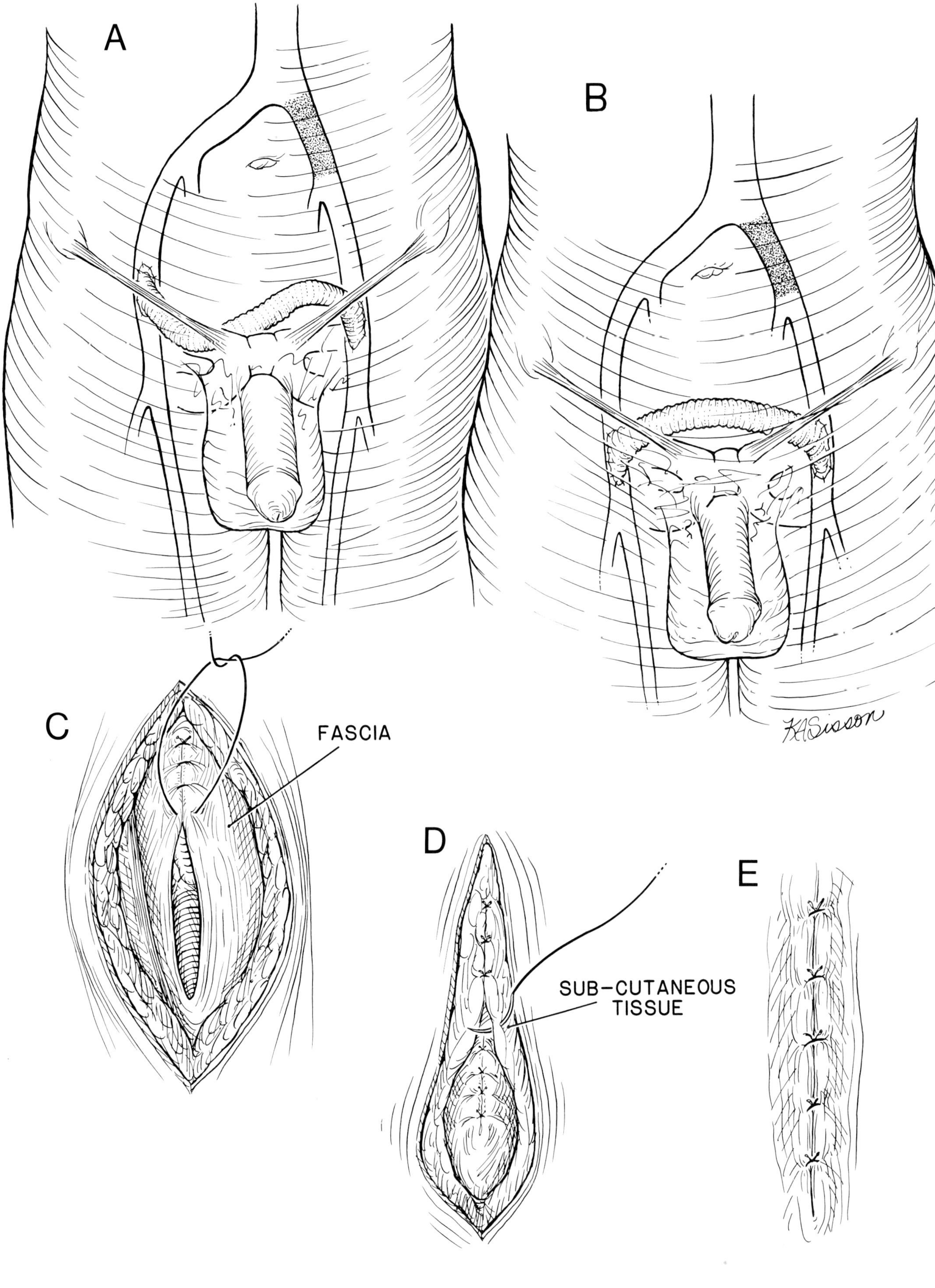
A
B
C
FASCIA
KASisson
D
E
SUB-CUTANEOUS
TISSUE

Pulses are then palpated distal to the anastomoses. If there is any concern about technical error, intra-arterial pressures are measured at the operating table. Operative arteriography is not routinely performed.

Heparin is not continued postoperatively. It may be reversed with protamine sulfate, if desired.

The need for meticulous hemostasis cannot be overstated. A wound complication in the groin puts the patient at risk for a graft infection, which is, of course, a risk to life as well as limb.

The wound is closed in three layers: fascia, subcutaneous tissue, and skin. In particularly obese patients, a two-layer subcutaneous closure may be required. The fascial layer is closed with interrupted 2–0 synthetic absorbable suture (Fig. 4C). The subcutaneous closure is accomplished with interrupted 3–0 synthetic absorbable suture (Fig. 4D), and the skin is closed with simple sutures of 4–0 nylon. Drains are not placed. The wounds are dressed with occlusive dressings and the procedure is concluded.

REFERENCES

1. Vetto RM: The treatment of unilateral iliac artery obstruction with a transabdominal subcutaneous, femoro-femoral graft. Surgery 52:342, 1962
2. Tyson RR, Reichel FA: Retropubic femoro-femoral bypass: A new route through the space of Retzius. Surgery 72:401, 1972
3. Flanigan DP, Pratt DG, Goodreau JJ, Burnham SJ, Yao JST, Bergan JJ: Hemodynamic and angiographic guidelines in selection of patients for femoro-femoral bypass. Arch Surg 113:1257, 1978
4. Brewster DC, Darling RC: Optimal methods of aorto-iliac reconstruction. Surgery 84:739, 1978

PORTAL HYPERTENSION

Mesocaval Shunt

John L. Cameron

The mesocaval interposition shunt was first reported in 1970.[1,2] The first large series of patients treated with interposition mesocaval shunts was reported by Drapanas in 1972. Currently, the standard means of constructing a mesocaval interposition shunt is to interpose a short, straight, Dacron graft between the anterior surface of the inferior vena cava just below the third portion of the duodenum and the posterior surface of the superior mesenteric vein. This results in an "H" configuration. Although reasonably easy to construct, at times one has to perform the anastomosis to a superior mesenteric vein that has already branched and is of small caliber. In addition, the superior mesenteric vein has to be rotated so that the graft can be anastomosed to the posterior aspect. I have modified this procedure to make it technically easier to perform and, hopefully, to increase the long-term patency rate.

As demonstrated in Figure 1, after opening the abdomen through a vertical midline incision, the transverse colon is retracted in a cephalad direction. The root of the transverse mesocolon is dissected, and the superior mesenteric vein is mobilized and cleaned on top of the third portion of the duodenum and the uncinate process of the pancreas to where the vein disappears behind the neck of the pancreas.

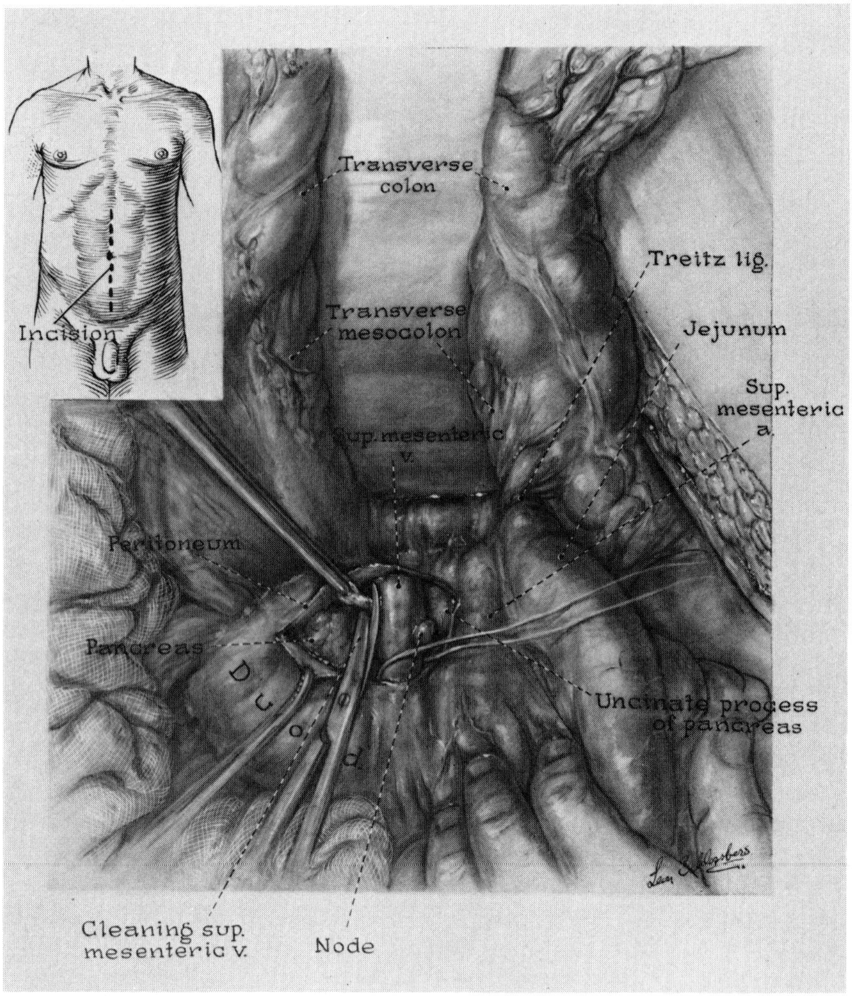

Fig. 1. The superior mesenteric vein is isolated on top of the uncinate process to the point where it passes posterior to the neck of the pancreas to join the splenic vein. The insert depicts the incision used for this operation. (Reprinted with permission.[4])

Ordinarily, the superior mesenteric vein would be cleaned and isolated in a more caudal location, just below the third portion of the duodenum. However, when one isolates and cleans the superior mesenteric vein in this more cephalad position (Figs. 1 and 2), one is always dealing with a vein of large caliber, to which the Dacron graft can easily be anastomosed. A 4- to 5-cm segment of superior mesenteric vein is completely isolated circumferentially. This often means dividing large mesenteric branches entering the superior mesenteric vein. The right colic and middle colic can be divided with impunity. In addition, the inferior mesenteric vein frequently enters the superior mesenteric vein before its junction with the splenic vein and, if need be, this can also be ligated and divided. Often, however, these large venous branches can be mobilized, preserved, and controlled during the anastomosis with vessel loops.

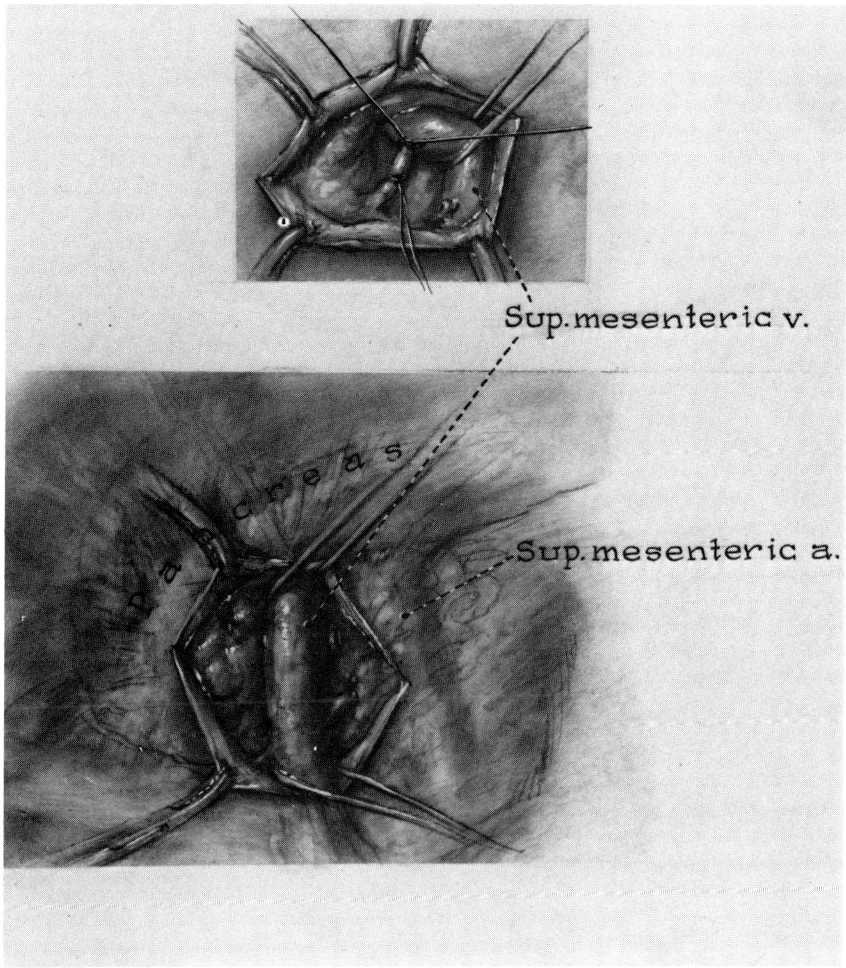

Fig. 2. Superior mesenteric vein is freed circumferentially on top of the third portion of the duodenum and on top of the uncinate process of the duodenum. (Reprinted with permission.[4])

Once a long segment of superior mesenteric vein is isolated, the junction between the second and third portions of the duodenum is visualized in the retroperitoneum. Even in obese individuals, there is usually a bare spot where the distal second and proximal third portions of the duodenum can be identified through the retroperitoneal fat. The duodenum is extensively mobilized and the inferior vena cava identified (Fig. 3). The duodenal mobilization should be extended over to the left side of the mesenteric vessels to include the fourth portion of the duodenum and the ligament of Treitz. This will result in mobility of the duodenum in a cephalad direction, so that obstruction by the Dacron graft is not a possibility. The inferior vena cava does not need to be cleaned circumferentially. The anterior and lateral surfaces of the vena cava can be freed quickly and easily. It is also important to divide all soft tissues that reside between the inferior vena cava and the superior mesenteric vein. Often, the right colic artery will be encountered in this plane, and if need be it can be divided after a test interval of bulldog clamping.

Once the inferior vena cava is appropriately mobilized, it is partially occluded by a Statinsky clamp and an ellipse of vein excised. An end-to-side anastomosis is then carried out utilizing an 18-mm knitted Dacron graft. Because of the low-pressure venous system, these grafts generally do not require preclotting.

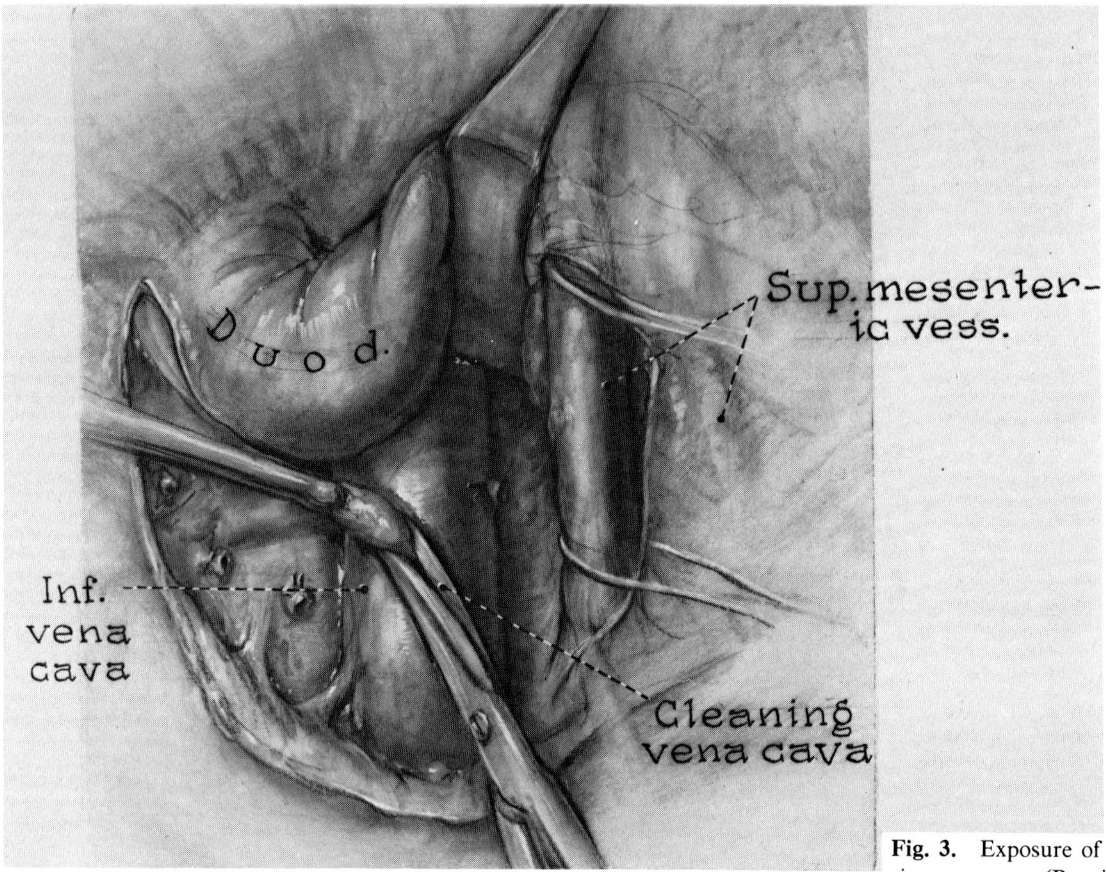

Fig. 3. Exposure of anterior wall of the inferior vena cava. (Reprinted with permission.[4])

The anastomosis is performed with continuous 5–0 prolene sutures (Fig. 4). After the anastomosis is completed, a DeBakey clamp is placed across the graft just above the anastomosis and the Statinsky is loosened to be certain that the anastomosis is secure. The Statinsky clamp is then reinserted. The superior mesenteric vein is then totally occluded. Straight and acutely curved Cooley clamps are often ideal for this purpose. Smaller branches entering the superior mesenteric vein that have not been divided can be controlled with vessel loops. An ellipse is then cut from the anterior surface of the superior mesenteric vein. The Dacron graft is then stretched up over the third portion of the duodenum in a cephalad direction so it can be anastomosed to the superior mesenteric vein on top of the uncinate process. The graft should not be stretched as tautly as for an arterial anastomosis or the venous pressure may not adequately distend the graft. Nevertheless, if it is too long it will bow. Next, the Dacron graft has to be cut on the bevel, since it will approximate the superior mesenteric vein at an acute angle. An anastomosis is then performed between the end of the Dacron graft and the side of the superior mesenteric vein using continuous 5–0 prolene. The right lateral wall of the anastomosis has to be made from within the lumen of the superior mesenteric vein.

When the anastomosis is completed (Fig. 5), the graft actually conforms to a "C" configuration. The Cooley clamps are removed first, leaving the Statinsky clamp in place. The graft rapidly fills with blood, and most of the air is expressed. The graft can then be needled to be certain that all the air is gone before removing the Statinsky clamp. I call this anastomosis the mesocaval "C" graft. Mesenteric venous pressures can be measured directly by sticking the superior mesenteric vein before and after constructing the shunt. An easier method is to wait until the shunt is open and then measure the superior mesenteric vein pressure with the Dacron graft open and occluded.

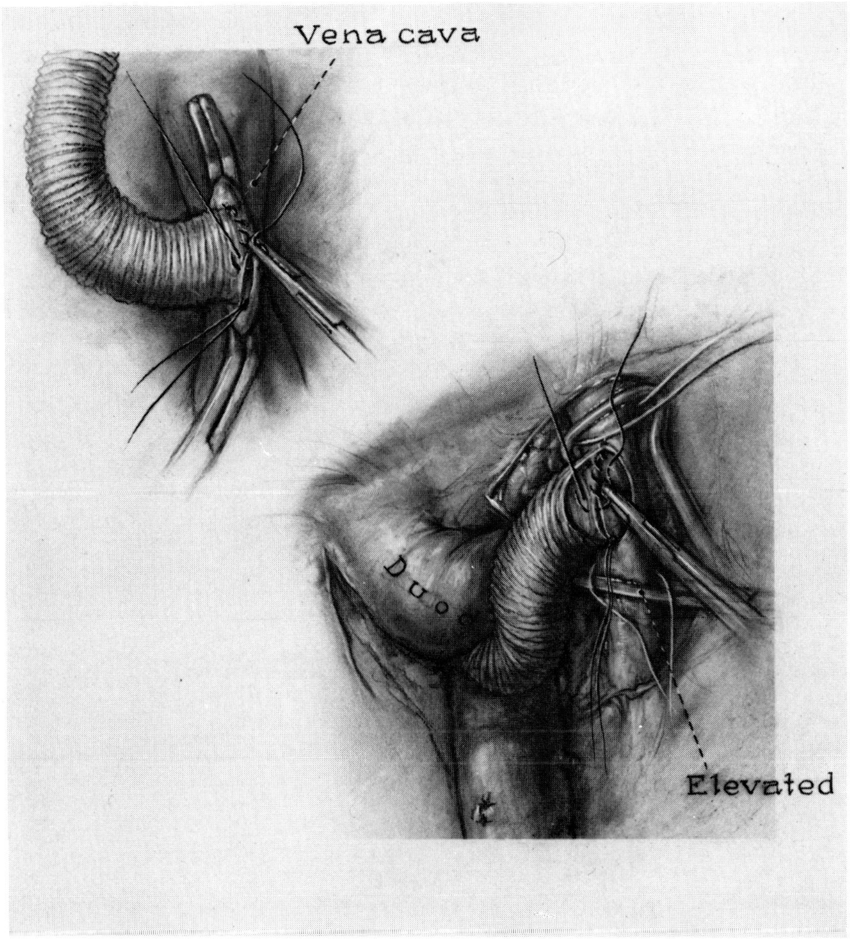

Fig. 4. Eighteen-millimeter knitted Dacron graft is anastomosed to inferior vena cava and to the superior mesenteric vein with continuous 5–0 prolene. (Reprinted with permission.[4])

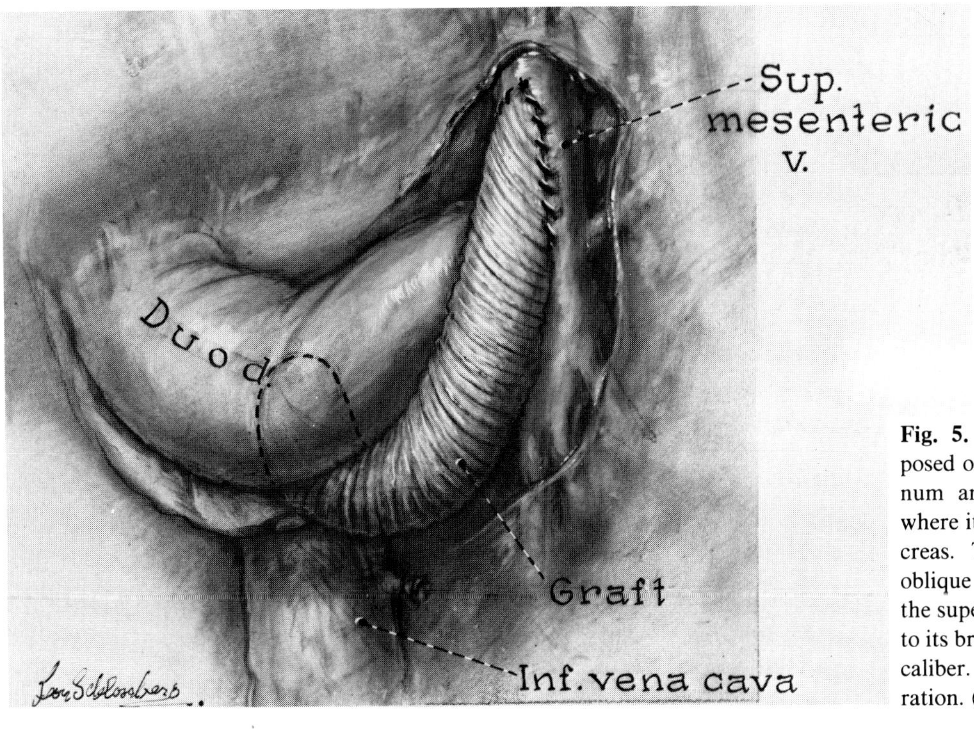

Fig. 5. The superior mesenteric vein is exposed on top of the third portion of the duodenum and the uncinate process to the point where it disappears behind the neck of the pancreas. This allows one to perform a large oblique anastomosis between the prosthesis and the superior mesenteric vein at a point cephalad to its branches, where the vein is always of large caliber. Thus the graft assumes a "C" configuration. (Reprinted with permission.[5])

The mesenteric "C" shunt is technically easier to perform than the mesocaval "H" graft, since the anastomosis is being performed to the superior mesenteric vein on the anterior and thereby more accessible portion of the vein. In addition, since the graft meets the superior mesenteric vein at an acute angle, the anastomosis is oblique and therefore larger. The vein itself is also of larger diameter in this location. Figure 6 demonstrates the differences between the mesocaval "H" and mesocaval "C" grafts. The mesocaval "H" graft is anastomosed to the inferior vena cava at approximately the level of the third portion of the duodenum and travels straight anteriorly, to be anastomosed to the posterior surface of the superior mesenteric vein. The superior mesenteric vein has frequently branched at this point and is small in caliber. In contrast, the mesocaval "C" graft is anastomosed to the inferior vena cava at approximately the same level as the "H" graft, but then it is swung up on top of the third portion of the duodenum and the uncinate process to be anastomosed to the superior mesenteric vein just prior to its disappearance behind the neck of the pancreas. At this location, the superior mesenteric vein is always of large caliber. The anastomosis is performed in an oblique fashion and is always large.

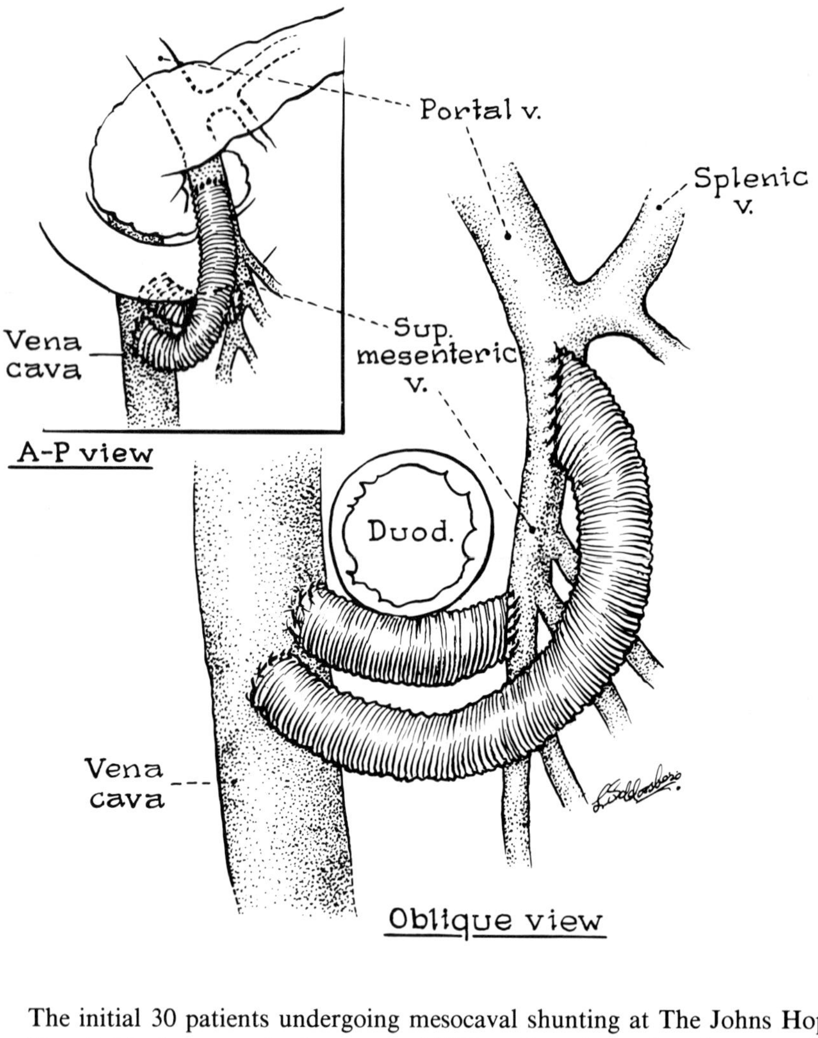

Fig. 6. Relative positions of the interposed prosthesis with the mesocaval "H" shunt and the mesocaval "C" shunt. The "C" shunt is anastomosed to the anterior surface of the superior mesenteric vein just before it joins the splenic vein and above all of its branches. The "H" shunt is anastomosed to the posterior surface of the superior mesenteric vein at the level of the duodenum and frequently at the site of branching. (Reprinted with permission.[6])

The initial 30 patients undergoing mesocaval shunting at The Johns Hopkins Hospital had the standard mesocaval "H" graft performed, and among this group of patients there are four known shunt thromboses. The subsequent 30 patients in the Hopkins series had their shunts performed in the mesocaval "C" fashion. There are no known shunt thromboses in this group. This operation is technically easy to perform and should result in a high long-term shunt patency rate.

REFERENCES

1. Lord JW, Rossi G, Daliana M, Rosati LM: Mesocaval shunt modified by the use of a teflon prosthesis. Surg Gynecol Obstet 130:525, 1970
2. Read RC, Thompson BW, Wise WS, Murphy ML: Mesocaval "H" venous homografts. Arch Surg 101:785, 1970
3. Drapanas T: Interposition mesocaval shunt for treatment of portal hypertension. Ann Surg 176:435, 1972
4. Zuidema G, Cameron JL, Zeppa R: Portal hypertension. II. Operative procedures. In Norsa PF (ed): Operative Surgery: Principles and Techniques. Philadelphia, Lea & Febiger, 1980, pp 652–655
5. Cameron JL, Zuidema GD, Smith GW, Harrington DP, Maddrey WC: Mesocaval shunts for the control of bleeding esophageal varices. Surgery 85:257–262, 1979
6. Cameron JL, Harrington DP, Maddrey WC: The mesocaval "C" shunt. Surg Gynecol Obstet 150:401–403, 1980

Placement of the LeVeen Shunt

Harry H. LeVeen

Since inception of the peritoneovenous shunt,[1] a number of variations in technique have been divised, a fraction of which have been published. The author prefers the internal jugular vein for access to the vena cava, nonetheless, a number of other veins have been used for access, especially in patients where the internal jugular is not patent or available. The access to the superior vena cava via the jugular vein on the right side was chosen because it is a straight line to the superior vena cava and the possibility of malposition is reduced. Malpositions are nonetheless possible when the venous tubing is introduced into the internal jugular vein. The tubing can enter the subclavian vein rather than the superior vena cava, especially if the head is laterally flexed onto the left shoulder. Although the standard internal jugular vein approach is the one recommended for most situations, it should be understood that the operation is really a peritoneovenous shunt and that any access vein to the superior vena cava will be successful. When no access veins are available in the upper half of the body, the author has, on nine occasions, threaded the venous tubing up the inferior vena cava through the saphenofemoral junction. In this approach, the valve is separated from the venous tubing, and one end of the venous tubing is attached to a spinal monometer. In the inferior vena cava, the pressure will be about 30 cm of water, rising with inspiration. When the diaphragm is passed, the pressure drops and becomes even more negative with inspiration. The venous tubing is visualized on x-ray by the injection of a radio-opaque dye before fixing the position of the tubing. The valve is reattached and placed in the lower quadrant. The patient should be heparinized for 2 weeks. The author knows of one case where access was made into the right atrium by thoracotomy.

The proper positioning of the patient on the table will facilitate the approach to the jugular vein. The shoulders are elevated to extend the head. A sheet is placed under both shoulders and the headboard is dropped (Fig. 1). The patient can be rotated on the table so that when the abdominal incision is made it will be uppermost, to avoid undue spilling of ascitic fluid in the operative field.

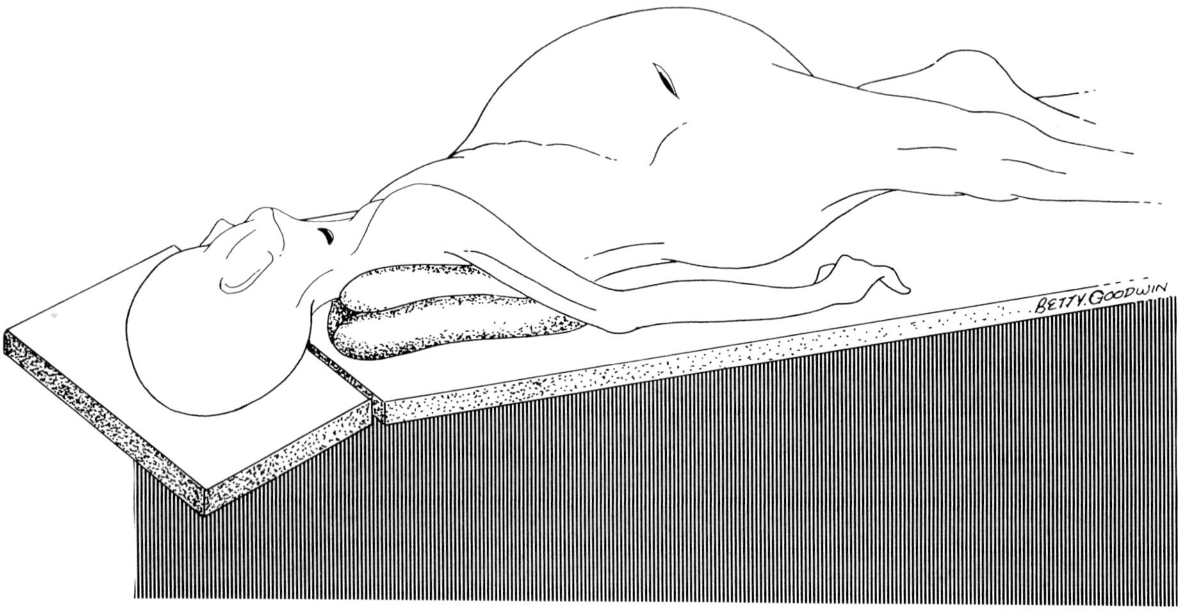

Fig. 1. Proper patient positioning facilitates placement of the shunt.

The abdominal incision is made about 3 or 4 fingerbreadths beneath the costal margin at the anterior axillary line. The abdominal muscles are split in a McBirney fashion to expose the transversalis fascia and transversus muscle, which are left intact to give support to the peritoneum. A double pursestring suture is then placed (Fig. 2A). A stab wound is made in the center of the pursestring (Fig. 2B), and the abdomen is aspirated with a Pool suction tip. (Fig. 2C). Aspiration of the peritoneal fluid will reduce the total amount of ascitic fluid that enters the venous system and, in the author's experience, has diminished the occurrence of disseminated intravascular coagulation. As much as 10,000 to 15,000 cc of fluid have been aspirated from the peritoneal cavity. This can induce hypovolemic shock, since reduction of the hydrostatic fluid pressure in the peritoneal cavity causes the visceral surfaces to weep and the otherwise compressed splanchnic vessels to dilate and fill with blood. Therefore, plasma and saline solution may be required during the period of aspiration to combat the hypovolemia. When this precaution is taken, no untoward effects have occurred. When sufficient fluid has been aspirated, the collecting tube is thrust into the abdomen in the direction of the lower pelvis (Fig. 2D). The collecting tube is too long as supplied by the manufacturer, and approximately 4 inches are cut from its tip unless the patient is very tall. Failure to cut off a portion of the abdominal collecting tubes may cause lower abdominal pain from pressure on the peritoneum or a viscus. This has disappeared upon subsequent shortening of the peritoneal collecting tube. The pursestring sutures are pulled tightly (Fig. 2E) around the neck of the valve, leaving the valve in the extraperitoneal position. A stab wound is made in the muscle, and the venous tube is brought through the stab wound (Fig. 2F). The muscle is then closed with interrupted nonabsorbable sutures (Fig. 2G).

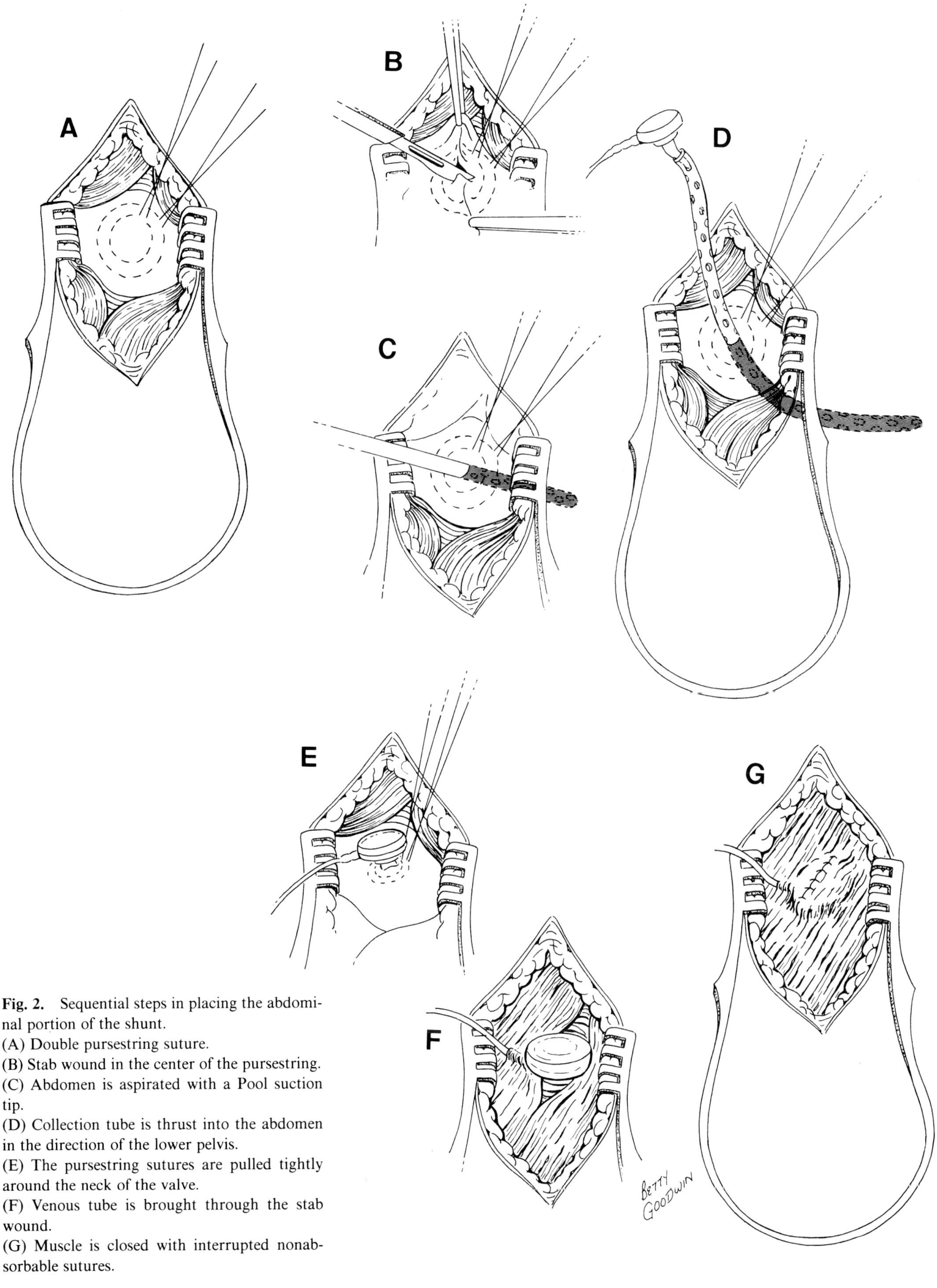

Fig. 2. Sequential steps in placing the abdominal portion of the shunt.
(A) Double pursestring suture.
(B) Stab wound in the center of the pursestring.
(C) Abdomen is aspirated with a Pool suction tip.
(D) Collection tube is thrust into the abdomen in the direction of the lower pelvis.
(E) The pursestring sutures are pulled tightly around the neck of the valve.
(F) Venous tube is brought through the stab wound.
(G) Muscle is closed with interrupted nonabsorbable sutures.

Attention is next directed to the neck, where a transverse incision is made between the two heads of the sternomastoid approximately 2½ fingerbreadths above the clavicle. The venous tubing may be pulled into the neck with an alligator forceps or by a special tube-passing instrument. The tube-passing instrument is rapid and useful in performing saphenofemoral bypass grafts, in addition to its use in pulling the venous tube into the neck wound. It is essential that the tunnel through the subcutaneous tissue be as small as possible to avoid accumulation of ascitic fluid around the tubing or possibility of hematoma. The rigid tube-passer is pushed upward through the subcutaneous tissue of the chest into the neck wound. The bullet tip of the tube-passer is grasped between the fingers and the rigid outer tube is withdrawn from the wound, allowing the bullet tip with its attached flexible innercore to remain in the subcutaneous tissue. The venous tubing is then attached to the nipple-like abdominal end of the flexible inner core and pulled through the subcutaneous tissue into the neck wound (Fig. 3). The use of a tube-passer is rapid, simple, and causes a minimal amount of trauma. If a tube-passer is not available, a rectal biopsy forceps or alligator forceps is passed through the subcutaneous tissue into the neck. A long No. 2 silk or other heavy suture is grasped in the jaws of the biopsy forceps or alligator forceps and pulled from the neck wound into the abdominal wound. The venous tubing is then secured to this heavy suture and pulled into the neck wound (Fig. 4). The alligator forceps or tube-passer can be pushed through the subcutaneous tissue without additional local infiltration of anesthetic agent. However, extra sedation may be necessary during this interval of the operation. The patients tolerate this maneuver without major discomfort.

Fig. 3. The tube-passing instrument eases placement of the shunt tubing.

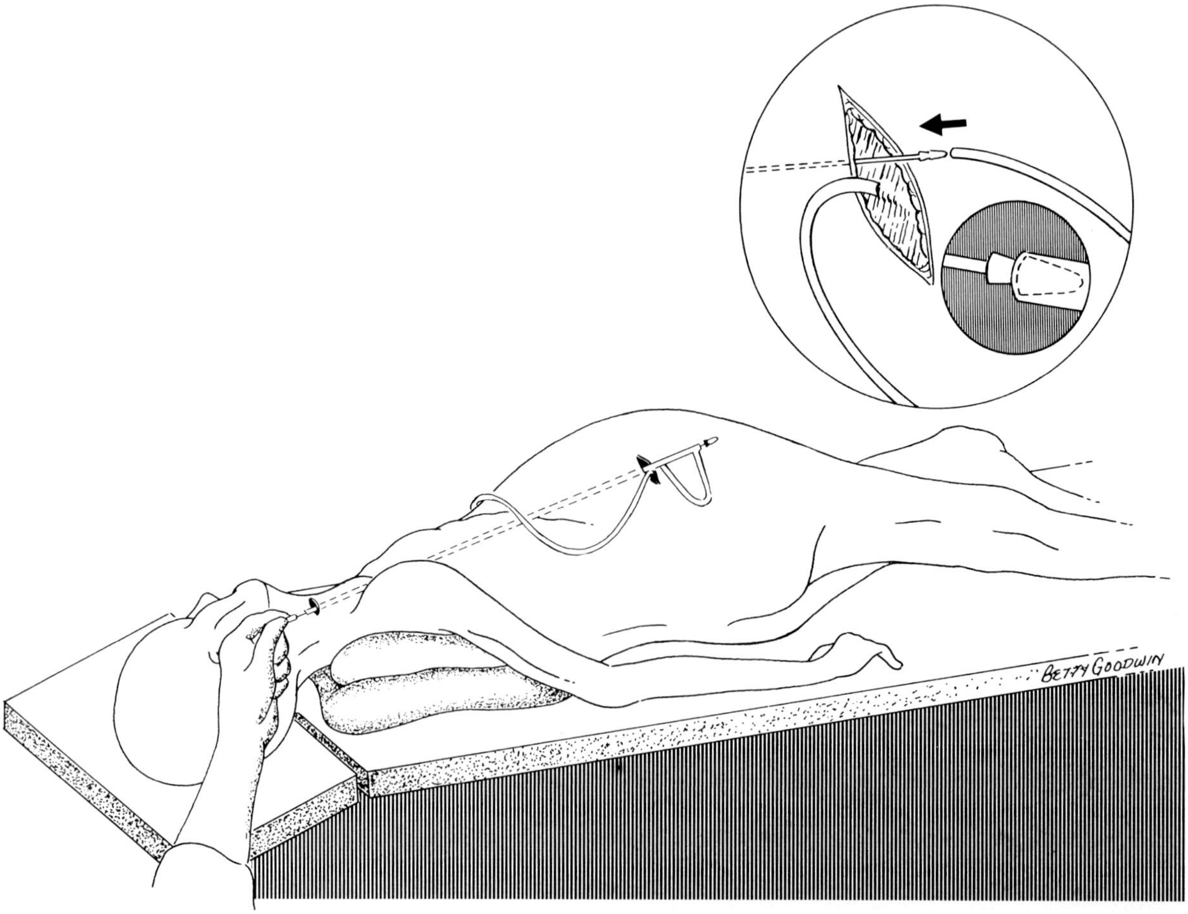

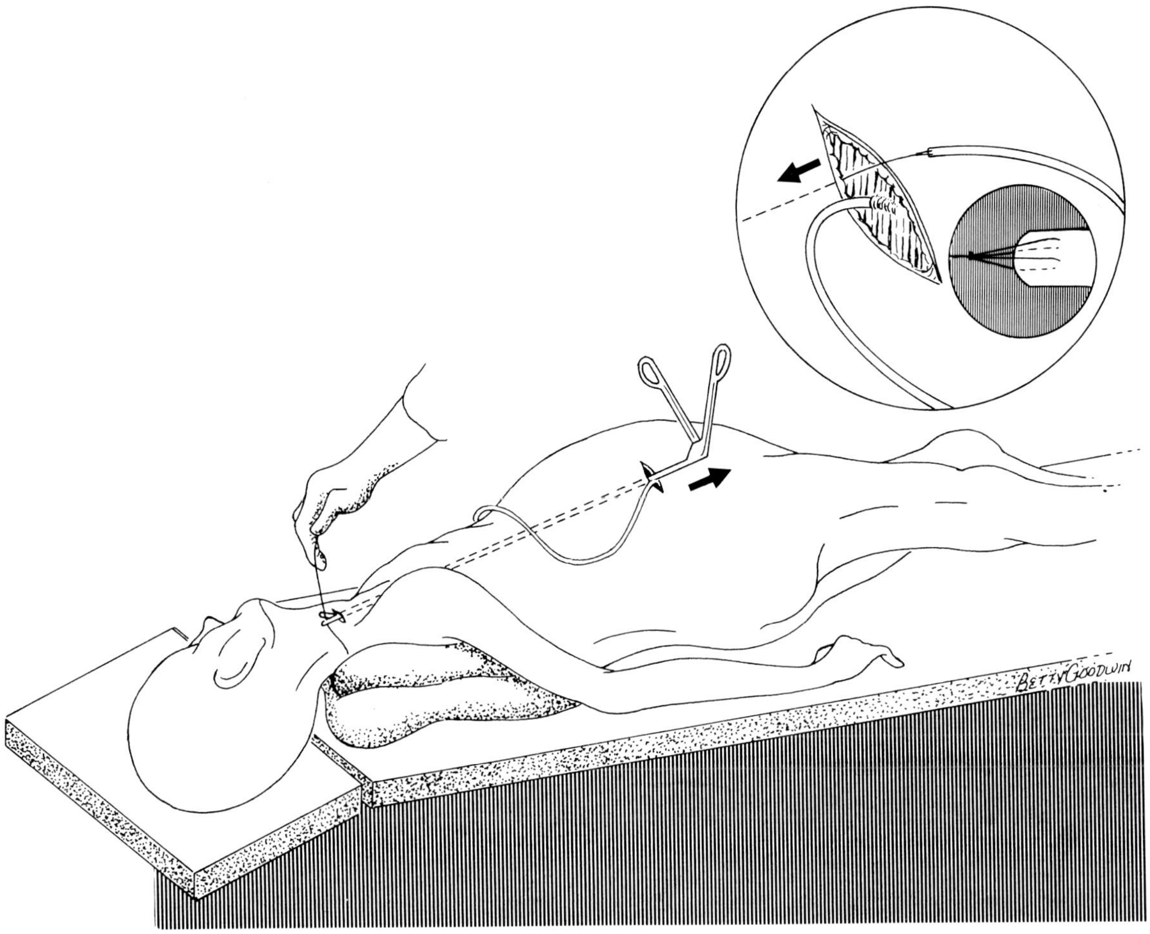

Fig. 4. A long alligator biopsy forcep in useful if a shunt-passing instrument is unavailable.

The venous tube can be introduced into the jugular vein in different ways. The simplest and quickest way, as suggested by Dr. Vincent Piccone, is to utilize a pacemaker-lead introducer. This apparatus consists of a tubular piece containing an obturator-type cannula in its center. The obturator cannula has a fine central hole, which allows it to follow a guide wire. The thin guide wire is introduced into the vein through a needle, which is withdrawn (Fig. 5). The introducer is then passed over the guide wire to dilate the small hole made by the needle and guide wire into a sizable orifice. This dilation is made by a rotary motion (Fig. 6A). After the cannula has been introduced for a distance into the vein, the obturator of the cannula is withdrawn (Fig. 6B). Then the venous tubing is quickly introduced through the sheath of the introducer to replace the obturator (Fig. 6C). After a good portion of the tubing has been introduced, the sheath around the tubing is peeled off (Fig. 6D) and the introducer is totally removed, leaving only the venous tubing in the vein. No sutures are used.

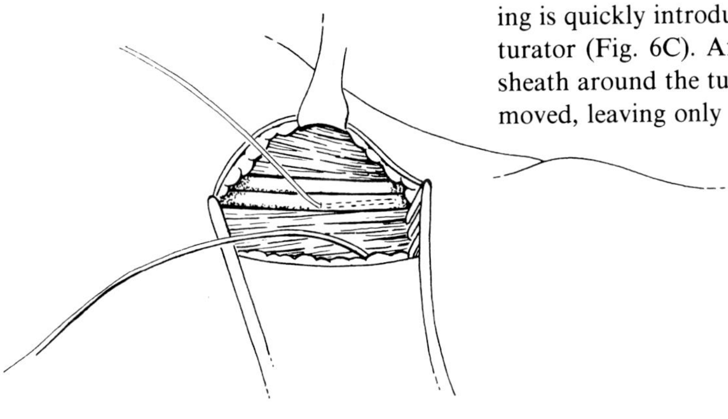

Fig. 5. Introduction of venous tube into the jugular vein by use of a thin guide wire, which is introduced into the vein through a needle.

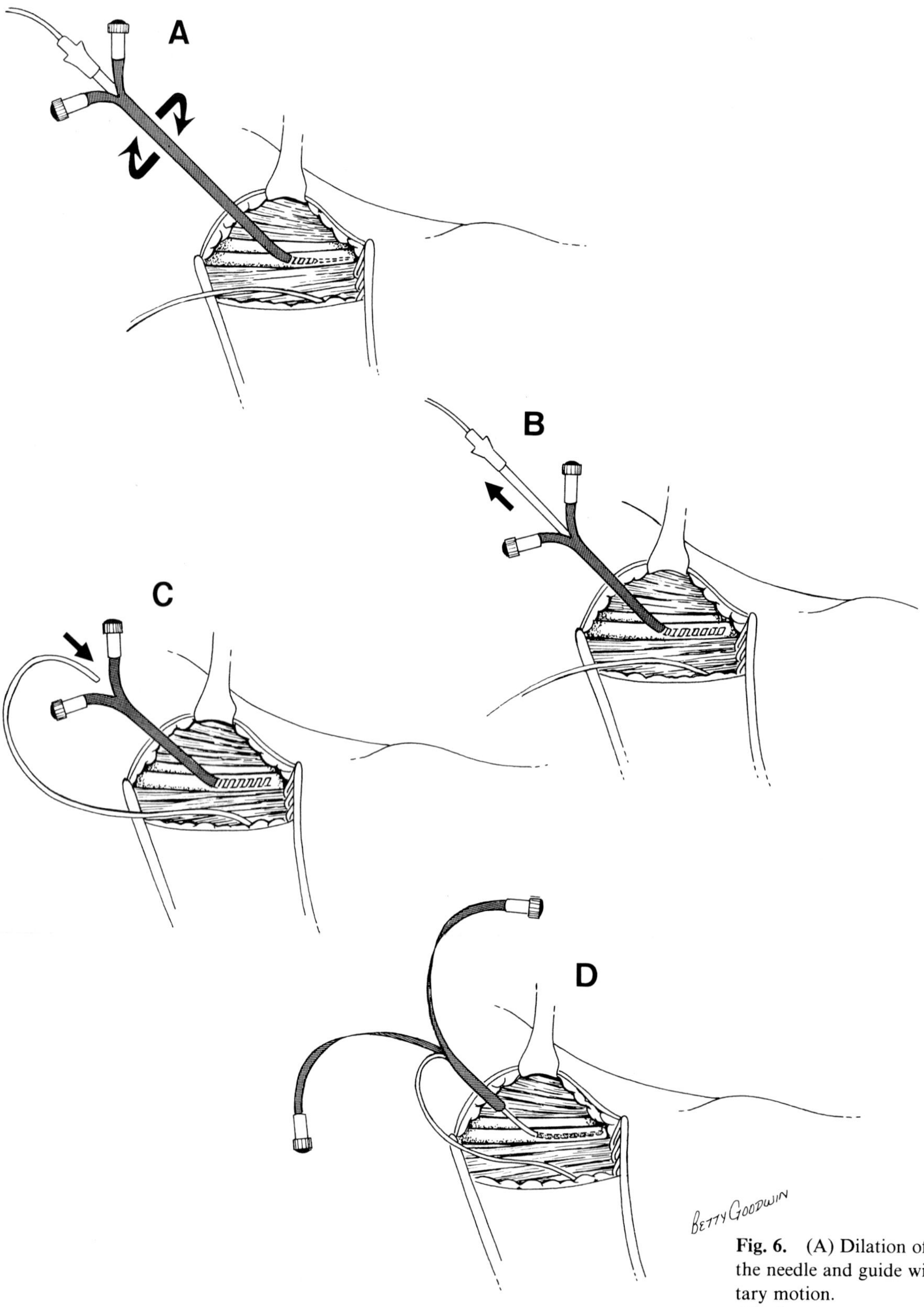

Fig. 6. (A) Dilation of the small hole made by the needle and guide wire is performed by a rotary motion.
(B) The obturator of the cannula is withdrawn after the cannula has been introduced a distance into the vein.
(C) Venous tubing is quickly introduced through the sheath of the introducer to replace the obturator.
(D) The sheath around the tubing is peeled off.

Another method to introduce the venous tubing into the vein is to place a pursestring suture in the vein and make a stab wound into the center of the pursestring. The traction sutures are placed above and below the pursestring to occlude the vessel (Fig. 7, top) while the tubing is being introduced into the vein. The traction suture is relaxed to allow passage of the tube. Before introduction of the tubing, the distance from the venotomy site to the second rib must be measured and the excess tubing excised (Fig. 7, bottom). The tubing must reach the superior vena cava, must not be so short that it remains in the jugular vein, and must not be overly long so that it extends beyond the heart into the inferior vena cava. Also, an extra length of tubing can carry the tip into the pulmonary artery, where it will not function. The tubing should be either in the superior vena cava or in the right atrium, but nowhere else.

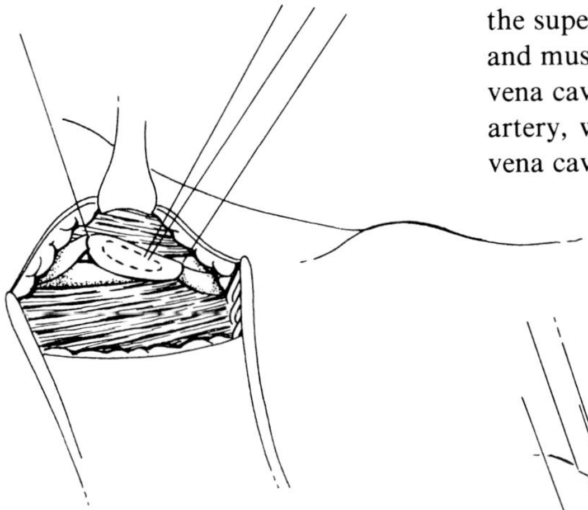

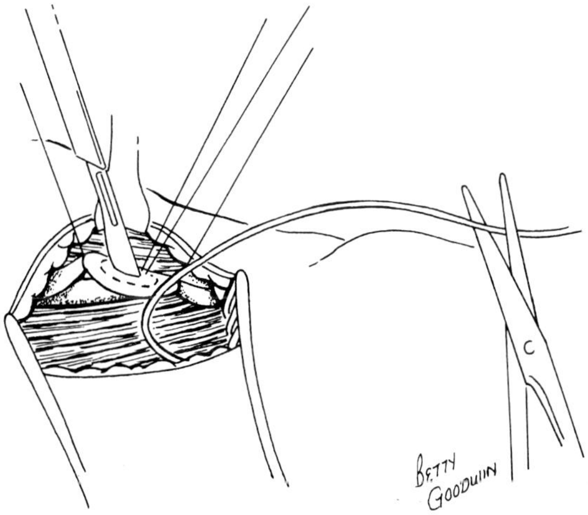

Fig. 7. A pursestring suture may be used, if desired, to close vein wall closely around the shunt tubing. (Top) Traction sutures are placed above and below the pursestring suture to occlude the vessel.
(Bottom) the distance from the venotomy side to the second rib must be measured and the ex cess tubing excised.

Still another method is to place simple traction sutures around the jugular vein below and to tie off the jugular vein above. A longitudinal venotomy is made in the jugular vein. After the tubing is introduced, it is secured with a circumferential tie around the tube and the vein below the venotomy. Care must be taken with this technique to avoid the vagus nerve, which contains the recurrent laryngeal nerve, compression of which will produce unilateral vocal cord paralysis. After the valve has been placed, the author prefers to inject either methelene blue or indigo carmine dye into a straight portion of the venous tubing just above the valve. The patient is then asked to take a deep breath to observe whether the dye travels up the tubing into the neck (Fig. 8).

If the shunt is functional, the dye will be seen to flow into the jugular vein on inspiration. The puncture of the venous tubing should be made with a 25-gauge or smaller needle, so as not to induce any leaks in the tubing. After it has been ascertained that the valve is functional, the wounds are irrigated with an aminoglycoside solution such as gentamycin and closed tightly with interrupted and continuous suture materials. It is essential that the skin closure be absolutely watertight. Any leakage of ascitic fluid through the skin wound may cause a fatal infection, since these wounds communicate with the peritoneal cavity and the circulation. Because these patients have so little subcutaneous fat, even a stitch infection could initiate fatal sepsis. The author prefers a subcuticular skin closure with absorbable continuous polyglycocolic acid suture. All patients are placed on antibiotics preoperatively with a penicillianase-resistant penicillin. The wounds are thoroughly irrigated at the time of surgery with an aminoglycoside antibiotic. Because these precautions were taken and the wounds were made watertight, the author has not seen an infection in more than 150 cases.

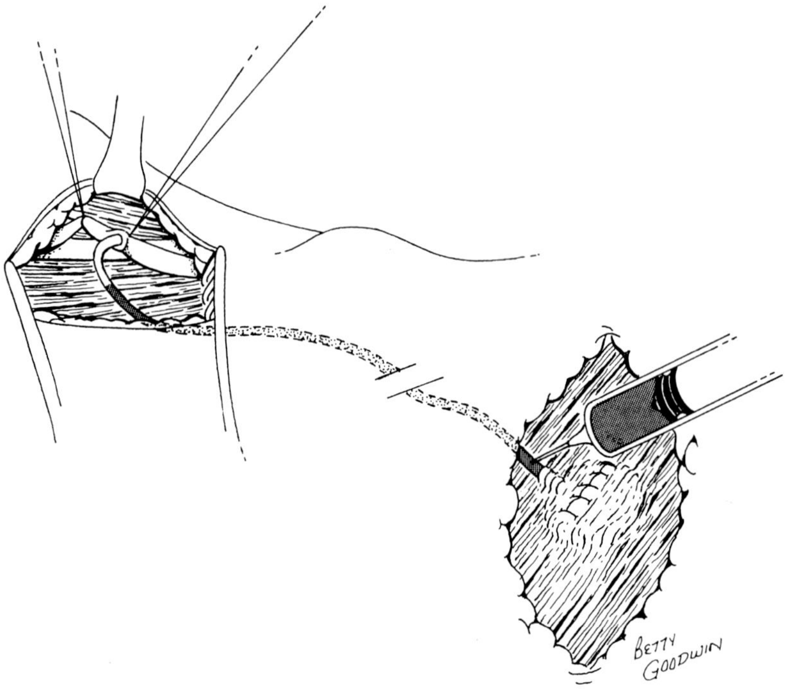

Fig. 8. A contrast medium injection into the shunt allows an intermediate check on shunt function.

POSTOPERATIVE ORDERS

Postoperatively, the patient must be given sufficient furosamide to produce sustained diuresis during the period of maximum ascitic fluid inflow. The patient must be weighed daily and urinary output charted. On the second or third day, the patient is taught to inspire against a resistance by breathing through a bottle with a constricted inflow placed about 10 cm below the fluid level of the bottle. The patient is also fitted with a Velcro elastic abdominal binder and taught to do the breathing exercises lying flat with the abdominal binder applied four times daily for 10 to 15 min. As the abdomen regains its tone, it may be unnecessary to continue the breathing exercises. If urinary volume is excessive, electrolytes should be monitored to guard against a serious drop in serum potassium. The use of spironolactone further prevents an abrupt fall in the serum potassium concentration. If there is any leakage of ascitic fluid from the wound in the postoperative period, extra sutures must be placed immediately to prevent the further escape of ascitic fluid. Complications in the postoperative period include disseminated intravascular coagulation, which can usually be treated with platelets and epsilon-amino-caproic-acid (EACA). Fibrinogen and heparin can be added if needed. If the disseminated intravascular coagulation is life-threatening, the shunt should be interrupted and the peritoneal cavity washed out with saline before the shunt is restarted. A mild coagulopathy appearing on the third day may need no therapy. Severe coagulopathies are usually seen within the first 24 hours. The tendency to coagulopathy disappears by the seventh day. Although the coagulation parameters are often impaired by surgery and split products can be identified both in the ascitic fluid and the blood, patients do not exhibit any serious bleeding tendencies.

REFERENCES

LeVeen HH, Wapnick S, Diaz D, Grosberg S, Kinney, M: Ascites: Its correction by periotoneovenous shunting, Curr Probl Surg 26:1–61, 1979

The Sugiura Operation for Portal Hypertension and Bleeding Esophageal Varices

George Johnson, Jr., Blair A. Keagy

Attempts to ablate esophagogastric varices, the collateral venous circulation around the liver, or the major contributions to the portal venous system have been periodically tried since Guido Banti first presented the concept in 1883.[1] Simple transesophageal or transgastric ligation of bleeding varices is technically easy but has an unacceptable rate of rebleeding.[2–4] It is presently advocated only as a temporary means of controlling massive hemorrhage prior to an elective shunting procedure.

More extensive interruption of the portasystemic collateral circulation that develops in the region of the esophagogastric junction has been repeatedly attempted. Hassab[5,6] suggested that the predisposition to variceal rupture is due to hypoxia caused by venous congestion of the gastroesophageal mucosa. Hassab employed exterior devascularization of the cardia of the stomach and the abdominal portion of the esophagus to "decongest" this area. A significant fall in portal blood flow and pressure was found, which Hassab attributed to ligation of the left gastric and splenic arteries. Hassab's patients had a low incidence of rebleeding and encephalopathy.

Our experience with this type of operative approach is based on a prospective series of ablative operations performed on 60 consecutive patients in the 1960s and 1970s.[7–9] There was a high immediate postoperative mortality and significant incidence of rebleeding in this group, but no encephalopathy was noted and the long-term survival was similar to that following a portacaval shunt.

The technique advocated by Sugiura and Futagawa[10–12] combines many aspects of the operations advocated by Womack and Hassab as well as the addition of an extensive transthoracic external devascularization and transection of the distal esophagus. The goal of this operation is paraesophagogastric devascularization from the inferior pulmonary vein to the cardia of the stomach, transection of the esophagus and its submucosal varices, reanastomosis of the esophagus, splenectomy, selective vagotomy, and pyloroplasty. The technique has a low mortality, low incidence of rebleeding, no encephalopathy, and no interference with hepatic metabolism.

This type of procedure has been performed sporadically in the United States, although the excellent results reported by Sugiura and Futagawa[10–12] have not been duplicated in this country. Based on our experience with the Womack ablative procedure, we feel this type of operation should be reserved for those patients in whom there is no vein suitable for a shunt operation, and those patients in whom encephalopathy is likely to occur and will be poorly tolerated. Hypersplenism, as evidenced by thrombocytopenia, leukopenia, and an enlarged spleen, will usually be controlled by this procedure. The Sugiura operation may be contraindicated in obese or poor-risk patients, since it is associated with a considerable amount of operative trauma. Again, based on our experience with the Womack procedure, it will not help ascites and, initially at least, will make it worse.

The operation is best done in two stages. Sugiura and associates recommend that the thoracic stage be done first in those patients in whom bleeding from esophageal varices is a problem. The second, or abdominal stage, can be performed in a month to 6 weeks following the thoracic operation. Two stages allow the esophageal anastomosis to heal before completely ligating the blood supply to the upper stomach. The originators of this procedure noted an esophageal leak in only 19 of 265 (7 percent) of their patients, but esophageal leak has been a major complication in this country.

The following illustrations demonstrate the technique used in completing the Sugiura procedure.

Fig. 1.
(A) The patient is positioned for a left posterior lateral thoracotomy. Sugiura suggests entering the chest through the sixth intercostal space with optional posterior transection of the sixth and seventh ribs for additional exposure. We found that a seventh interspace incision or subposterial resection of the seventh rib is more optimal. There will often be collateral veins on the chest wall, so it is necessary to carefully occlude the bleeding points.
(B) The inferior pulmonary ligament is divided to the level of the inferior pulmonary vein, and the lung is retracted superiorly. The pleura overlying the esophagus is incised, and the edges are retracted with silk sutures. The vagus nerves are identified and preserved.
(C) Using blunt and sharp dissection, the esophagus is freed from its bed and encircled with a Penrose drain. In the actively bleeding patient, hemorrhage can usually be controlled with traction of the esophagus, so this portion of the procedure should be completed with some dispatch in the acutely bleeding patient.

Many collateral veins resembling a vein plexus paralleling the vagus nerves can be seen around the esophagus as well as numerous vessels on the muscularis. These vessels connect freely to the esophageal mucosa and must be doubly ligated and divided. The larger vessels are secured with transfixion sutures. There are usually 30 to 50 of these shunting veins, and this devascularization is carried out for a length of 12 to 18 cm and as far as possible to the upper stomach.
(D) The paraesophageal dissection is complete with identification, ligation, and division of the numerous veins on the esophagus. Metal clips are left as markers for the lowest portion of devascularization.

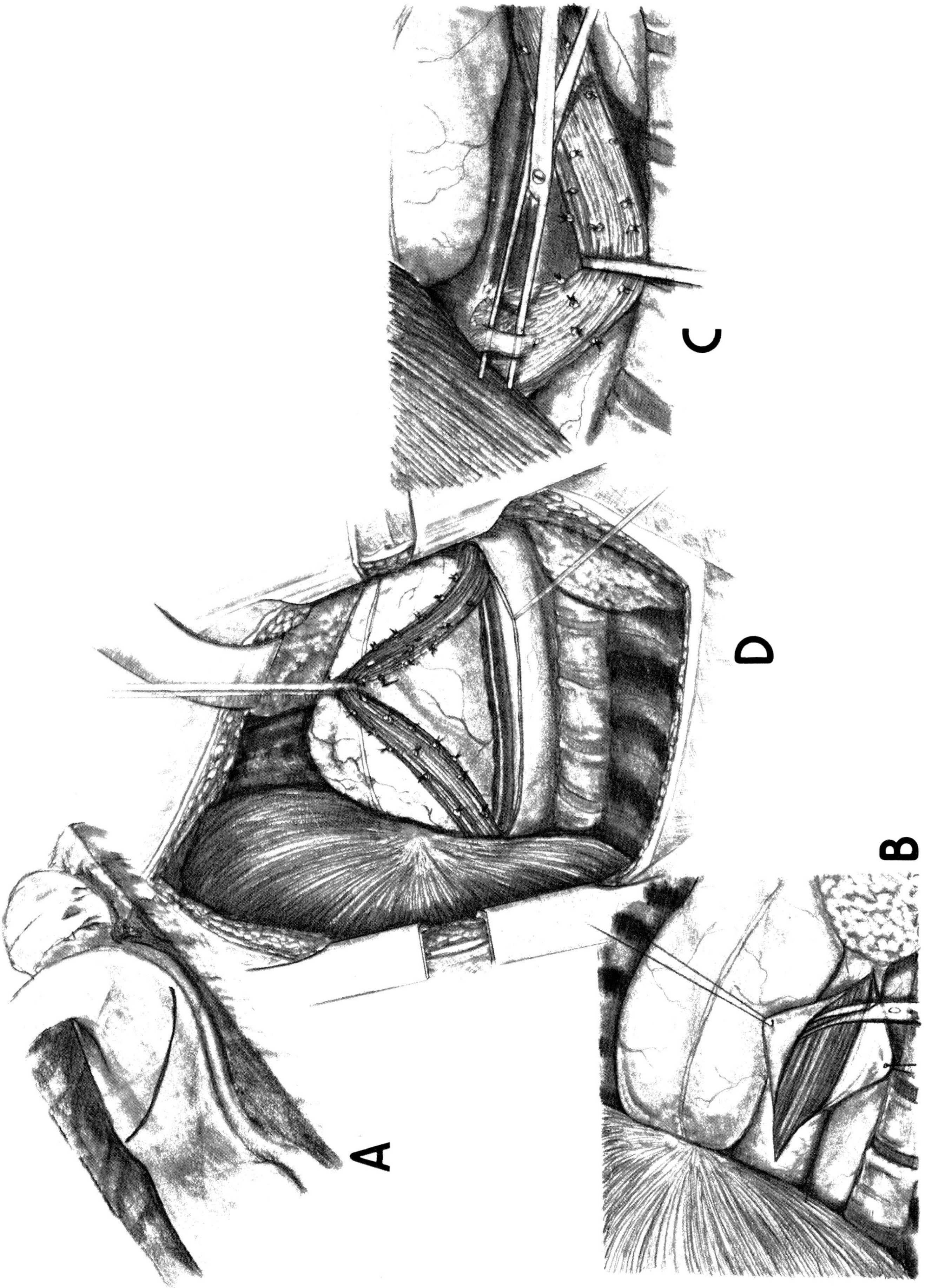
A
B
C
D

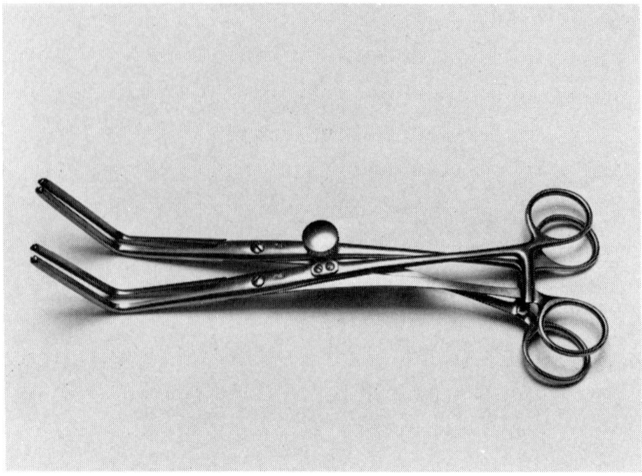

Fig. 2. Special clamps developed by Sugiura and associates[10–12] are applied to the esophagus. They are extremely valuable during this part of the operation. They can be attached to each other, and an assistant can hold the clamps as one.

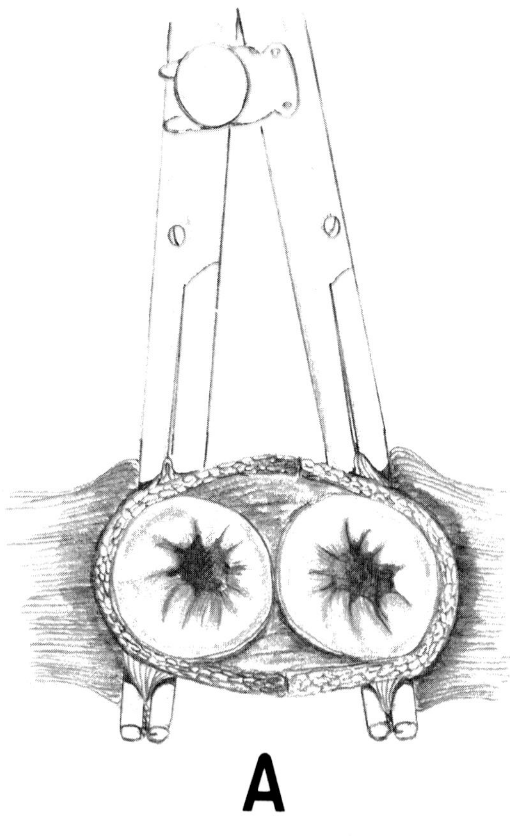

A

Fig. 3.
(A) One clamp is placed at the esophagogastric junction and the other 7 to 8 cm proximal to it. They are approximated and secured to relieve tension on the esophageal suture line. The esophagus is transected between the clamps at the level of the diaphragm. The anterior three quarters of the muscularis is divided, and the mucosa is then divided circumferentially. This maneuver completely transects the veins in the mucosa and submucosa of the esophagus, leaving the posterior portion of the muscularis intact. Sugiura and Futagawa[10–12] feel this is extremely important, in order to preserve some of the esophageal blood supply. No bleeding occurs during the subsequent anastomosis because of the noncrushing clamps. The divided varices are not ligated.
(B) A continuous suture of 5–0 braided, polyglycolic (Dexon "S") is used to reapproximate the mucosa. This anastomosis was initially done with 70 to 90 interrupted sutures. Sugiura and Futagawa now use a continuous suture technique in the interest of conserving time. The bites are small in an effort to prevent recanalization of the esophageal veins.
(C) The mucosal anastomosis has been completed. Interrupted sutures are used to reinforce the anastomosis as indicated.
(D) The muscularis is then approximated with interrupted sutures of 4–0 monofilament silicone-treated polyester fiber (Ti-Cron). Meticulous hemostasis is obtained. A nasogastric tube is passed into the esophagus for postoperative suction and nutrition. The pleura is reapproximated over the anastomosis, and thoracotomy tubes are placed. They are removed as soon as the drainage has ceased, usually in 12 to 24 hours. The chest wall is closed in the usual fashion.

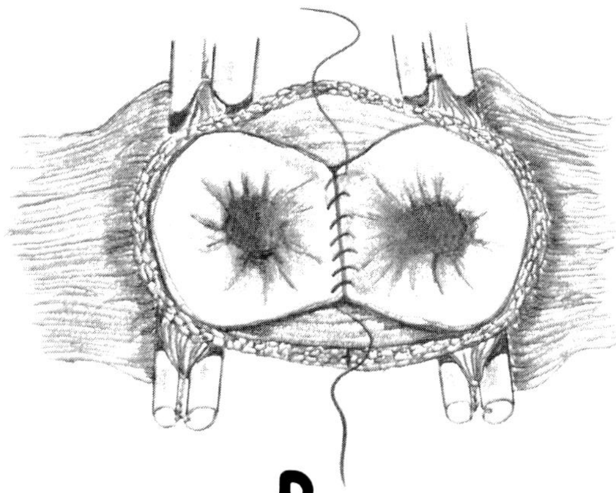

B

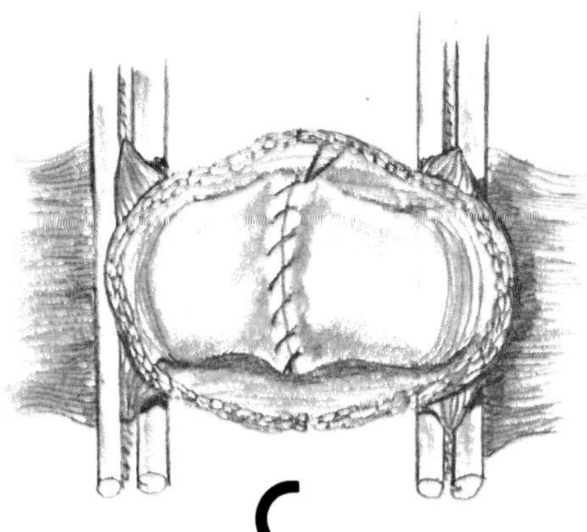

C

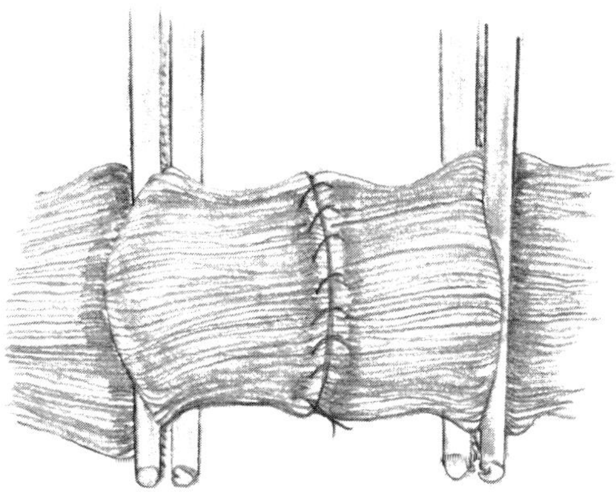

D

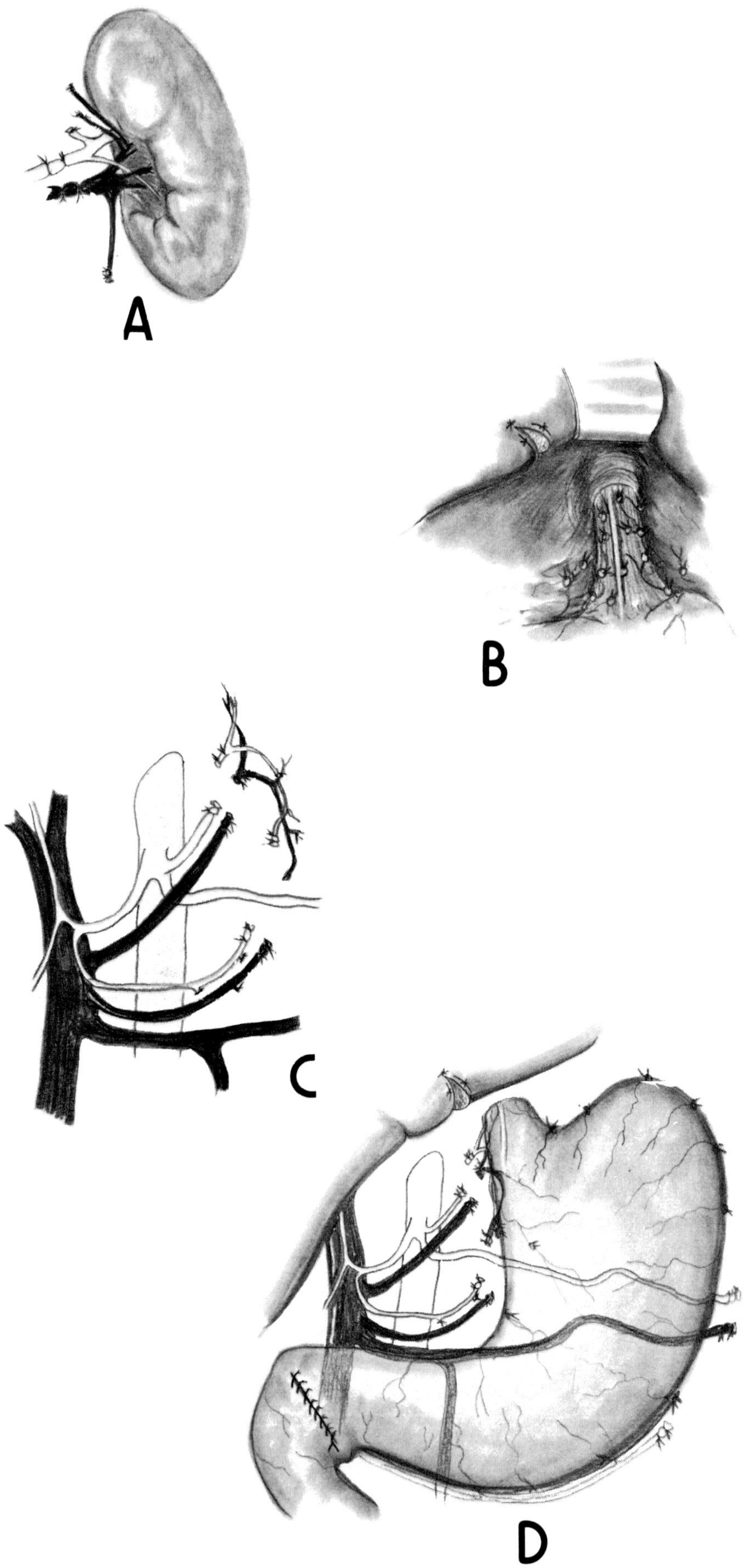

Fig. 4. The abdominal portion of the operation is usually delayed 4 to 6 weeks following the thoracic portion of the procedure. While Sugiura and Futagawa[10–12] employ a midline incision with extension to the left (trap door type), a long midline incision is perfectly adequate. It is very important to obtain a liver biopsy at this stage and portal manometrics and angiography as might be indicated.
(A) A splenectomy is performed. We frequently isolate and tie the splenic artery along the superior border of the pancreas prior to dissecting around the spleen, since bleeding can sometimes be quite troublesome. Cautery is used to divide the peritoneum. One has to be very careful, since the vessels in this area have a high venous pressure and there is frequently a coagulopathy. The extensive collateral circulation surrounding the capsule of the spleen may also add to the difficulty. These vessels will frequently require multiple ligatures or metallic clips. The short gastric vessels are clamped and divided and the stomach side transfixed. The stomach may become distended following the procedure and simple ties will be pushed off. Finally, the splenic artery and vein are isolated, clamped, divided, transfixed, and the spleen is removed.
(B) The stomach is pulled inferiorly exposing the esophagus and the paraesophageal structures. An extensive devascularization of this area is then carried out. Most of this tissue contains small vessels that need to be exposed and tied before being divided. The thoracic esophagus is pulled into the abdomen until the previous area of esophageal dissection is encountered. Due to the intimate association of the gastric vagus nerve, it is divided during this procedure. The dissection then continues inferiorly along the lesser and greater curvatures of the stomach.
(C) The vessels along the lesser curvature are meticulously identifed, dissected, tied, transfixed, divided, and a portion of them excised. This includes the coronary and left gastric vessels. The dissection is carried down to the junction of the proximal two thirds with the distal one third of the stomach. Devascularization is facilitated by division of the anterior gastric vagus nerves.
(D) On the greater curvature, the dissection is carried down to the junction of the upper two thirds and the lower one third of the stomach. Transfixion sutures, on the stomach side especially, should be used liberally since meticulous hemostasis is essential to this operation. A pyloroplasty is performed. No drains are required unless there is concern regarding damage to the pancreas at the time of splenectomy.

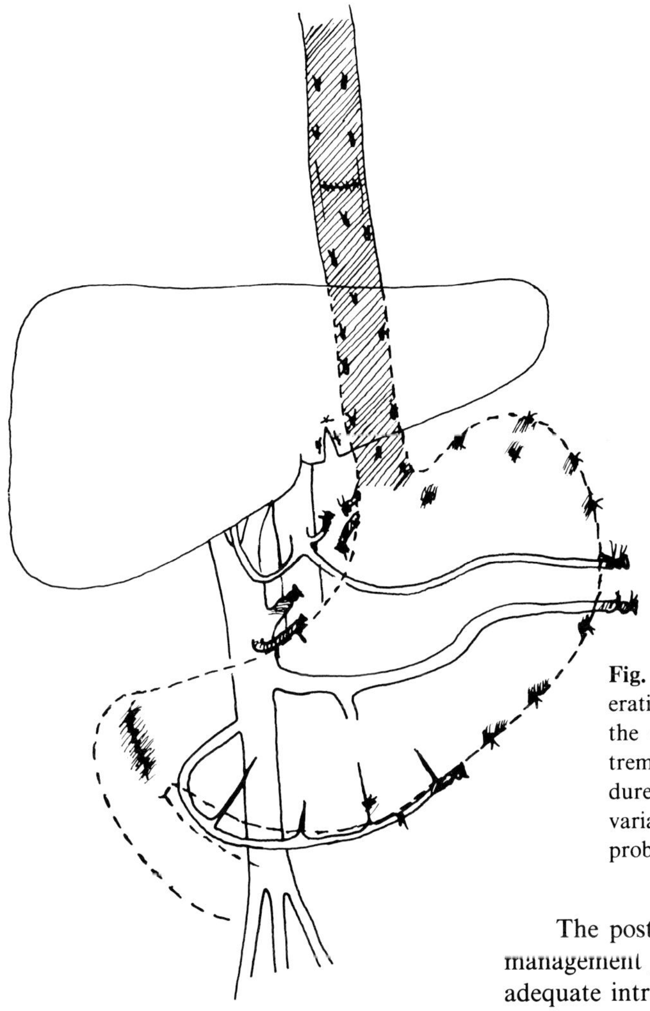

Fig. 5. This is a diagram of the completed operation. The anatomy of the venous drainage of the esophagogastric area, as elsewhere, is extremely variable. The devascularization procedure, however, is an en bloc dissection, and the variability of the blood supply should not be a problem.

The postoperative period following these procedures can present difficult management problems. Thus, there must be a careful balance in maintaining an adequate intravascular fluid volume without creating any more crystalloid excess than is required. The extensive dissection leads to a tendency to develop ascites, and fluid restriction within the confines of maintaining adequate hemodynamics is essential. While there are many methods of managing these patients, we depend considerably on monitoring the hemodynamics to include pulmonary wedge pressure, cardiac output, urine output, arterial blood pressure, central venous pressure, and body weight. Sugiura and Futagawa[10–12] recommend maintaining the red-cell volume as monitored by the hematocrit or hemoglobin at a normal range. We find that this frequently causes hypervolemia and do not feel it necessary for healing of the esophagus. Previously albumin was given frequently, but we have assiduously avoided this because of the cost and lack of confirming data that it is essential. Following the thoracic stage, the nasogastric tube is left in place for at least a week, following which a gastrografin swallow is obtained to document that there is no leak from the esophagus. The patient is given nutrition via the nasogastric tube as soon as gastrointestinal function has returned. The patient is then started slowly on oral feedings.

Following the abdominal part of the operation, the nasogastric tube is removed as soon as the patient has appropriate gastrointestinal function. Hyperalimentation is often used in Japan between the thoracic and abdominal portions of the operation to maintain adequate nutrition and keep the patient in nitrogen equilibrium for the second procedure.

This operation offers a method of surgical treatment of esophageal varices which does not cause encephalopathy or hepatic failure. Although the low operative mortality and incidence of rebleeding have not yet been duplicated in the United States, this approach deserves further consideration. It may be that modification and continued experience will result in improved results.

REFERENCES

1. Banti G: Anemia splenica. Arch Seula Anat Patol (Firenze) 2:53, 1883
2. Walker RM: Esophageal transection for bleeding varices. Surg Gynecol Obstet 118:323–329, 1964
3. Wirthlin LS, Linton RR, Ellis DS: Transthoracoesophageal ligation of bleeding esophageal varices; A reappraisal. Arch Surg 109:688, 1974
4. Cooperman A, Herman RE: Ligation procedures in the management of portal hypertension. Surgery 81:382–384, 1977
5. Hassab MA: Gastroesophageal decongestion and splenectomy in the treatment of esophageal varices in bilharzial cirrhosis: Further studies with the report on 355 operations. Surgery 61:169–176, 1967
6. Hassab MA: Nonshunt operations in portal hypertension without cirrhosis. Surg Gynecol Obstet 131:648, 1970
7. Peters RM, Womack NA: Surgery of vascular distortions in cirrhosis of the liver. Ann Surg 154:432, 1961
8. Johnson G Jr, Womack NA, Gabriele OF, Peters RM: Control of the hyperdynamic circulation in patients with bleeding esophageal varices. Ann Surg 169:661–671, 1979
9. Johnson G Jr: Nonshunt operations: Techniques and results, in Rutherford RB (ed): Vascular Surgery. Philadelphia, WB Saunders Co, 1977, pp 913–916
10. Sugiura M, Futagawa S: A new technique for treating esophageal varices. J Thorac Cardiovasc Surg 66:677, 1973
11. Sugiura M, Futagawa S: Further evaluation of the Sugiura procedure in the treatment of esophageal varices. Arch Surg 112:13–17, 1977
12. Futagawa S, Sugiura M, Hidat K, Shima F: Emergency esophageal transection with paraesophagogastric devascularization for variceal bleeding. World J Surg 3:229–234, 1979

Mesoatrial Shunt

John L. Cameron

Over the past decade, therapy for the Budd-Chiari syndrome has increasingly included portosystemic decompression. Because the hepatic veins are obstructed in this disease, sinusoid pressure is extremely high, resulting in pressure necrosis of hepatocytes. Long-term survival in the majority of patients with the Budd-Chiari syndrome is only possible if the portal vein is converted into an outflow tract by a portal systemic anastomosis.

Our preferred operative procedure for the Budd-Chiari syndrome is the mesocaval interposition graft. We feel it has an advantage over the side-to-side portocaval shunt in that marked hepatomegaly and caudate lobe hypertrophy are generally present. This makes access to the portal vein always difficult, and occasionally the construction of a side-to-side portocaval shunt is impossible. With the mesocaval interposition procedure, one works with the superior mesenteric vein and inferior vena cava below the transverse colon and transverse mesocolon, well away from the hypertrophied liver. If the superior mesenteric vein and the inferior vena cava are patent, the mesocaval shunt is always possible and usually easy. On occasion, however, the thrombotic process that involves the hepatic veins extends into the inferior vena cava and results in complete occlusion of this vessel. In other instances marked caudate lobe hypertrophy results in such compression to the inferior vena cava that it is functionally obstructed. In this subgroup of patients with the Budd-Chiari syndrome who have venous hypertension in their infradiaphragmatic vena cava, the usual portal-systemic decompression procedures are not applicable. In this situation the mesoatrial shunt can be performed. This allows one to decompress the liver via a shunt that connects the mesenteric venous system to the right atrium.

SURGICAL PROCEDURE

The patient is placed on the operating table in the supine position, and the abdomen and chest are prepped and draped appropriately. The abdomen is entered through a long midline incision. The transverse colon and transverse mesocolon are retracted in a cephalad direction, and the superior mesenteric vein is identified in the root of the transverse mesocolon. There are no good landmarks to identify the superior mesenteric vein in this location, and one must make a transverse incision in the peritoneum and dissect until the vein is identified. Once the superior mesenteric vein is identified, it is cleaned circumferentially on top of the duodenum and on top of the uncinate process of the pancreas to the point where it passes posterior to the neck of the pancreas (Fig. 1). The superior mesenteric vein is isolated in this proximal location, so that one is dealing with a vein of large caliber. Once the vein is isolated, a long (16-mm) Dacron graft is cut on the bevel and anastomosed end-to-side to the superior mesenteric vein with continuous 5–0 prolene. The superior mesenteric vein is totally occluded during the anastomosis with straight and acutely curved Cooley clamps. In cleaning this segment of superior mesenteric vein, any of the several large branches that enter this segment can be ligated and divided. The middle colic vein frequently has to be sacrificed because of its takeoff from the anterior portion of the superior mesenteric vein. An elipse of the anterior wall of the superior mesenteric vein should be removed prior to the anastomosis.

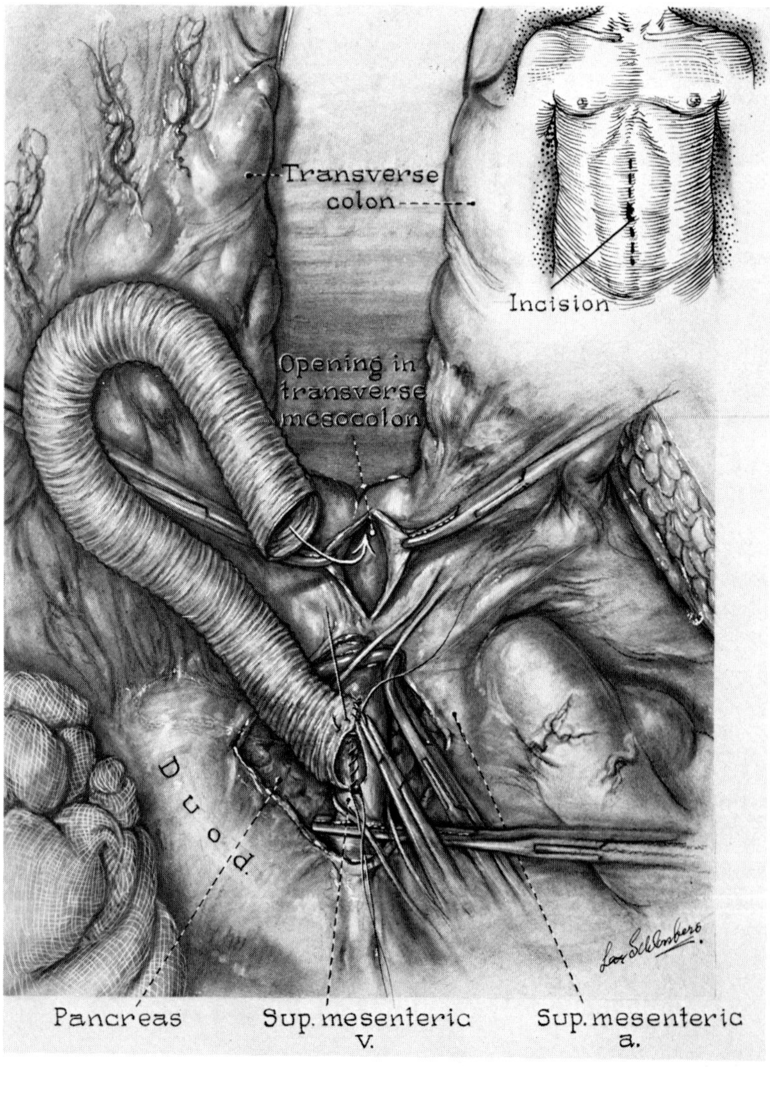

Fig. 1. A Dacron graft is anastomosed end-to-side to the superior mesenteric vein. The graft is then passed through the transverse mesocolon under the transverse colon. (Reprinted with permission.[1])

After the anastomosis has been completed, a DeBakey clamp is placed above the anastomosis, and the Cooley clamps are removed to be certain that the anastomosis is secure. The Cooley clamps are then replaced and the DeBakey is removed. The dacron graft is then tunneled through the root of the transverse mesocolon, through the greater omentum, and anterior to the body of the stomach (Fig. 2). The graft is then passed into the mediastinum directly beneath the xiphoid, after removing a small portion of the diaphragmatic insertion. During this portion of the procedure, a second team is performing a right-anterior thoracotomy. Once the right chest is opened, the right mediastinal pleura is divded and the Dacron graft pulled into the right pleural cavity. A portion of the right atrium is partially occluded with a Statinsky clamp, and after removing an elipse of artial wall an end-to-side anastomosis is performed using continuous 4–0 prolene (Fig. 3). Once the anastomosis is completed, the Statinsky clamp is removed from the atrium and the graft is allowed to fill retrograde back to the superior mesenteric vein anastomosis. It is not necessary to preclot the 16-mm knitted Dacron graft used for this procedure because of the low pressure system to which it is anastomosed. The graft fills quickly and most of the air bleeds out through the pores of the graft. Trapped air can be looked for by inserting a 19-gauge needle at several locations along the graft. The Cooley clamps are then removed from the superior mesenteric vein and antegrade flow is initiated from the mesenteric venous system through the long Dacron graft into the right atrium.

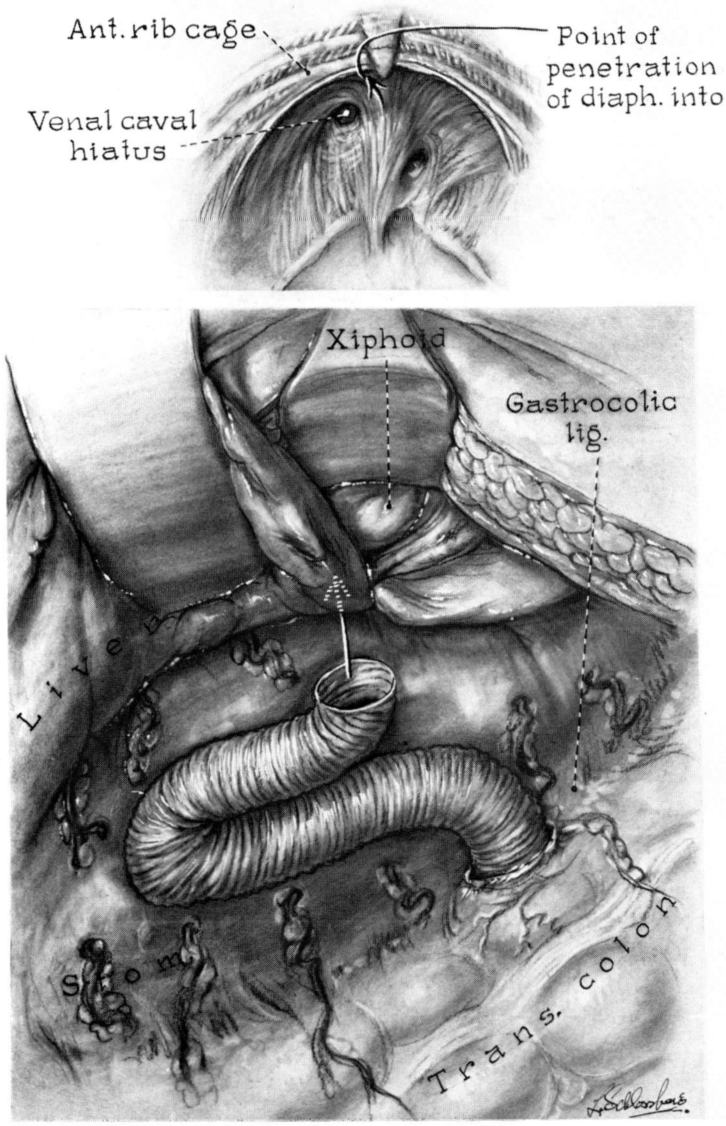

Fig. 2. The graft passes posterior to the transverse colon and anterior to the stomach before entering the anterior mediastinum under the xiphoid. (Reprinted with permission.[1])

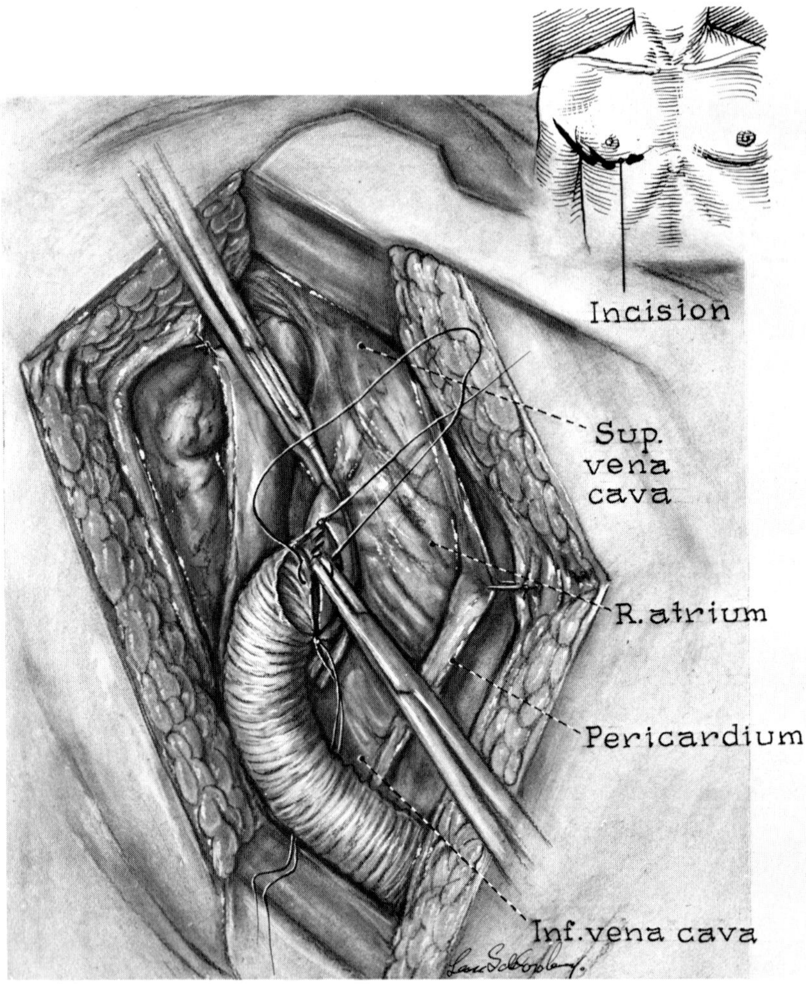

Fig. 3. The graft enters the right pleural cavity from the anterior mediastinum and is anastomosed end-to-side to the right atrium. (Reprinted with permission.[1])

Prior experience with the mesocaval shunt has demonstrated that a Dacron graft placed in the venous system can maintain long-term patency when anastomosed between the high-pressure portal system and the low-pressure systemic venous circulation. The 16-mm Dacron graft used in the mesoatrial shunt is longer than that used in the mesocaval shunt and is also of somewhat smaller caliber. However, since the long graft passes from the positive pressure of the peritoneal cavity up through the mediastinum into the negative pressure pleural cavity, flow through the graft should be enhanced by the significant pressure gradient.

We have one patient who, 3½ years after construction of a mesoatrial shunt, remains asymptomatic and has angiographic demonstrated shunt patency.

REFERENCE

1. Cameron JL, Maddrey WC: Mesoatrial shunt: A new treatment for the Budd-Chiari syndrome. Ann Surg 187:402, 1978

DIRECT VENOUS RECONSTRUCTIVE SURGERY

Venous Reconstructive Surgery

W. Andrew Dale

Reconstruction of large and medium-sized veins has lagged considerably behind arterial repair, for several reasons. First, it is difficult to maintain patency of any type graft placed into the low-pressure venous system. Second, operation is usually unnecessary because veins obstructed by thrombosis generally recanalize spontaneously. While no actual data are available, it is suspected that only 1 to 2 percent of deep venous thromboses remain occluded and thus become candidates for reconstruction. The final reason for this lag is the failure to identify suitable candidates by phlebography and to recognize the possibilities for bypasses.

Our interest in these problems in the 1960s led to considerable experience with the experimental animals indicating that properly placed grafts would remain open in the venous system.[1–3] Clinical experience has accumulated slowly since then, but our approximate 75 percent success rate[4] has been confirmed by others,[5,6] and at present there is little doubt that venous reconstruction is useful for properly selected patients.

Details of etiology, diagnosis, and nonoperative management have been discussed previously and are specifically omitted from this presentation. The operations themselves are not extremely difficult and, even if they fail, are not expected to produce a high complication rate nor make the overall limb situation worse.

CROSSOVER SAPHENOUS-TO-FEMORAL-VEIN GRAFT

Complete phlebography is essential to selection of a site for anastomosis and is performed preoperatively along with ambulatory venous pressure studies.[7]

The initial portion of the operation consists of dissection of the common femoral or superficial femoral vein on the affected side (Fig. 1). This dissection passes through edematous tissue in which a good many venous collaterals lie. These are preserved where possible and carefully tied with absorbable suture material (3–0 Dexon) when necessary. The femoral vein lying just medial to the artery may be encased in a fibrotic fascial sheath, and its walls are often thickened. The lumen may contain postphlebitic webs and bands. If the proximal portion of the femoral system in the groin is not patent by phlebogram, a more distal site in the midthigh should be selected. Occasionally the only patent vein is the saphenous; it may be used for the anastomosis.

The involved side is dissected first, in order that oozing from the wound may subside completely while the saphenous vein is being dissected from the other side and prior to intraoperative heparinization.

The saphenous vein is dissected for whatever length is necessary to provide a long crossover bypass graft. Branches are tied with 4–0 silk and the vein is gently distended with heparinized saline, while its proximal end in the groin is occluded with a delicate serrefine clamp. The anterior aspect of the vein is marked to prevent twisting or angulation during the remainder of the procedure. A suprapubic tunnel is developed in the subcutaneous tissue by blunt dissection and the vein graft pulled through this.

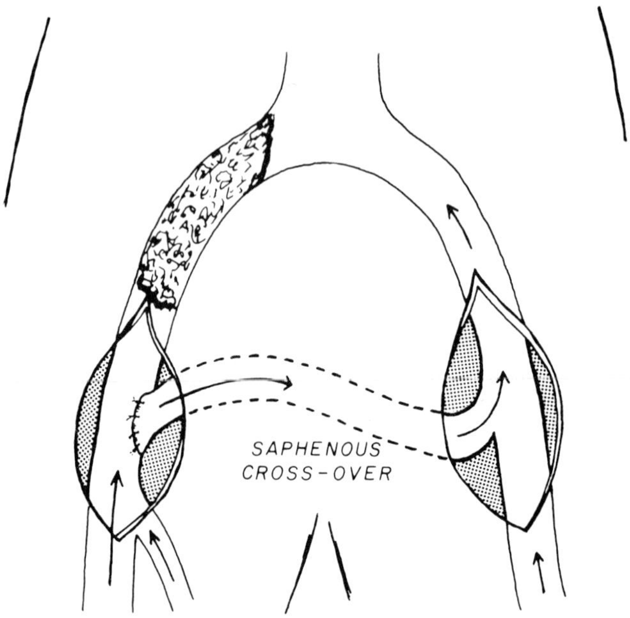

Fig. 1. The saphenous crossover vein graft provides a bypass from the obstructed venous system across the suprapubic area to the patent contralateral vein (with permission from Archives of Surgery[4]).

A special U-shaped venous clamp (Codman & Shurtleff Inc, Randolph, Mass) (Fig. 2) is used to occlude the femoral vein during the anastomosis, so that an extensive dissection of a long segment of that vein is not necessary. The crossed-over saphenous vein is anatomosed as an onlay to the selected site in the femoral vein using continuous 6–0 prolene. The anastomosis should be approximately three times the diameter of the femoral vein.

Systemic heparinization (100 units/kg) is provided throughout the procedure before the occluding venous clamp is placed. It is not necessary to reverse this, since venous anastomoses do not bleed as do arterial ones. It should also be remarked that, while blood immediately flows up into the venous crossover graft, the vein does not become distended as does an arterial bypass. This may be disappointing to the operator who is expecting a much more dramatic filling.

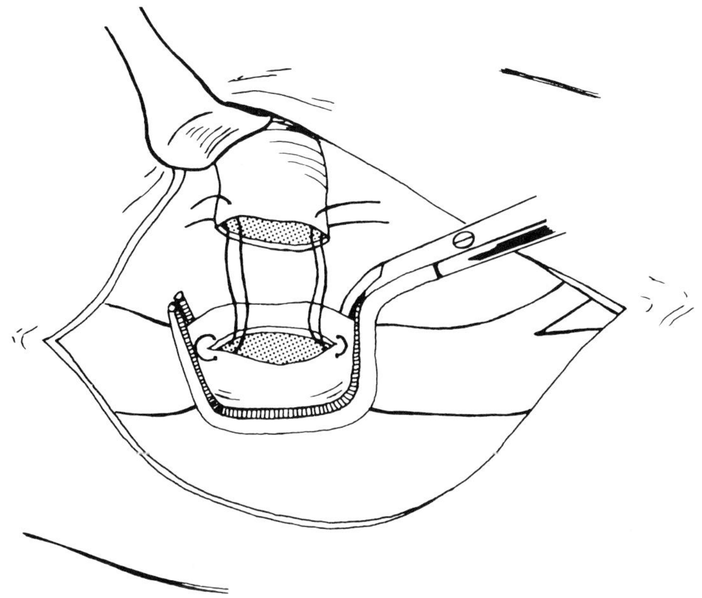

Fig. 2. The U-shaped clamp allows isolation of the common femoral artery during the anastomosis without the necessity to completely dissect around it and consequent danger to the veins that enter from the posterior aspect (not shown here) (with permission from Archives of Surgery[4]).

Wounds are closed with continuous 3–0 Dexon in the subcutaneous tissue and skin with removable clips or interrupted Dacron sutures.

The postoperative dressing consists of Ace bandages wrapped firmly from toes to the proximal thigh over absorbent cotton to provide some degree of pressure during the postoperative period. The foot of the bed is elevated and the patient is asked either to lie with the legs elevated or to walk, but to avoid sitting or prolonged standing during the first 7 to 10 postoperative days. A thigh-length stocking is therafter fitted and used for at least one year postoperatively to encourage venous flow out of the extremity.

The procedure requires 1½ to 2 hours and is easily done under spinal anesthesia. We have experienced no mortality and only an occasional complication or seroma or hematoma, which should be prevented by proper intraoperative hemostasis and the use of a suction drain for 24 to 48 hours if there is any evidence of continued ooze as the wound is being closed. Figure 3 shows a successful crossover graft postoperatively.

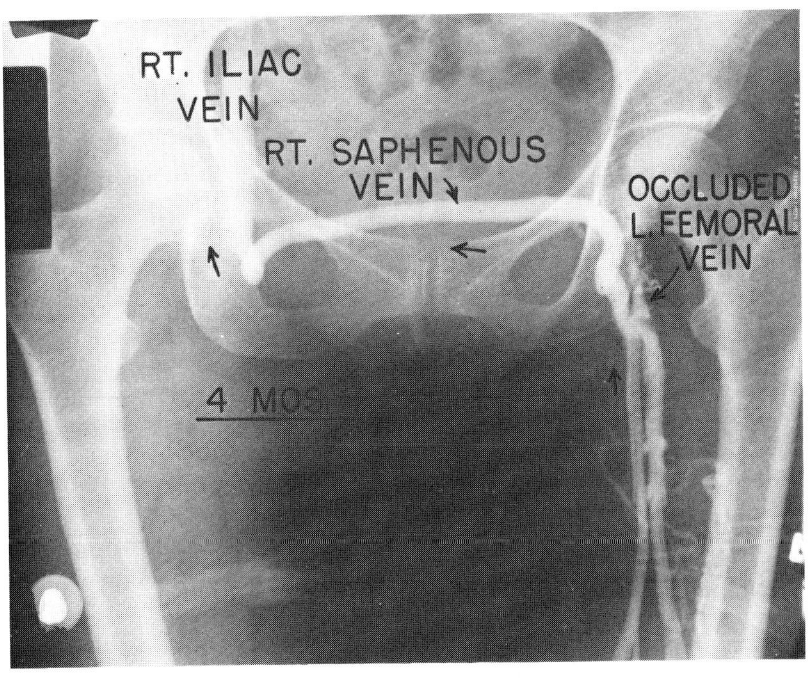

Fig. 3. A patent crossover vein graft 4 months after placement (with permission from Archives of Surgery[4]).

SAPHENOUS BYPASS OF THE OCCLUDED SUPERFICIAL FEMORAL VEIN

The superficial femoral vein is a common site of continued venous occlusion after deep venous thrombosis. If this is persistent and symptomatic, a bypass may be constructed using the ipsilateral saphenous vein (Fig. 4). Comprehensive preliminary phlebography will provide information regarding the obstructed as well as patent areas.

The ipsilateral saphenous vein is dissected as it lies along the medial aspect of the proximal calf, and enough branches are divided between 4–0 silk ligatures to allow the distal end to be swung into the deeper tissues to be anastomosed to the underlying popliteal vein below the knee joint. Alternatively, the saphenous vein may not be divided but simply anastomosed side-to-side; however, this requires dissection of a longer length of saphenous vein. It is not yet known whether this is better than the end-to-side anastomosis shown in Figure 4.

The popliteal vein below the knee is easily accessible through the same medial calf approach used for the distal end of a femoropopliteal arterial anastomosis. After the fascia is opened, the gastrocnemius muscle may be dropped away posteriorly, and the artery and vein are found lying in an easily opened tissue plane. The vein is dissected sufficiently to allow the special U-clamp to be placed.

The saphenous vein is carefully oriented to prevent twisting and is anastomosed to the side of the popliteal vein with continuous 6–0 prolene.

The tissues are closed with continuous Dexon in the subcutaneous fat and either skin clips or 4–0 Dacron. An Ace bandage dressing from toes to groin is placed to cover the wound and also to partially immobilize the knee, although early ambulation is encouraged.

This operation may be combined with a proximal crossover saphenous-to-femoral-vein graft when that is also indicated. The saphenofemoral anastomosis alone requires about an hour. Spinal anesthesia is particularly suitable. Postoperatively the pressure dressings are continued and the foot of the bed is elevated for 7–10 days, but the patient is also encouraged to walk about freely and may be discharged from the hospital at an early time (Fig. 5).

BRACHIAL TO JUGULAR BYPASS FOR SUBCLAVIAN AND AXILLARY VENOUS OCCLUSION

Occasional incidences of occlusion of the axillary and/or subclavian veins result from indwelling catheters, from injuries, and as acute manifestations of the shoulder-girdle compression (thoracic-outlet) syndrome. Most of these venous occlusions progress to spontaneous recanalization, but occasional ones persist, producing pain and swelling in the upper extremity, which may be correctible by a venous shunt.

Complete phlebography of both of the upper extremities will outline the area of venous occlusion. Injection of the contrast material into the cephalad aspect of the external jugular vein will demonstrate its relationship to the overall collateralization and allow prediction as to whether or not it is suitable terminus for the bypass. Its use is particularly appealing because it is quite superficial and the dissection is easy.

A patent portion of the brachial vein in the upper arm is selected and approached by a medially placed incision (Fig. 6). The neurovascular bundle is exposed just posterior to the biceps and the vein teased away from the adjacent nerves and the brachial artery.

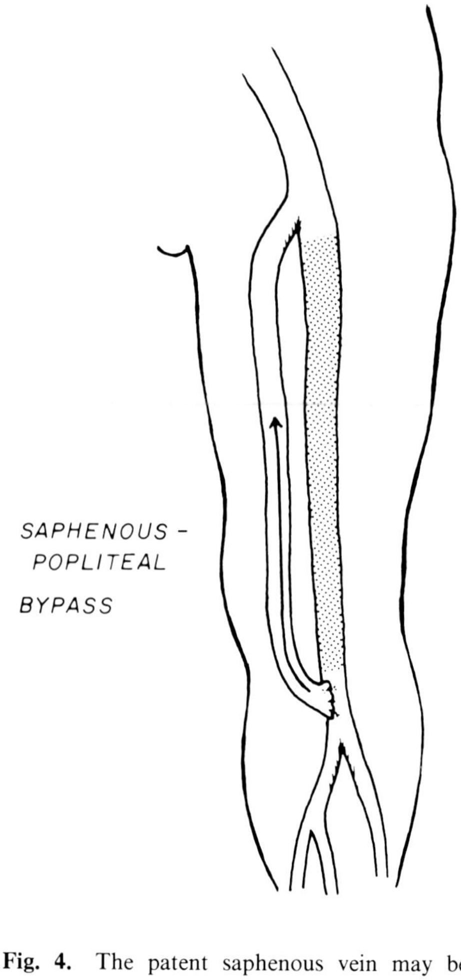

Fig. 4. The patent saphenous vein may be transplanted to the patent popliteal vein to bypass an occluded segment of superficial femoral vein (with permission from Archives of Surgery[4]).

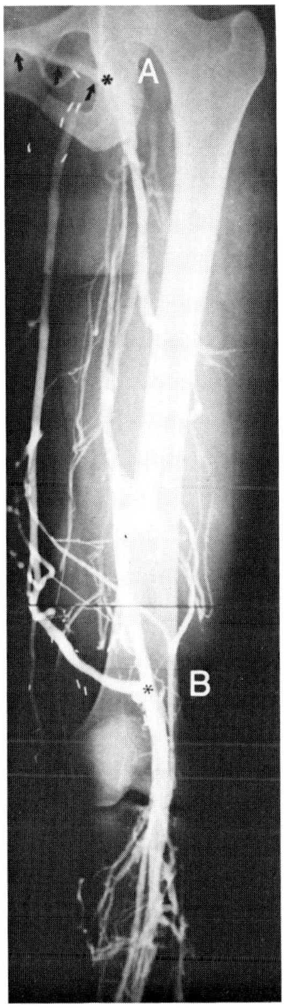

Fig. 5. (A) The site of anastomosis of the saphenous vein to the popliteal vein to bypass the occluded superficial femoral vein.
(B) The beginning of the crossover vein graft to transfer blood around the proximally occluded external iliac vein (with permission from Archives of Surgery[4]).

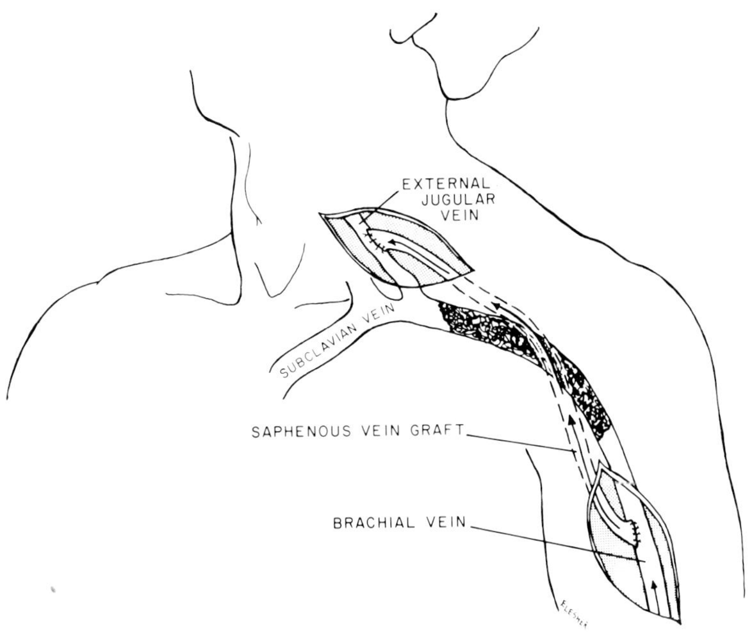

Fig. 6. A free saphenous vein graft is used to carry blood between the patent brachial and external jugular veins to bypass the subclavian and/or axillary venous occlusion.

A saphenous vein graft is removed from the groin, all branches are tied with 4–0 silk, and it is gently distended with heparinized Ringer's solution. After reversal of the graft to point the valves correctly, the originally distal end is anastomosed to the side of the brachial vein using continuous 6–0 prolene. The anastomosis should be approximately three times the diameter of the brachial vein. If webs and intraluminal adhesions are discovered within the vein, these should be trimmed out prior to placement of the anastomosis.

The saphenous vein is then oriented longitudinally and tunneled to the neck in the subcutanous tissue overlying the upper arm and clavicle. The originally proximal end of the saphenous vein may then easily be anastomosed as an onlay to the external jugular vein in the neck, again using continuous 6–0 prolene.

This procedure is an easy one and, should it fail, is not expected to worsen the overall situation. The key to the entire operation is comprehensive preoperative phlebography to localize proper sites for the anastomoses.

BYPASS OF INFERIOR VENA CAVA TO FEMORAL VEIN BY ARM VEIN

The completely occluded inferior vena cava with attendant ambulatory venous hypertension of the lower extremities usually causes severe disability due to edema, pain, varicose veins, and the other sequelae of long continued ambulatory venous hypertension of the lower extremities.

Attempts to replace the inferior vena cava directly by an intra-abdominal procedure have to date usually failed, with the exception of occasional replacements for trauma or venous resections accompanying tumor dissection. These no doubt represent special circumstances where the replacement graft is relatively short, whereas the graft necessary for the postphlebitic syndrome would be expected to course for the long distance between the femoral system in the groin and the more proximal reaches of the inferior vena cava near the renal vein.

In an effort to provide a feasible alternative, we have dissected a vein out of the soft tissues of the upper extremity, tunneled it inferiorly in the subcutaneous tissue of the chest and abdominal wall, and made an anastomosis to the femoral vein in the groin.

This long bypass is certainly not proven at present. Three patients have agreed to the procedure with full understanding that we lack information regarding long-term results. In the first individual, previous phlebitis in the arm veins necessitated several resections and anastomoses, which may have contributed to complete failure of the bypass. In the second attempt the vein in the arm proved to be entirely too small, and the procedure was abandoned without setting up a bypass. The third effort was successfully completed and the patient made an uneventful recovery. At time of writing, the postoperative phlebogram has not been obtained. If successful for several months, a second stage for the other side is planned.

The arm-to-groin venous bypass is presently a nonestablished operation that may be considered because of its relative simplicity and lack of overall risks but whose long-term outlook is not known.

ILIAC VENOTOMY FOR VEIN COMPRESSION

Occasionally the aorta and the right iliac artery compress the underlying left common iliac vein, with resultant fibrosis and/or venous thrombosis (Fig. 7).[8–10] Our experience with eight cases and review of the literature indicate that some of these are severe enough in terms of edema and discomfort to warrant operation. Two different procedures may be useful. A crossover saphenofemoral vein graft can be used to shunt blood around the compressed iliac vein. More recently, we have come to believe that a direct attack by transabdominal venotomy is preferable (Fig. 8).

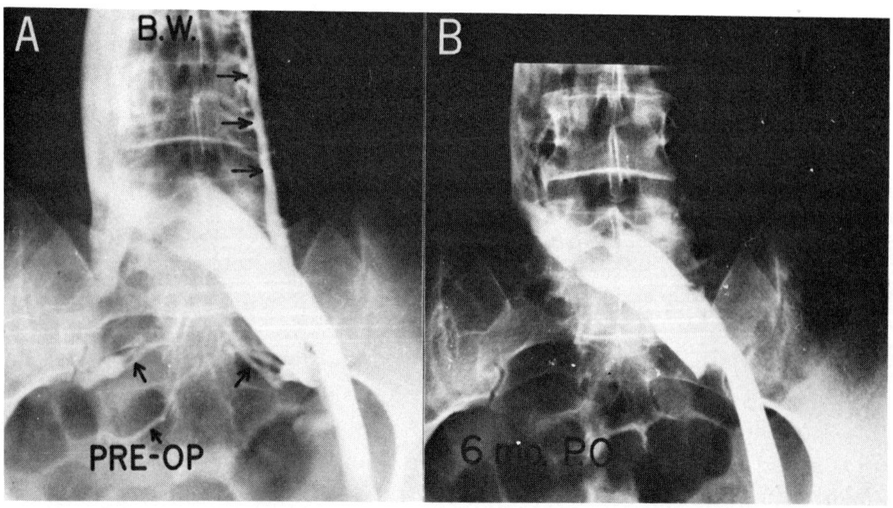

Fig. 7. (A) Stenosis of the left common iliac vein by the crossing right iliac artery is demonstrated in the preoperative phlebogram. The large collaterals are emphasized by the arrows. (B) Six months postoperatively, following venotomy and anterior patch graft, the vein is widely patent and the collaterals have disappeared.

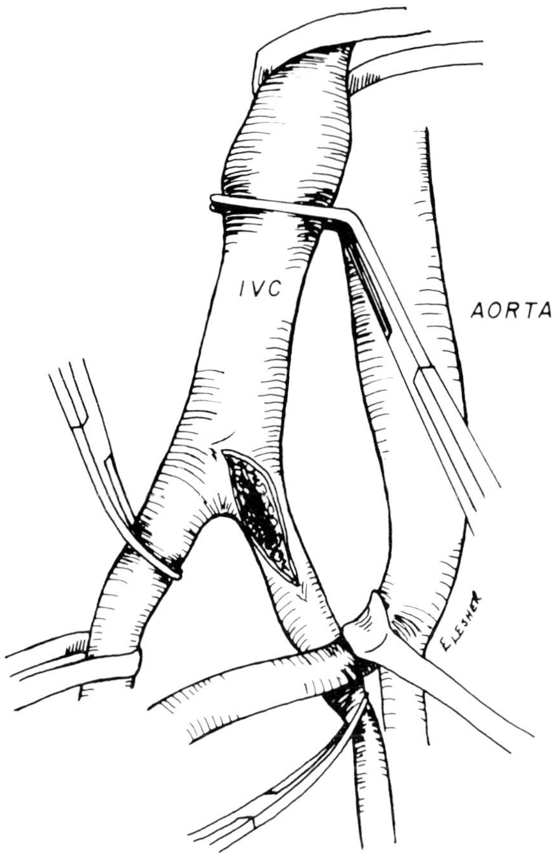

Fig. 8. Through a laparotomy incision, the aortic bifurcation and iliac arteries are elevated up off the underlying left common iliac vein. An anterior venotomy allows intraluminal dissection of any webs found within. The venotomy may be closed with a venous patch graft (often conveniently removed from the dorsum of the hand or wrist).

After appropriate phlebologic localization to indicate compression of the left common iliac vein with collateralization carrying blood around this segment, a laparotomy is performed through a midline incision centered on the vena caval confluence located at the level of the umbilicus. The intestines are temporarily eviscerated, and the retroperitoneal space is entered. The aorta and common iliac artery are carefully dissected so that they may be elevated up off the underlying iliac veins. After systemic heparinization, the vascular clamps are placed. An opening is made on the anterior surface of the vein to allow internal webs and strictures to be removed. The venotomy is then closed with a venous patch graft using continuous 6–0 prolene. Since only a short segment of vein is needed, it is taken from the dorsum of the hand or forearm rather than disturbing the saphenous vein in the groin (since the latter might be needed later for some other procedure).

The remaining problem is whether to allow the elevated iliac artery simply to lie back on top of the vein and perhaps recreate the original problem, whether to elongate it by interpolating a short segment of synthetic graft, or whether to elevate it permanently over a silastic bridge.[11] In our experience with four cases, neither the silastic bridge nor elongation by placement of a graft has been used. From a theoretic standpoint, we prefer elongation rather than placement of any firm material in direct contact with an artery, where it might provoke erosion and bleeding.

No one yet has any large experience with this problem. As experience accumulates, further changes in the operative indications and the indicated procedure may occur.

Our experience with reconstructions of major veins is shown in Table 1. There were no deaths, and complications were uncommon. Particularly notable is the low rate of deep vein thrombosis (4 of 65 patients). These operations are helpful to selected patients.

Table 1
Peripheral Venous Reconstructions*

Type of Reconstruction	No.	Excellent	Partial	Failure
Saphenous to iliac or femoral crossover graft	50	30	9	11
Saphenous to popliteal anastomosis	6	3	—	3
Brachial to jugular	2	2	—	0
Brachial to femoral transplant	3	1	—	2
Iliac venotomy and patch graft	4	3	0	1
Total	65	39	9	17

* SVC, IVC and portal reconstructions are omitted.

REFERENCES

1. Dale WA, Scott HW: Grafts of the venous system. Surgery 53:52, 1963
2. Dale WA: Thrombosis and recanalization of veins used as venous grafts. Angiology 12:603, 1961
3. Dale WA, Harris J: Cross-over vein grafts for iliac and femoral venous occlusion. Ann Surg 168:319, 1968
4. Dale WA: Reconstructive venous surgery. Arch Surg 114:1312, 1979
5. Husni EA: Clinical experience with femoro-popliteal reconstruction, in Bergan JJ, Yao JST (eds): Venous Problems. Chicago, Year Book Publishers, 1978, pp 485–491
6. Smith DE, Trimble C: Surgical management of obstructive venous disease of the lower extremity, in Rutherford RB (ed): Vascular Surgery. Philadelphia, WB Saunders Co, 1977, pp 1247–1268
7. Lewis MR, Dale WA: Phlebography as a clinical tool. Surg Gynecol Obstet, 133:301, 1971
8. McMurrich JP: The occurence of congenital adhesions in the common iliac veins and their relation to thrombosis of the femoral and iliac veins. Am J Med Sci 135:342, 1908
9. Cockett FB, Thomas ML: The iliac compression syndrome. Br J Surg 52:816, 1965
10. Rigas A, Vomvoyannis A, Tsardakas E: Iliac compression syndrome. J Cardiovasc Surg 11:389, 1970
11. Trimble C, Bernstein E, Pomerantz M, Eiseman B: A prosthetic bridging device to relieve iliac venous compression. Surg Forum 23:249, 1972

Technique of Surgical Reconstruction of Femoral Vein Valves

Robert L. Kistner, Eugene B. Ferris

The purpose of reconstructive surgery in the femoral venous system is to restore competence to veins rendered incompetent either by primary valve disease or by previous phlebitis.[1,2] The important principle is to provide at least one competent valve for the major venous pathway of the extremity. Depending upon circumstances, the major venous pathway in any given instance could be the superficial femoral vein, the greater saphenous vein, the profunda femoris vein, or any combination of these. The patient who is a candidate for this type of surgery should have severe symptoms of venous insufficiency, including severe aching, incapacitating swelling, advanced stasis changes, or recurrent ankle ulceration. These symptoms may occur singly or in combination. When, with accurate diagnostic means, the patient with these symptoms is found to have major incompetent venous segments, the restoration of competence to as many segments as possible will usually be sufficient to restore the leg to a compensated state of venous drainage.

Diagnostic maneuvers must include ascending and descending venography. On the basis of these studies, the patency and competence of the superficial femoral, profunda femoris, and greater saphenous veins will be determined. Whether the problem originates from postphlebitic veins or from primary valve incompetence will also be determined.

The operative approach is planned only after the anatomic and functional status of the patient has been studied thoroughly. In the patient who has primary valve incompetence in a single system (usually the superficial femoral system), the choice of operative approach can be either primary valve repair or vein segment transposition. In the patient whose incompetent segment is due to the postphlebitic state, the operation will usually be vein segment transposition because the valves in the involved vein segment will have been destroyed. An operation combining valve repair and vein segment transfer is also possible.

VALVE REPAIR SURGERY

Valve repair is performed through a long longitudinal incision over the femoral vein (Fig. 1). The femoral vein is exposed from the level of the saphenofemoral junction superiorly down to the junction of the upper and middle thirds of the superficial femoral vein at the midthigh. This long exposure has been necessary to identify the valves that are present and to provide adequate exposure for the venotomy. The preoperative descending venogram will be the basic guide as to which valve will be repaired. The valve we have usually chosen for repair has been the highest valve in the superficial femoral vein, but there have been instances when the second valve in the superficial femoral vein was a better valve for repair.

When the venous segment is exposed, the adventitia is carefully cleaned and the vein is closely inspected until the outline of the valve cusp insertion is found through the intact vein wall. This insertion appears as a white line around the circumference of the vein; it has a semilunar shape with the convexity directed downward. In some patients, the sinus of the valve is very prominent and it is easy to find the valve; in others, the sinus is difficult to see and great care must be taken to find the precise line of insertion of the valve cusp.

When the valve cusp insertion is found, it can be traced around to the commissure where the two cusps of the bicuspid valve meet. A 6–0 marking suture is placed through the intact vein wall precisely at the apex of the commissure (Fig. 1a). This is a critical point, because the marking suture will guide the line of the venotomy incision. If a mistake is made in the placement of this suture, the venotomy will transect the cusp in the midportion of its insertion and will destroy any opportunity to repair the valve. The location of the commissure is usually in an eccentric position on the circumference of the vein and is not located in a direct anterior-posterior orientation.

Using the marking suture as a guide, a point is chosen inferior to the valve on a direct line leading up to the commissure. The initial venotomy is performed inferior to the valve, and the vein is emptied of blood (Fig. 1b). Traction sutures are placed on each wall of the vein. The blood is carefully drained out of the valve cusps so that they lie flattened against the side wall of the vein, to avoid injury to the cusps during venotomy. With the sides of the vein held open by traction sutures, the incision is carried directly up to the marking suture at the apex, actually cutting the suture and then extending the incision into the common femoral vein. At this point, two more traction sutures are placed in the lateral walls of the vein above the level of the valve. The completed venotomy needs to be 6 to 8 cm long, allowing 3 to 4 cm both above and below the valve to provide clear exposure for repair.

When the vein is laid open in this fashion, the valve cusps can be carefully inspected. The morphologic finding in primary valve incompetence is an elongated or stretched valve cusp, which can be seen lying in vertical folds across the face of the vein (Fig. 1c). On initial inspection, the valve cusp may appear normal, because it is a gossamer-thin membrane that shows no sign of previous inflammation or disease. However, inspection of the leading edge of the valve cusp reveals these vertical folds, which represent stretching of the cusp. When the cusp is filled with blood, the stretched cusp permits prolapse of the leading edge, thereby producing an incompetent valve.

Fig. 1. Valve repair is performed through a long longitudinal incision over the femoral vein.
(a) A marking suture is placed through the intact vein wall precisely at the apex of the commissure.
(b) The initial venotomy is performed inferior to the valve, and the vein is emptied of blood.
(c) Vein laid open showing valve cusps with vertical folds.

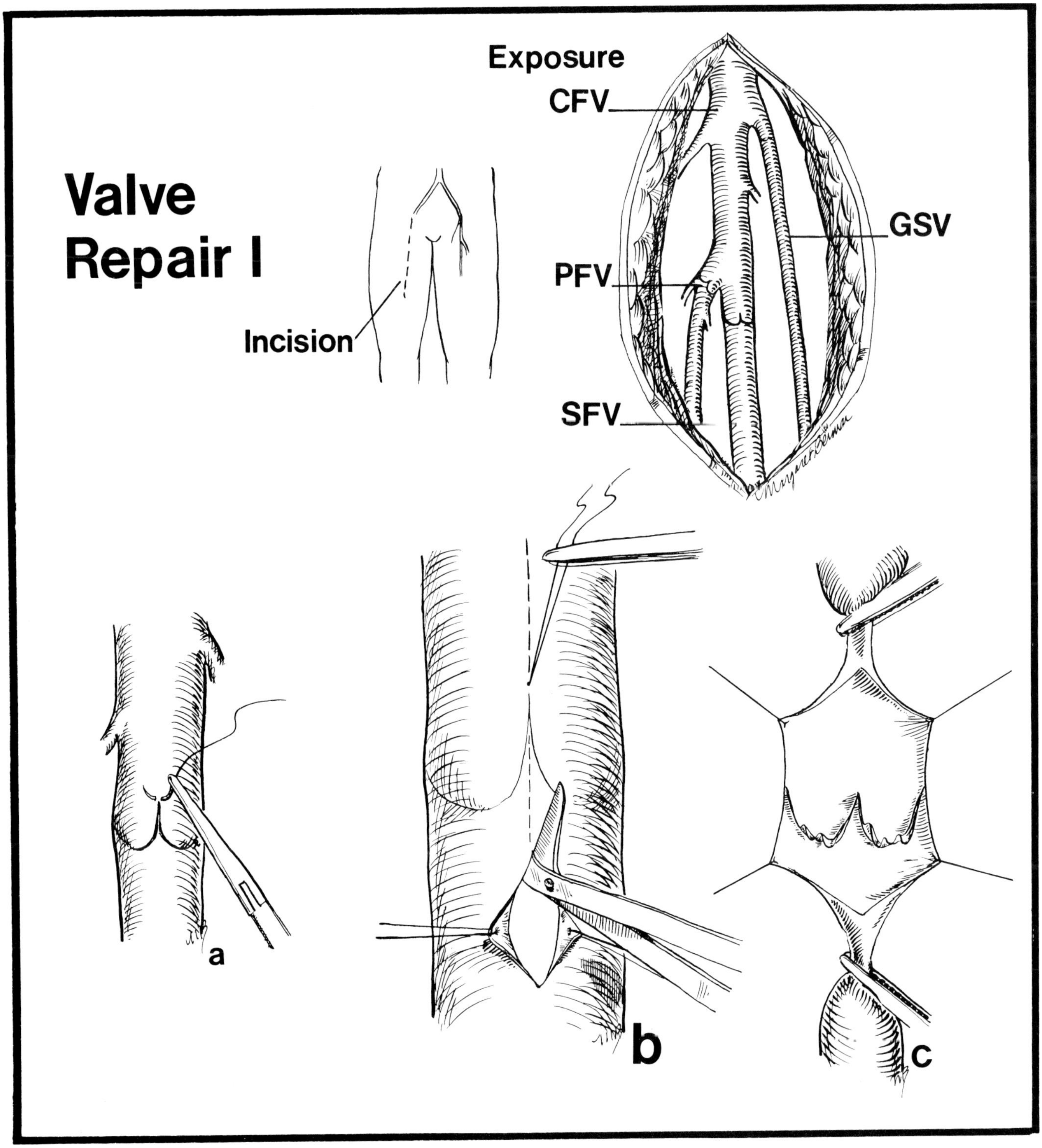
Valve
Repair I
Incision
Exposure
CFV
GSV
PFV
SFV
a
b
c

Repair of the valve consists of placement of multiple interrupted sutures of 7–0 monofilament, each suture being placed so as to serially shorten the leading edge of the valve cusp (Fig. 2). Loupe magnification is used (3.5×). Each suture is introduced from the outside of the vein wall at the level of the apex of a commissure to the inside of the vein (Fig. 2a).

The next step is to draw the leading edge of the valve cusp up to the commissure so as to shorten the edge by 1 or 2 mm and then pass the needle through the edge of the valve cusp and out through the vein wall from inside the vein to the outside (Fig. 2b). This is done at the same level where the suture had been introduced originally into the vein.

With the two ends of the suture on the outside of the vein wall, this suture is tied down so as to form a single interrupted suture, which shortens the leading edge of the valve cusp by 1 to 2 mm (Fig. 2c). The rest of the repair is a repetition of this process of placing interrupted sutures. They may be placed at any commissure point, that is, on either lateral wall of the venotomy where one of the cusps can be shortened, or on the posterior wall where the two cusps meet and both cusps can be shortened with a single interrupted suture (Fig. 2c). Multiple sutures may be placed at a single commissure. Repeated sutures are placed until the leading edge of the valve cusp has been shortened sufficiently to allow it to lie across the face of the vein in a gentle arc (Fig. 2d). The decision as to when the valve cusp has been sufficiently shortened is made by observing that all of the vertical folds have been removed from the valve. If shortened too much, the edge will be taut like a bowstring, and if too little, it will be lax with persisting vertical folds.

When the two cusps have been adequately shortened, the venotomy is carefully closed. The initial suture is placed at the level of the commissure so as to exactly coapt the commissure on either side of the venotomy (Fig. 2e).

The vein is closed with 7–0 monofilament suture carefully placed to avoid deforming the valve cusp. If the upper half of the venotomy is closed first, the competence of the valve can be checked by simply opening the proximal venous segment and observing the valve as it fills with blood (Fig. 2f). If the repair has been ideal, the cusp will fill with blood and there will be no reflux. When the venotomy is completely closed, the valve is inspected again for leakage. This is done by clamping the vein distally and then milking the blood through the valve. In a valve that has had an ideal repair, it will not be possible to force blood back through the valve even with vigorous proximal milking maneuvers that exert pressure of the distending blood on the valve from above (Fig. 2, bottom). In our experience it has not always been possible to obtain a perfectly functioning valve, and there have been times when we have accepted a slight leakage of the valve following repair. If gross leakage of the valve persists, it is necessary to reopen the venotomy and improve the repair or choose another valve for repair. If there is no other valve for repair and a poor repair has been obtained, the next choice would be to abandon the procedure of valve repair and perform a vein segment transposition. In our experience, it has been possible to obtain an adequate repair of the valve structure in more than 80 percent of the cases in which the pathology was one of primary valve incompetence.

The wound is closed with interrupted sutures for the fascia and subcutaneous tissue and running subcuticular for the skin. All valve repairs have been performed with the patient under intravenous heparinization. Our practice has been to maintain the patient on intravenous heparin during the early postoperative period. Continuous heparin has been used in a dose sufficient to alter the activated partial thromboplastin time enough to show a definite heparin effect. We do not use high doses of heparin because our major postoperative morbidity has been due to wound hematomas (approximately 30 percent). There have been no instances of postoperative venous thrombosis of a repaired segment, as proven by ascending and descending venography on all valve repair patients.

Fig. 2. Valve repair consists of placement of multiple interrupted sutures, each being placed so as to serially shorten the leading edge of the valve cusp.
(a) Each suture is introduced from the outside of the vein wall at the level of the apex of a commissure to the inside of the vein.
(b) The needle is passed through the edge of the valve cusp and out through the vein wall from inside to outside.
(c) The suture is tied down to form a single interrupted suture.
(d) Repeated sutures are placed until the leading edge of the valve cusp has been shortened sufficiently to allow it to lie across the face of the vein in a gentle arc.
(e) The venotomy is closed. The initial suture is placed at the level of the commissure so as to exactly coapt the commissure on either side of the venotomy.
(f) Closure of venotomy.
Lower Panel: Milking maneuvers to determine competence of valve.

Valve Repair II

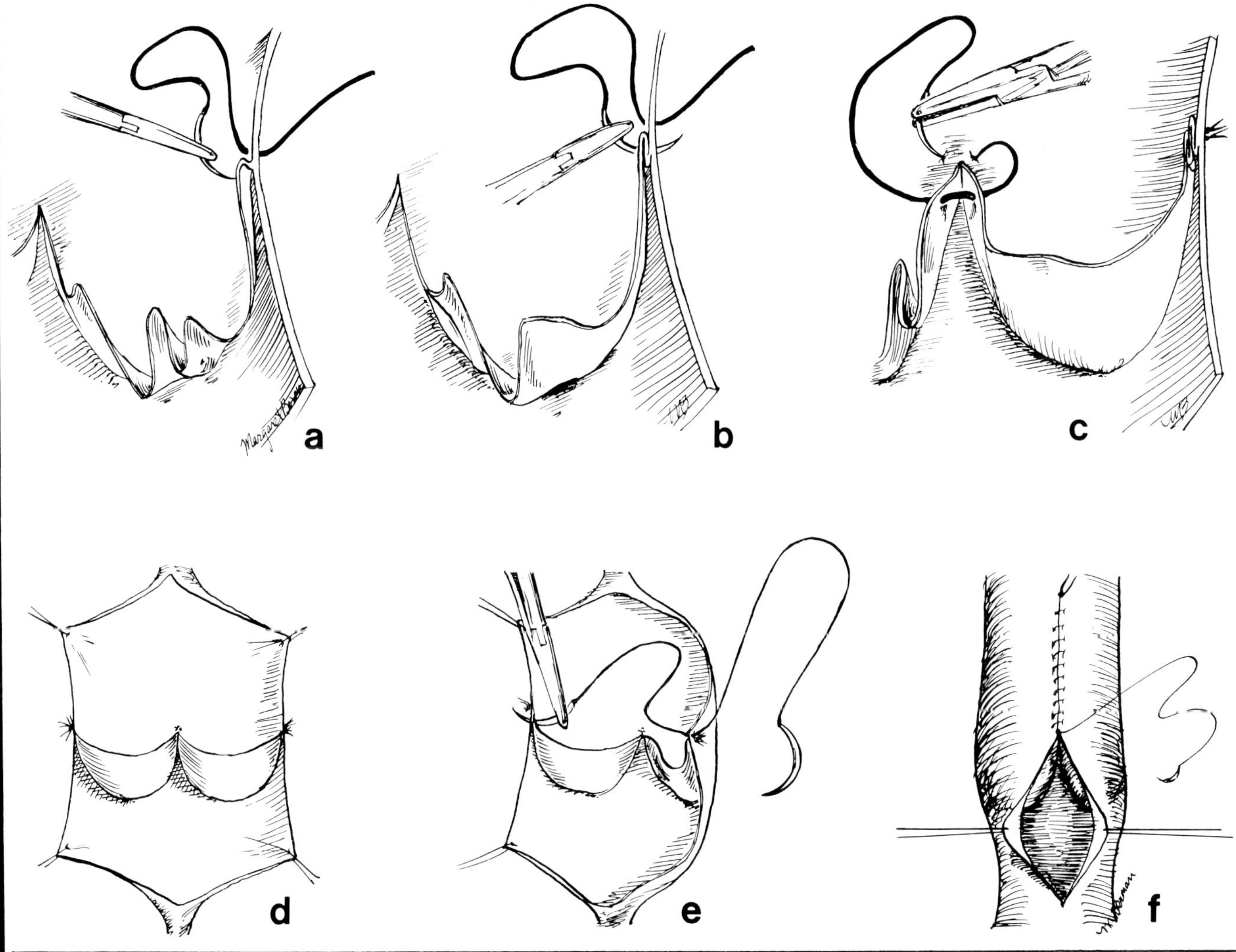

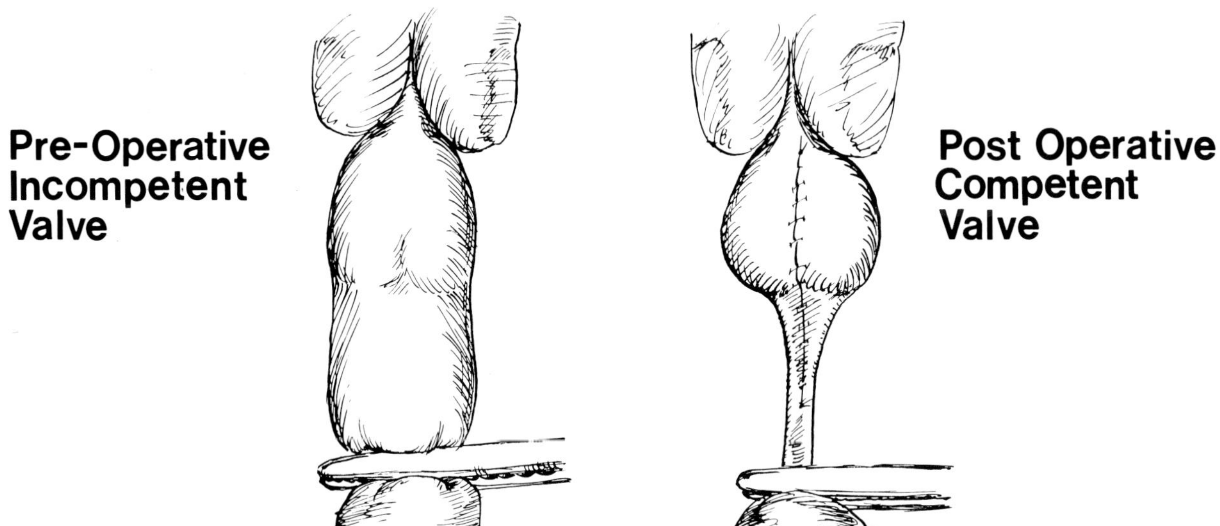

VEIN SEGMENT TRANSPOSITION

For those patients who do not have a repairable valve, such as the patient with the postphlebitic recanalized venous system, the procedure of vein segment transposition has been devised. The principle in this procedure is the same as that of primary valve repair, which is to provide a functionally competent proximal valve for the major venous outflow tract of the extremity. Ascending venography is used to determine the patent segments, whether they be superficial femoral, profunda femoris, saphenous vein, or any combination of these. Descending venography is used to determine in each segment whether the vein has a proximal competent valve.

The surgical procedure requires exposure of the common femoral vein, greater saphenous vein, and the superficial and profunda femoris veins. The incision is similar to the incision described for the primary valve repair.

After the venous segments have been dissected, they are carefully inspected to determine the presence and function of valves. This is accomplished by clamping the vein distally, emptying the segment by milking blood up through the vein, and observing whether or not there is free reflux back down the vein. This procedure is carried out separately for each segment. When all of the segments have been dissected, the location of valves determined, and the relative degree of competence of the valves has been checked, the procedure can be composed.

The anastomoses between segments can be done either end-to-end or end-to-side. Since the important principle is to provide a competent proximal valve for the venous drainage, the segment chosen for the proximal outflow end will be the one containing the demonstrated competent valve. Gentle occluding bulldog clamps are placed on the veins proximally and distally. Anastomoses are performed in a conventional technique, using continuous sutures placed in an over-and-over fashion, usually using 6–0 or 7–0 monofilament suture. When a significant discrepancy exists in the size of segments, the anastomosis is tailored by a long oblique cut of the two ends to be anastomosed.

The operation is done with the patient under intravenous heparinization. The heparin is not reversed at the end of the procedure. The patient is given 500 cc of Dextran 70 later on in the day of surgery and for the next two postoperative days. No further anticoagulation is used.

Figure 3 illustrates a typical surgical procedure in which the greater saphenous vein is used as the outflow vessel for a recanalized superficial femoral vein. In this instance, the saphenous vein has a competent proximal valve as determined both by descending venography preoperatively and by milking maneuvers at surgery (Fig. 3a). After dissection of both the saphenous vein and the superficial femoral vein, the greater saphenous vein is transected at the point where it can be approximated easily to the superficial femoral vein (Fig. 3b). The superficial femoral vein is transected flush at its juncture with the common femoral vein. The common femoral vein is oversewn with a running 5–0 suture so that a blind cul-de-sac is not left as a postoperative nidus for thrombosis. The end-to-end anastomosis is then performed between the superficial femoral and greater saphenous veins, with running sutures placed in over-and-over fashion and interrupted at three points around the circumference of the vein (Fig. 3c). The distal transected end of the greater saphenous vein can be placed end-to-side into the superficial femoral vein if the saphenous system is deemed large enough to merit its salvage (Fig. 3d).

Fig. 3. Greater saphenous vein is used as the outflow vessel for a recanalized superficial femoral vein.
(a) Anatomic relationships of venous segments.
(b) Greater saphenous vein is transected at the point where it can be approximated easily to the divided superficial femoral vein.
(c) End-to-end anastomosis, with running sutures placed in over-and-over fashion and interrupted at three points around vein circumference.
(d) The distal transected end of the greater saphenous vein can be placed end-to-side into the superficial femoral vein.

Vein Segment Transposition I

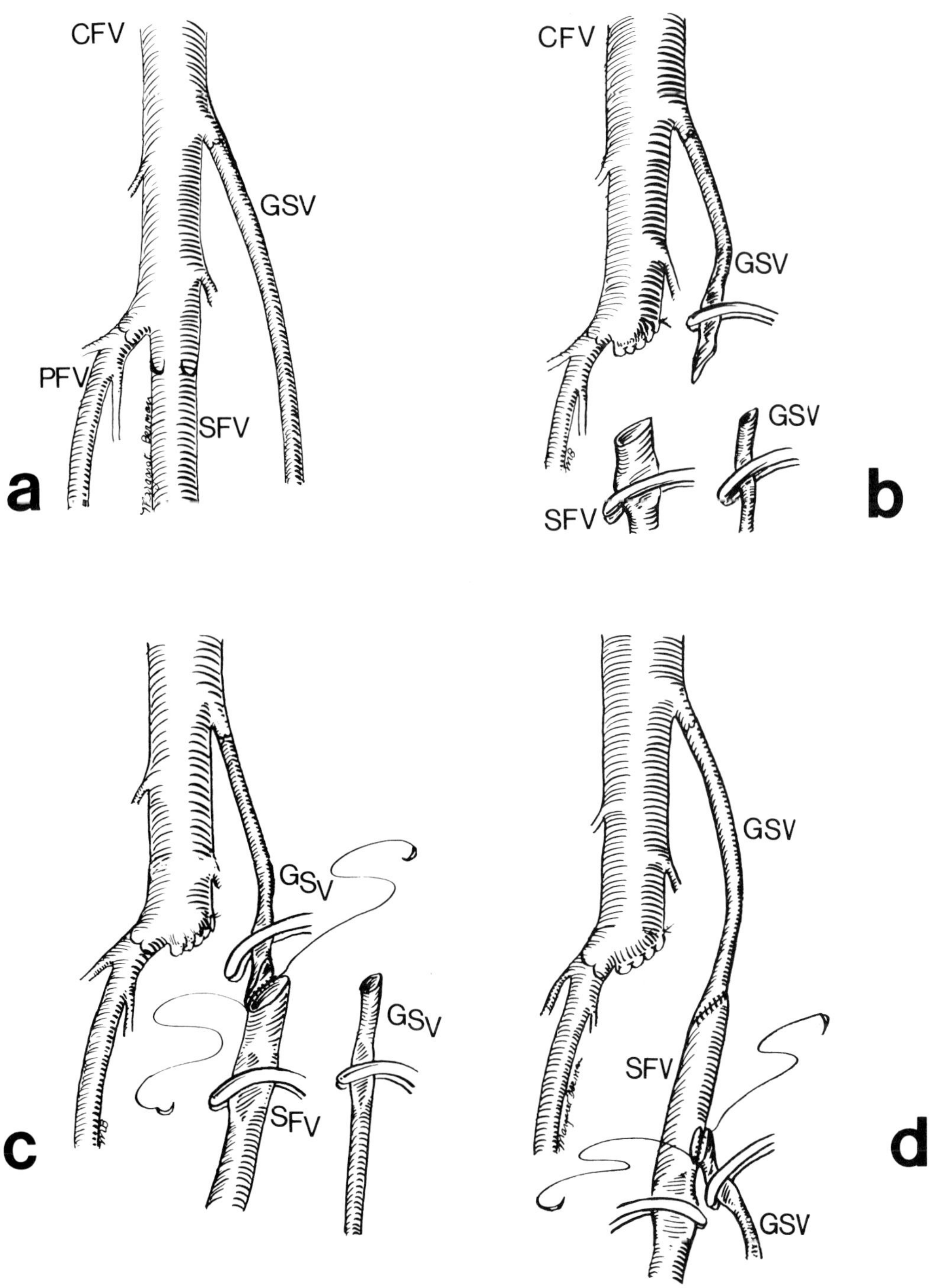

Variations of this operation are illustrated in Figure 4. It will be noted that the greater saphenous, superficial femoral, or profunda femoris vein may be used as a major outflow tract for either or both of the other two veins. In the surgical experience of our cases so far, we have had instances of the use of each segment as the major outflow tract and find that any segment works as well as the other. In over half the cases we have performed multiple anastomoses, usually utilizing end-to-end anastomosis for the main portion of this segment transposition and often employing an end-to-side anastomosis to add the third vessel into the outflow tract.

In a patient in whom multiple segments are incompetent, it is possible to combine valve repair and vein segment transposition to produce a competent system (Fig. 4d).

Fig. 4. Various types of procedures for transposition of vein segments to produce a competent valvular system.
(a) Superficial femoral vein transposed to profunda femoris vein and end-to-side anastomosis of greater saphenous vein to superficial femoral vein.
(b) Transposition of incompetent profunda femoris vein to competent superficial femoral vein.
(c) Transposition of profunda femoris vein to competent saphenous vein with end-to-side anastomosis.
(d) Transposition of superficial femoral vein to greater saphenous vein with simultaneous repair of incompetent saphenous valve.

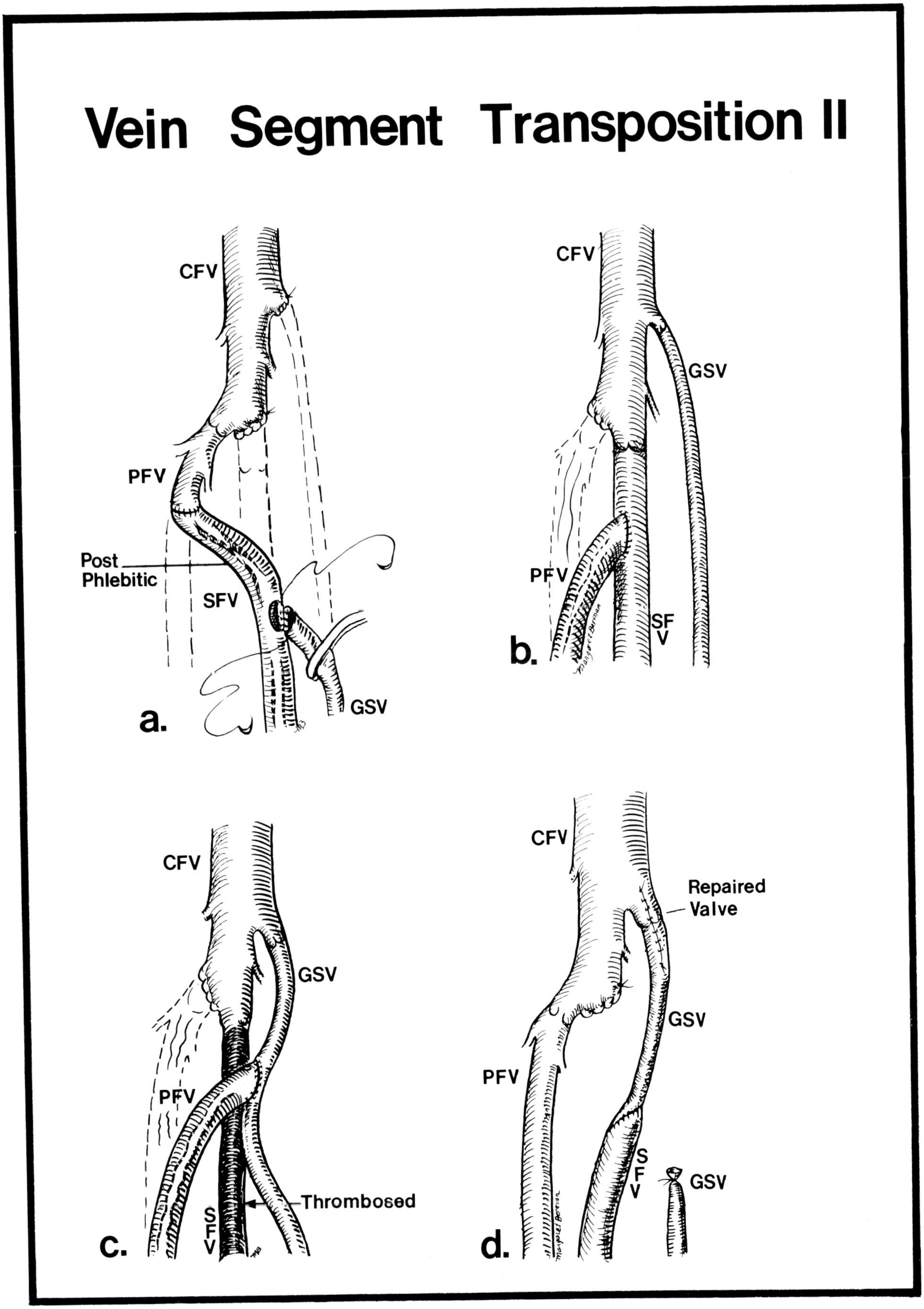
Vein Segment Transposition II
CFV
PFV
Post
Phlebitic
SFV
GSV
a.
CFV
GSV
PFV
SF
V
b.
CFV
GSV
PFV
S
F
V
Thrombosed
c.
CFV
Repaired
Valve
GSV
PFV
S
F
V
GSV
d.

REFERENCES

1. Kistner RL: Surgical repair of the incompetent femoral vein valve. Arch Surg 110:1336, 1975
2. Kistner RL, Sparkuhl MD: Surgery in acute and chronic venous disease. Surgery 85:31, 1979

Correction of Deep Venous Insufficiency by Valvular Transposition

Luis A. Queral

Loss of valvular integrity in the veins of the lower extremity is responsible for the postphlebitic syndrome. Such venous insufficiency inhibits the physiologic muscle pump mechanism of blood return to the heart. Resultant ambulatory venous hypertension causes edema, stasis dermatitis, and distal leg ulceration.

A variety of surgical procedures aimed at correcting venous insufficiency have been proposed. Most involve the removal and/or ligation of abnormal veins. However, none of these techniques has achieved permanent success. Perhaps a more physiologic approach to the problem is surgical restoration of valvular competency. This was first proposed by Kistner,[1,2] who described dramatic relief of symptoms after direct repair of an incompetent superficial femoral valve. An alternate method of establishing a competent and functional valve in the deep veins of the lower extremity, at the groin level, is transposition. This technique has been shown to be hemodynamically sound.[3]

SURGICAL PROCEDURE

The patient is placed in a supine position, and the groin is thoroughly prepped with Betadine soap solution. General anesthesia has been routinely employed, but a spinal anesthetic is a reasonable alternative. A review of the topographic anatomy of the femoral vessels is suggested prior to draping the operative field (Fig. 1A). A vertical incision approximately 8 cm in length is utilized. The incision parallels the course of the pulsatile artery, and its upper limit overlies the inguinal ligament. The greater saphenous vein is encountered in the subcutaneous tissues (Fig. 1B). Numerous tributaries are individually ligated, and the saphenous vein is dissected proximally until the saphenofemoral junction is identified. The major veins are exposed with the aid of a self-retaining retractor (Fig. 1C).

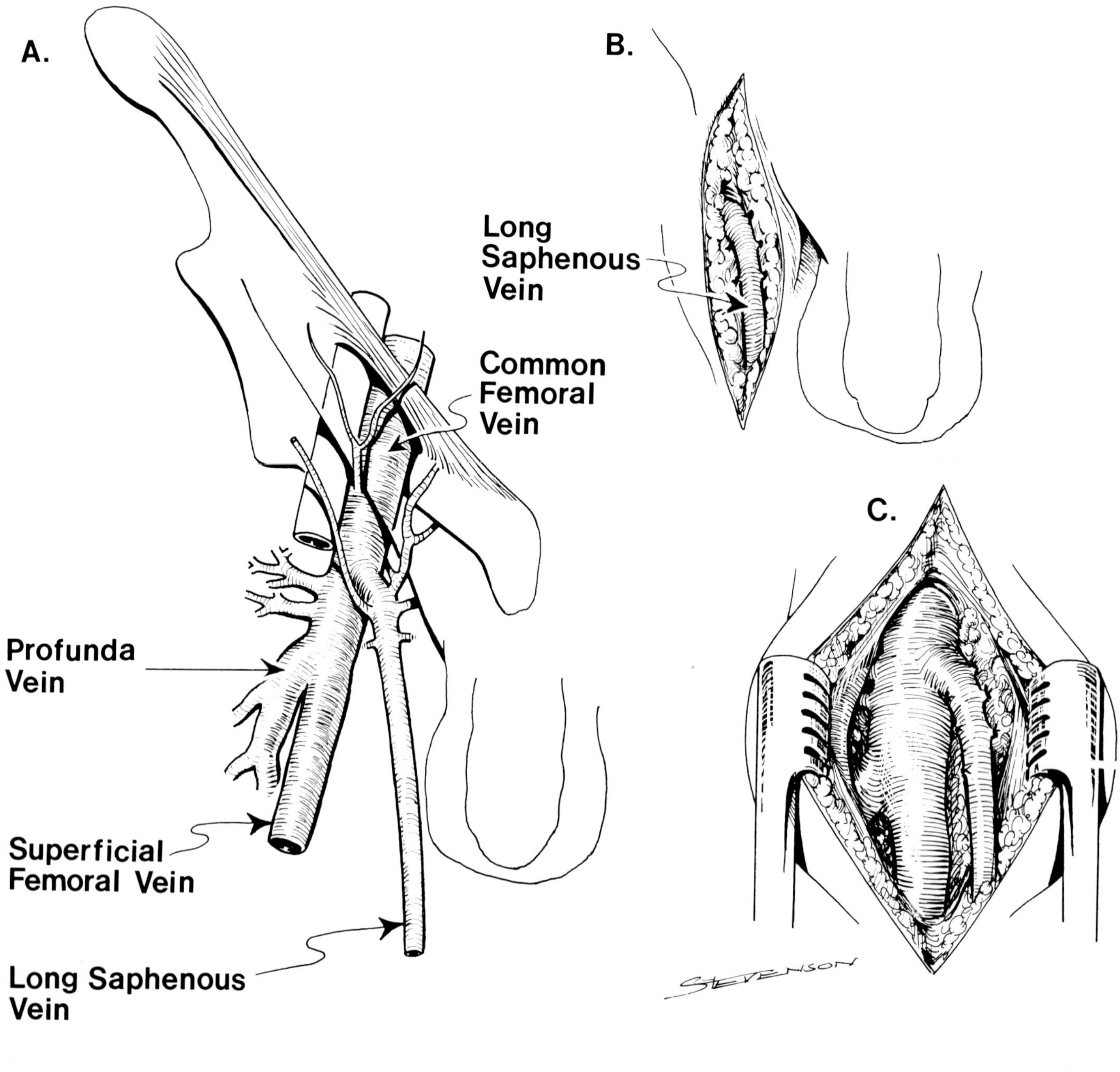

Fig. 1. (A) Topographic anatomy of the femoral vessels.
(B) The greater saphenous vein is encountered in the subcutaneous tissues.
(C) Use of a self-retaining retractor aids exposure of the saphenofemoral junction.

Elastic vessel loops are placed around the common femoral, superficial femoral, profunda femoris, and saphenous veins. (Fig. 2A). This must be done with great care and gentleness because of the fragile nature of the vessels. A judicious combination of sharp and blunt dissection appears to be most satisfactory. Small branches arising from the major channels can be suture-ligated. Digital examination of the greater saphenous vein (Fig. 2B) is then performed to confirm the competency of its valves. The vein is emptied of blood by a "milking maneuver," and the direction from which it refills is noted. This is done by alternatively releasing the proximal and distal ends. A competent saphenous vein fills only from its distal end. The patient is systemically anticoagulated with heparin, and the saphenous vein is transected (Fig. 2C). The distal end requires ligation, but the proximal end bleeds little because of the competent valves.

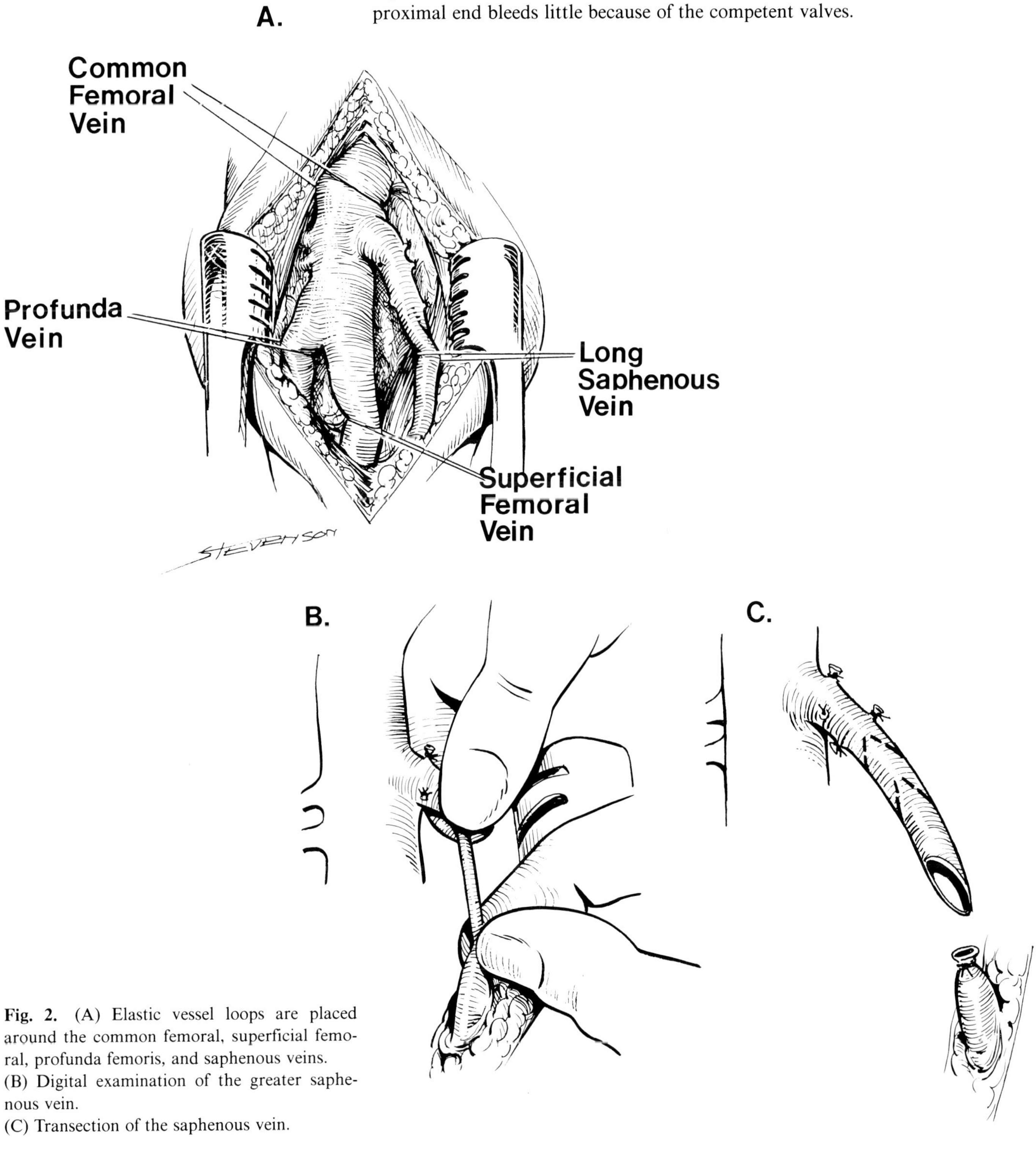

Fig. 2. (A) Elastic vessel loops are placed around the common femoral, superficial femoral, profunda femoris, and saphenous veins.
(B) Digital examination of the greater saphenous vein.
(C) Transection of the saphenous vein.

The transected saphenous vein can be anastomosed to the superficial femoral vein in an end-to-end or end-to-side fashion (Fig. 3 A and B). If the end-to-end technique is utilized, the proximal portion of the superficial femoral vein must be oversewn. Conversely, when the end-to-side anastomosis is performed, the superficial femoral vein can just be ligated. Both techniques appear to be equally effective. The anastomosis is done with 7–0 prolene suture material after the superficial femoral vein is either tenderly clamped or doubly looped with the silastic strands. The saphenous vein is spatulated to achieve a "toe-to-heel" distance that is roughly $1\frac{1}{2}$ times larger than the diameter of the superficial femoral vein. Those patients whose greater saphenous vein is either incompetent or missing can undergo a profunda venous transposition (Fig. 3C). The superficial femoral vein is anastomosed in an end-to-side manner to the profunda femoris vein just distal to a competent valve. The anastomosis is also performed with 7–0 prolene suture material. Magnification loops (2 to 3×) are helpful in ensuring precise endothelial anastomotic approximation. All of these transposition variations place a competent valve in the deep-venous system.

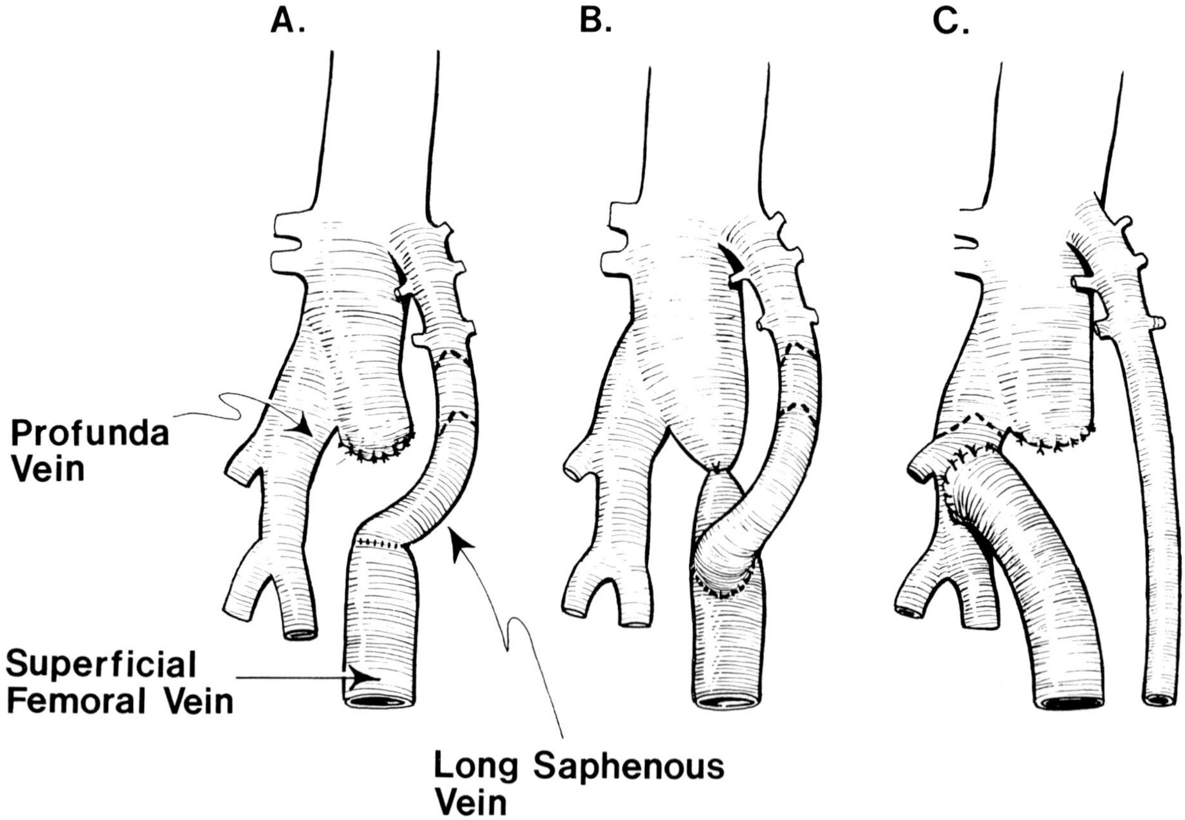

Fig. 3. The transected saphenous vein can be anastomosed to the superficial femoral vein in (A) end-to-end fashion or (B) end-to-side fashion. (C) Profunda venous transposition.

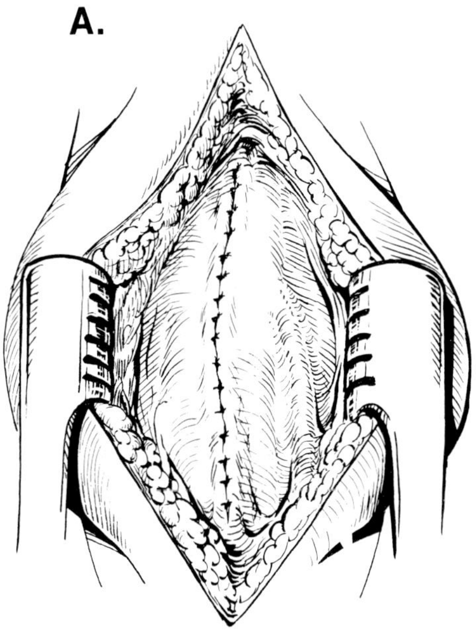

Closure of the wound after termination of the transposition is an important part of the procedure. Great care must be taken to avoid hematoma formation. The wound is approximated in layers with interrupted sutures of an absorbable material like polyglycolic acid (Fig. 4A), and meticulous care is taken to ensure absolute hemostasis (Fig. 4B). A wound hematoma is a serious complication because the external compression on the low-pressure venous system will cause thrombosis of the transposition. A subcuticular skin closure (Fig. 4C) also minimizes the likelihood of subcutaneous hemorrhage. Finally, the procedure is terminated with a compression dressing of elastic adhesive (Fig. 4D).

Postoperative care consists of strict bed rest for 48 hours with the leg elevated. A continuous infusion of low-molecular-weight Dextran (500 ml/24 hr) is utilized until the patient has been orally anticoagulated with warfarin. Ambulation is begun on the third postoperative day, and the patient is generally discharged on the seventh day after surgery. Elastic support stockings are prescribed prior to discharge, and the anticoagulation regimen is maintained for 3 months.

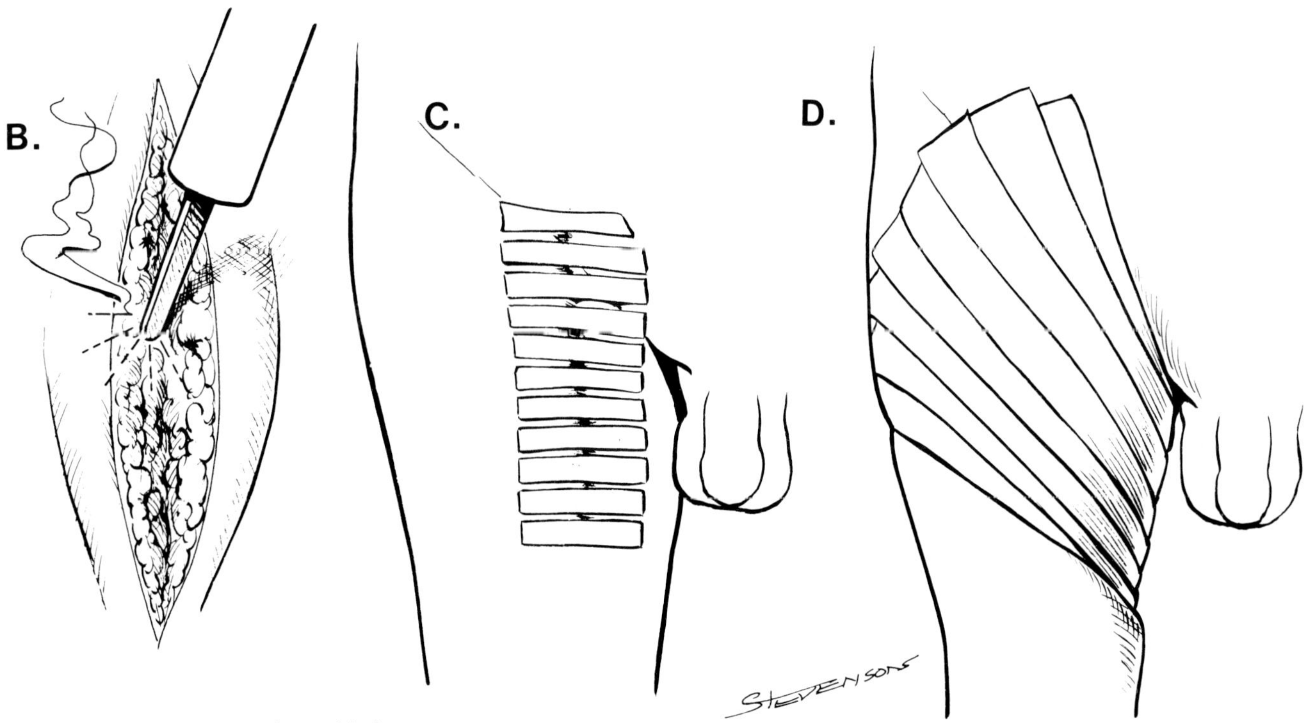

Fig. 4. (A) The wound is approximated in layers with interrupted sutures of an absorbable material like polyglycolic acid.
(B) Meticulous care is taken to ensure absolute hemostasis.
(C) Subcuticular skin closure minimizes likelihood of subcutaneous hemorrhage.
(D) The procedure is terminated with a compression dressing of elastic adhesive.

REFERENCES

1. Kistner RL: Surgical repair of the incompetent femoral vein valve. Arch Surg 100:1336–1342, 1975
2. Kistner RL, Sparkuhl M: Surgery in acute and chronic venous disease. Surgery 85:31, 1979
3. Queral LA, Whitehouse WM Jr, Flinn WR, Neiman HL, Yao JST, Bergan JJ: Surgical correction of chronic deep venous insufficiency by valvular transposition. Surgery 87:688, 1980

Spiral Vein Grafting: The Technique

Creighton B. Wright, Donald B. Doty

The most satisfactory substitute for vein is autogenous vein. Unfortunately, there are usually major size discrepancies involved in consideration of substitution for superior vena cava, inferior vena cava, portal vein, iliac vein, etc. Whereas the greater saphenous vein is a good substitute for small arteries and the superficial femoral and popliteal veins, its use as an interposition conduit in large veins has frequently been unsatisfactory. Initial attempts at panelling of saphenous vein, although successful in experimental settings, have not been widely utilized clinically.[1] Transposition of the internal jugular vein for mesocaval shunting and for other short segment venous transposition has been accomplished. Other conduits of biologic or nonbiologic origin have had an inconsistent but generally poor patency in venous systems.[2–7] This paper presents the technique of spiral formation of large venous conduits initially reported in experimental preparations by Chiu and for superior vena cava substitution at the University of Iowa.[8,9] The problem, diagnosis, and nonoperative management of superior vena cava obstruction are discussed in the references (Fig. 1).[2,9,10]

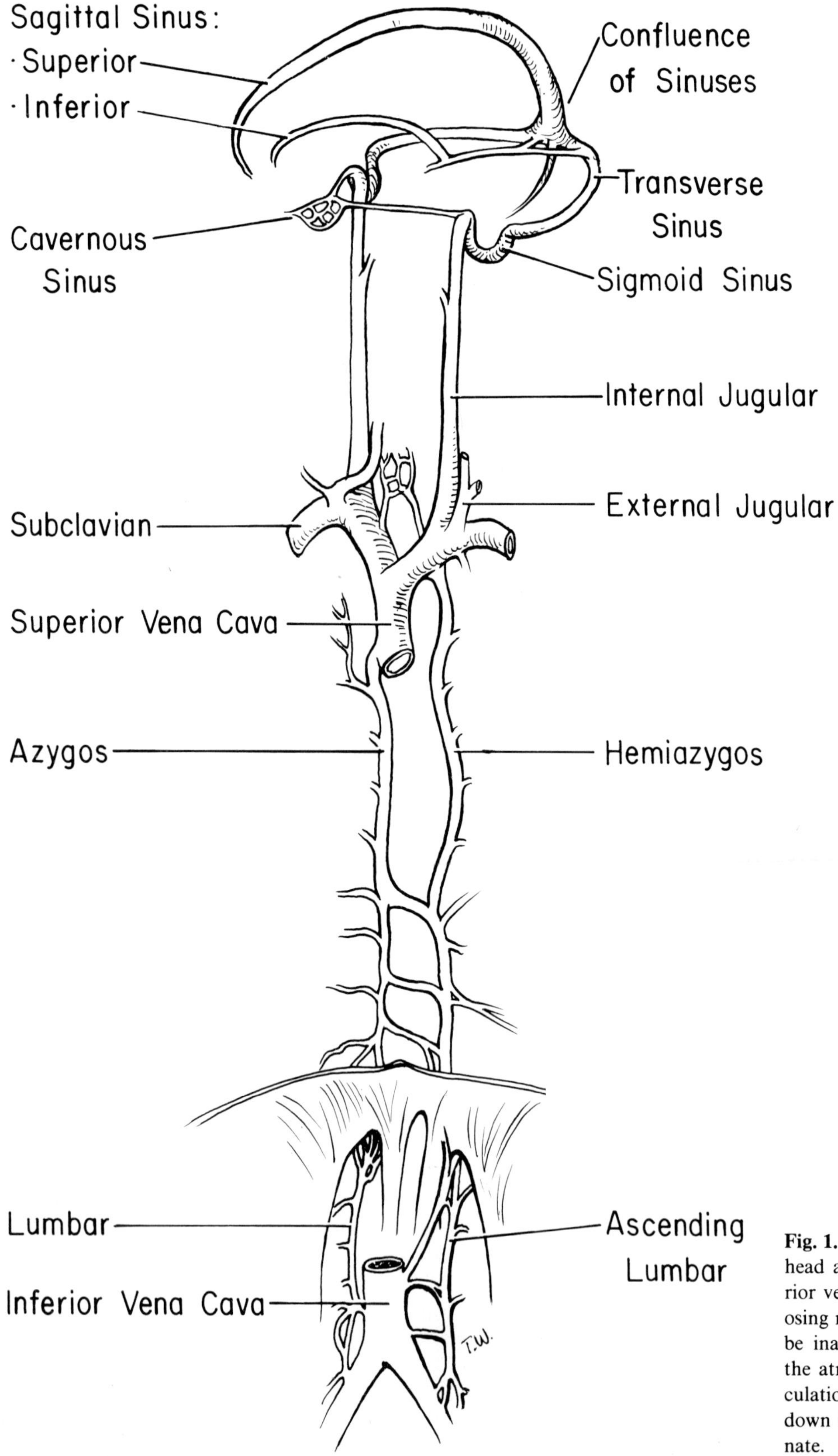

Fig. 1. The venous collateral circulation of the head and trunk. In particular, when the superior vena cava is involved with tumor or sclerosing mediastinitis, the azygous collaterals may be inadequate. Bypass from the innomiate to the atrium allows drainage of the cerebral circulation across the confluence of sinuses and down the left internal jugular into the innominate.

SURGICAL TECHNIQUE FOR SUPERIOR VENA CAVA BYPASS

A median sternotomy incision is made and the innominate vein exposed and dissected circumferentially. The pericardium is opened through a vertical incision and retracted laterally with silk stay sutures. If necessary for tissue histologic confirmation, the right upper mediastinum can be explored and appropriate biopsies taken. Measurement of length from innominate vein to atrial appendage is made and the size of the stent chosen.

Simultaneously, the greater saphenous vein is exposed, its branches are ligated with fine (4–0) silk, irrigated, distended with heparinized saline, and split longitudinally over the required length. The vein is then wrapped around the previously chosen stent of appropriate size (for superior vena cava a No. 40 French chest tube is suitable). A continuous anastomosis of 6–0 or 7–0 polypropylene is then carried out until adequate length of conduit has been constructed (Fig. 2).

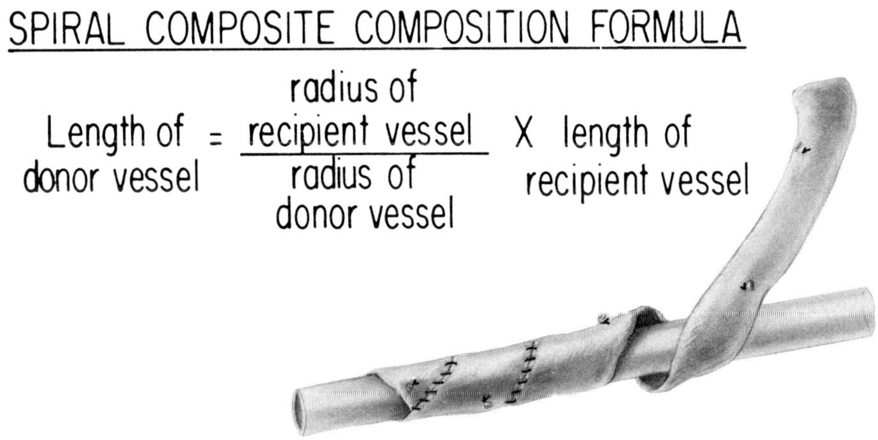

Fig. 2. A longitudinal section of saphenous vein, split and wrapped about a No. 40 French argyle mediastinal tube with beginning of anastomosis with running 6–0 prolene. Subpart of this figure demonstrates the length relationships of the spiral composite versus the original length of saphenous vein required.

Systemic heparin (2 mg/kg) is administered intravenously. The innominate vein anastomosis is constructed end-to-end after ligation and division of the innominate vein (Fig. 3). This is preferred over end-to-side in order to maintain maximal flow and decrease required conduit length (Fig. 4). The anastomosis is performed with 6–0 prolene using loupes for magnification (2.5 to 3.5 $\times$). Using a partial-occlusion clamp, the right atrial appendage is excluded, the trabeculated portion excised, and an end-to-end anastomosis constructed with fine prolene. Flow is restored through the conduit, which can easily be checked by "stripping" the conduit or by using the Doppler probe intraoperatively. Emphasis must be placed on meticulous technique for construction of both the conduit and the venous anastomoses. Fibrous adventitial strands must not be allowed in the suture lines. Pursestringing at the anastomoses will cause thrombosis. Leaks are of course annoying and may lead to buildup of an internal as well as external thrombus at the site. The pericardium is not closed. The median sternotomy is closed with peristernal wire and subcutaneous and subcuticular 3–0 continuous vicryl. The leg wound is closed with subcutaneous and subcuticular 3–0 continuous vicryl. Drainage tubes are left in the mediastinum. Aspirin (600 mg bid) and Persantine (50 mg orally tid) have been administered postoperatively to decrease platelet aggregation. Postoperative patency can be assessed by measurement of upper compartment venous pressure, by Doppler venous examination, by venography, and also very accurately and easily by radioisotope venography.

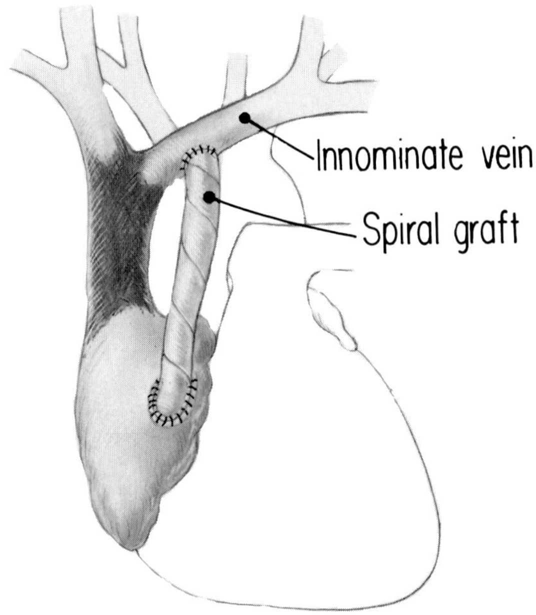

Fig. 3. An end-to-side anastomosis of the innominate vein to the spiral graft. Although this technique can be used, additional length of spiral conduit is required ordinarily. In addition, total flow is more likely to be routed through an end-to-end anastomosis and improve patency.

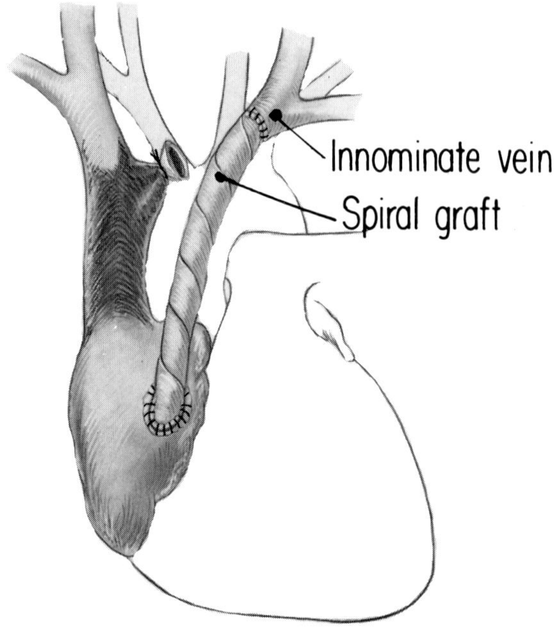

Fig. 4. The end-to-end innominate vein to spiral graft anastomosis, which is the preferred technique.

SUMMARY

The present paper describes a technique for creation of venous conduits of variable size, making a spiral anastomosis of autogenous saphenous vein. Multiple prior attempts at venous substitution have shown the regular superiority of autogenous saphenous vein, but the residual problem of size discrepancy has persisted. The panelling technique had never achieved great use, and the internal jugular vein, although used by some, is thin-walled, relatively difficult to handle, and may not be as versatile as the spiral conduit. The basic techniques are simple, well known to cardiovascular surgeons, and may potentially be applicable not only for superior vena cava syndrome but also for other large-vessel venous replacements for trauma, cancer, or portal hypertension surgery.

REFERENCES

1. Earle AS, Horsley JS, Villavicencio JL, Warren R: Replacement of venous defects by venous autografts. Arch Surg 80:119–127, 1960
2. Hiratzka LF, Wright CB: Experimental and clinical results of grafts in the venous system: A current review. J Surg Res 25:542, 1978
3. Hiratzka LF, Wright CB, Doty DB: Newer tissue and synthetic grafts in canine femoral veins (Manuscript in preparation)
4. Rich NM, Hobson RW II, Wright CB, Swan KG: Techniques of venous repair, in Swan KG (ed): Venous Surgery in the Lower Extremities. St. Louis, Warren H Green Inc, 1975, p 243
5. Bergan JJ, Yao JST (eds): Venous Problems. Chicago, Year Book Medical Publishers Inc, 1978
6. Hobson RW II, Wright CB, Rich NM: Investigative aspects of venous reconstruction, in Venous Disease: Medical-Surgical Management. Mouton, The Hague, Netherlands, American-European Symposium on Venous Disease, Foundation of International Cooperation in the Medical Sciences, 1974
7. Wright CB, Hobson RW II, Giordano JM, DeWitt PL, Rich NM: Acute femoral venous occlusion: Management by segmental venous replacement in the dog. J Cardiovasc Surg 18:523, 1977
8. Chiu CJ, Terzis J, MacRae ML: Replacement of superior vena cava with the spiral composite vein graft. Ann Thorac Surg 17:555, 1974
9. Lochridge SK, Knibbe WP, Doty DB: Obstruction of the superior vena cava. Surgery 85:14, 1979
10. Doty DB, Baker WH: Bypass of superior vena cava with spiral vein graft. Ann Thorac Surg 22:490, 1976

a
b
c
d
e
f
g
0 h
1 i
8 2 j